Translational Research in Cardio-Oncology

Editors

RAGAVENDRA R. BALIGA
GEORGE A. MENSAH

HEART FAILURE CLINICS

www.heartfailure.theclinics.com

Consulting Editor
EDUARDO BOSSONE

Founding Editor
JAGAT NARULA

July 2022 • Volume 18 • Number 3

ELSEVIER

1600 John F. Kennedy Boulevard • Suite 1800 • Philadelphia, Pennsylvania, 19103-2899

http://www.theclinics.com

HEART FAILURE CLINICS Volume 18, Number 3
July 2022 ISSN 1551-7136, ISBN-13: 978-0-323-98747-9

Editor: Joanna Collett
Developmental Editor: Jessica Cañaberal

Heart Failure Clinics (ISSN 1551-7136) is published quarterly by Elsevier Inc., 360 Park Avenue South, New York, NY 10010-1710. Months of publication are January, April, July, and October. Business and editorial offices: 1600 John F. Kennedy Boulevard, Suite 1800, Philadelphia, PA 19103-2899. Periodicals postage paid at New York, NY, and additional mailing offices. Subscription prices are USD 277.00 per year for US individuals, USD 681.00 per year for US institutions, USD 100.00 per year for US students and residents, USD 300.00 per year for Canadian individuals, USD 701.00 per year for Canadian institutions, USD 315.00 per year for international individuals, USD 701.00 per year for international institutions, and USD 100.00 per year for Canadian and foreign students/residents. To receive student and resident rate, orders must be accompanied by name of affiliated institution, date of term, and the *signature* of program/residency coordinator on institution letterhead. Orders will be billed at individual rate until proof of status is received. Foreign air speed delivery is included in all *Clinics* subscription prices. All prices are subject to change without notice. **POSTMASTER:** Send address changes to *Heart Failure Clinics*, Elsevier Health Sciences Division, Subscription Customer Service, 3251 Riverport Lane, Maryland Heights, MO 63043. **Customer Service: 1-800-654-2452 (US and Canada). From outside of the US and Canada, call 314-447-8871. Fax: 314-447-8029. For print support, E-mail: JournalsCustomerService-usa@elsevier.com. For online support, E-mail: JournalsOnlineSupport-usa@elsevier.com.**

Reprints. For copies of 100 or more of articles in this publication, please contact the Commercial Reprints Department, Elsevier Inc., 360 Park Avenue South, New York, NY 10010-1710. Tel.: 212-633-3874; Fax: 212-633-3820; E-mail: reprints@elsevier.com.

Heart Failure Clinics is covered in *MEDLINE/PubMed (Index Medicus)*.

Contributors

CONSULTING EDITOR

EDUARDO BOSSONE, MD, PhD, FCCP, FESC, FACC
Director, Division of Cardiology, AORN Antonio Cardarelli Hospital, Naples, Italy

EDITORS

RAGAVENDRA R. BALIGA, MD, MBA, FACP, FRCP (Edin), FACC
Inaugural Cardio-Oncologist Professor, Attending Cardiologist, Division of Cardiology, The Ohio State University Wexner Medical Center, Columbus, Ohio, USA

GEORGE A. MENSAH, MD, FACC, FAHA
Director, Center for Translation Research and Implementation Science, National Heart, Lung, and Blood Institute, National Institutes of Health, Bethesda, Maryland, USA

AUTHORS

JUN-ICHI ABE, MD, PhD
Department of Cardiology, The University of Texas MD Anderson Cancer Center, Houston, Texas, USA

DANIEL ADDISON, MD
Cardio-Oncology Program, Division of Cardiology, The Ohio State University Medical Center, Division of Cancer Prevention and Control, Department of Internal Medicine, College of Medicine, The Ohio State University, Columbus, Ohio, USA

BISHOW B. ADHIKARI, PhD
Division of Cardiovascular Sciences, NHLBI, NIH, Bethesda, Maryland, USA

NIKHIL AGRAWAL, MD
Division of Cardiology, Department of Internal Medicine, McGovern Medical School, The University of Texas Health Science Center at Houston, Texas, USA

AARTI ASNANI, MD
Division of Cardiovascular Medicine, Department of Medicine, Beth Israel Deaconess Medical Center, Harvard Medical School, Boston, Massachusetts, USA

CRAIG BEAVERS, PharmD
University of Kentucky College of Pharmacy, Lexington, Kentucky, USA

CARMEN BERGOM, MD, PhD
Department of Radiation Oncology, Cardio-Oncology Center of Excellence, Alvin J. Siteman Center, Washington University in St. Louis, St Louis, Missouri, USA

ANNE BLAES, MD, MS
Division of Hematology/Oncology, University of Minnesota, Minneapolis, Minnesota, USA

MARY BRANCH, MD, MS
Section of Cardiovascular Medicine, Wake Forest University, Winston-Salem, North Carolina, USA

RANDALL BRENNEMAN, MD, PhD
Department of Radiation Oncology,
Washington University in St. Louis, St Louis,
Missouri, USA; Alvin J. Siteman Center,
Washington University in St. Louis, St Louis,
Missouri, USA

SHERRY-ANN BROWN, MD, PhD
Cardio-Oncology Program, Division of
Cardiovascular Medicine, Medical College of
Wisconsin, Milwaukee, Wisconsin, USA

ZSU-ZSU CHEN, MD
Division of Endocrinology, Diabetes, and
Metabolism, Department of Medicine, Beth
Israel Deaconess Medical Center, Harvard
Medical School, Boston, Massachusetts, USA

RICHARD K. CHENG, MD, MSC
Cardio-oncology Program, Division of
Cardiology, University of Washington, Seattle,
Washington, USA

AARON CHUM, BA
Cardio-Oncology Program, Division of
Cardiology, The Ohio State University Medical
Center, Dorothy M. Davis Heart and Lung
Research Institute, Columbus, Ohio, USA

JESSE D. COCHRAN, BS
Hematovascular Biology Center, Robert M.
Berne Cardiovascular Research Center,
University of Virginia School of Medicine,
Charlottesville, Virginia, USA

PATRICE DESVIGNE-NICKENS, MD
Division of Cardiovascular Sciences, NHLBI,
NIH, Bethesda, Maryland, USA

ANITA DESWAL, MD, MPH
Department of Cardiology, The University of
Texas MD Anderson Cancer Center, Houston,
Texas, USA

HARDEEP DHOLIYA, MD
Cardio-Oncology Program, Division of
Cardiology, The Ohio State University Medical
Center, Dorothy M. Davis Heart and Lung
Research Institute, Columbus, Ohio, USA

MAMADOU DIALLO, MD
Dorothy M. Davis Heart and Lung Research
Institute, The Ohio State University, Columbus,
Ohio, USA

EILEEN P. DIMOND, BSN, MSN
Division of Cancer Prevention, NCI, NIH,
Bethesda, Maryland, USA

JOEL FERRALL, BS
Dorothy M. Davis Heart and Lung Research
Institute, The Ohio State University, Columbus,
Ohio, USA

MICHAEL G. FRADLEY, MD
Medical Director, Thalheimer Center for
Cardio-Oncology, Assocaite Professor of
Medicine, Division of Cardiology, Department
of Medicine, Perelman School of Medicine at
the University of Pennsylvania, Philadelphia,
Pennsylvania, USA

JOHN ALAN GAMBRIL, MD
Department of Internal Medicine, Ohio State
University Wexner Medical Center, Cardio-
Oncology Program, Division of Cardiology, The
Ohio State University Medical Center,
Columbus, Ohio, USA

SARJU GANATRA, MD
Division of Cardiovascular Medicine,
Department of Medicine, Cardio-Oncology
Program, Lahey Hospital and Medical Center,
Burlington, Massachusetts, USA

MORIE A. GERTZ, MD, MACP
Roland Seidler Jr. Professor of the Art of
Medicine, Mayo distinguished Clinician,
Department of Medicine, Mayo Clinic
Rochester, Rochester, Minnesota, USA

AKASH GOYAL, MD
Cardio-Oncology Program, Division of
Cardiology, The Ohio State University Medical
Center, Dorothy M. Davis Heart and Lung
Research Institute, Columbus, Ohio, USA

ASHLEY N. GREENLEE, BS
Dorothy M. Davis Heart and Lung Research
Institute, The Ohio State University, Columbus,
Ohio, USA

THAI H. HO, MD, PhD
Division of Medical Oncology, Department of
Internal Medicine, Mayo Clinic, Phoenix
Arizona, USA

CEZAR ILIESCU, MD
Department of Cardiology, The University of
Texas MD Anderson Cancer Center, Houston,
Texas, USA

MENKA KHOOBCHANDANI, PhD
Department of Radiation Oncology,
Washington University in St. Louis, St Louis,
Missouri, USA

EFSTRATIOS KOUTROUMPAKIS, MD
Department of Cardiology, The University of
Texas MD Anderson Cancer Center, Houston,
Texas, USA

DANIEL J. LENIHAN, MD
International Cardio-Oncology Society,
Tampa, Florida, USA

**DARRYL P. LEONG, MBBS, MPH, MBiostat,
PhD**
The Population Health Research Institute and
Department of Medicine, McMaster University
and Hamilton Health Sciences, Hamilton,
Ontario, Canada

JING LIU, MD, PhD
Division of Cardiovascular Medicine,
Department of Medicine, Beth Israel
Deaconess Medical Center, Harvard Medical
School, Boston, Massachusetts, USA

ANNA MATZKO
Davis Heart and Lung Research Institute, The
Ohio State University, Columbus, Ohio, USA

KATARZYNA MIKRUT, MD
Cardio-Oncology Program, Division of
Cardiology, The Ohio State University Medical
Center, Columbus, Ohio, USA

LORI M. MINASIAN, MD
Division of Cancer Prevention, NCI, NIH,
Bethesda, Maryland, USA

JOSHUA D. MITCHELL, MD, MSCI, FACC
Cardio-Oncology Center of Excellence, Alvin J.
Siteman Center, Division of Cardiology,
Department of Medicine, Washington
University in St. Louis, St Louis, Missouri, USA

SOMAYYA J. MOHAMMAD, MS
Dorothy M. Davis Heart and Lung Research
Institute, The Ohio State University, Columbus,
Ohio, USA

SHARANYA MOHANTY, MD
Division of Cardiology, Tufts Medical Center,
Boston, Massachusetts, USA

MCKAY MULLEN, PhD
Stanford Cardiovascular Institute, Stanford
University

MICHAEL T. NAUGHTON
Dorothy M. Davis Heart and Lung Research
Institute, The Ohio State University, Columbus,
Ohio, USA

NICOLAS L. PALASKAS, MD
Department of Cardiology, The University of
Texas MD Anderson Cancer Center, Houston,
Texas, USA

BRIJESH PATEL, DO
Dorothy M. Davis Heart and Lung Research
Institute, Columbus, Ohio, USA; Cardio-
Oncology Program, Heart and Vascular
Institute, West Virginia University,
Morgantown, West Virginia, USA

JAGVI PATEL, BS
Division of Cardiovascular Medicine,
Department of Medicine, Beth Israel
Deaconess Medical Center, Harvard Medical
School, Boston, Massachusetts, USA

LAUREN N. PEDERSEN, PhD
Department of Radiation Oncology,
Washington University in St. Louis, St Louis,
Missouri, USA

NAGA VENKATA K. POTHINENI, MD
Kansas City Heart Rhythm Institute, Overland
Park, Kansas, USA

AKASH RASTOGI, BA
Division of Cardiology, Tufts Medical Center,
Boston, Massachusetts, USA

ROHITH REVAN
Dorothy M. Davis Heart and Lung Research
Institute, The Ohio State University, Columbus,
Ohio, USA

JUNE-WHA RHEE, MD
Department of Medicine, City of Hope Comprehensive Cancer Center, Duarte, California, USA

PATRICK RUZ, BS
Cardio-Oncology Program, Division of Cardiology, The Ohio State University Medical Center, Dorothy M. Davis Heart and Lung Research Institute, Columbus, Ohio, USA

ETHAN J. SCHWENDEMAN, BS
Dorothy M. Davis Heart and Lung Research Institute, The Ohio State University, Columbus, Ohio, USA

SHANE S. SCOTT, MS
Dorothy M. Davis Heart and Lung Research Institute, The Ohio State University, Columbus, Ohio, USA

NONNIEKAYE SHELBURNE, CRNP, MS, AOCN
Division of Cancer Control and Population Sciences, NCI, NIH, Bethesda, Maryland, USA

SCARLET SHI, PhD
Division of Cardiovascular Sciences, NHLBI, NIH, Bethesda, Maryland, USA

GABRIEL SHIMMIN, BS
Dorothy M. Davis Heart and Lung Research Institute, The Ohio State University, Columbus, Ohio, USA

ORLANDO SIMONETTI, PhD
Cardio-Oncology Program, Division of Cardiology, The Ohio State University Medical Center, Dorothy M. Davis Heart and Lung Research Institute, Departments of Internal Medicine and Radiology, The Ohio State University Medical Center, Columbus, Ohio, USA

SAKIMA A. SMITH, MD, MPH
Dorothy M. Davis Heart and Lung Research Institute, The Ohio State University, Division of Cardiology, Department of Internal Medicine, The Ohio State University College of Medicine, Columbus, Ohio, USA

MATTHEW STEIN
Dorothy M. Davis Heart and Lung Research Institute, The Ohio State University, Columbus, Ohio, USA

ASHLEY F. STEIN-MERLOB, MD
Division of Cardiology, Department of Medicine, UCLA-Cardio-Oncology Program, University of California, Los Angeles, Los Angeles, California, USA

SHWETABH TARUN, BA
Dorothy M. Davis Heart and Lung Research Institute, The Ohio State University, Columbus, Ohio, USA

JENICA N. UPSHAW, MD, MS
Medical Director, Cardio-Oncology Program, Division of Cardiology, Tufts Medical Center, Boston, Massachusetts, USA

HERMAN VAN BESIEN, MD
Hospital of the University of Pennsylvania, Department of Medicine, Perelman School of Medicine, University of Pennsylvania, Philadelphia, Pennsylvania, USA

KENNETH WALSH, PhD
Hematovascular Biology Center, Robert M. Berne Cardiovascular Research Center, University of Virginia School of Medicine, Charlottesville, Virginia, USA

WILSON LEK WEN TAN, PhD
Stanford Cardiovascular Institute, Stanford University

JOSEPH C. WU, MD, PhD
Stanford Cardiovascular Institute, Department of Medicine, Division of Cardiovascular Medicine, Department of Radiology, Stanford University, Stanford, California, USA

ERIC H. YANG, MD
UCLA Cardio-Oncology Program, Division of Cardiology, Department of Medicine, University of California, Los Angeles, UCLA Cardiovascular Center, Los Angeles, California, USA

YOSHIMITSU YURA, MD, PhD
Hematovascular Biology Center, Robert M. Berne Cardiovascular Research Center, University of Virginia School of Medicine, Charlottesville, Virginia, USA; Department of Cardiology, Nagoya University Graduate School of Medicine, Nagoya, Japan

SYED WAMIQUE YUSUF, MBBS
Department of Cardiology, The University of
Texas MD Anderson Cancer Center, Houston,
Texas, USA

TABORAH Z. ZARAMO, BS
Dorothy M. Davis Heart and Lung Research
Institute, The Ohio State University, Columbus,
Ohio, USA

Contents

The development of human-induced pluripotent stem cell-derived cardiac cell types has created a new paradigm in assessing drug-induced cardiotoxicity. Advances in genomics and epigenomics have also implicated several genomic loci and biological pathways that may contribute to susceptibility to cancer therapies. In this review, we first provide a brief overview of the cardiotoxicity associated with chemotherapy. We then provide a detailed summary of systems biology approaches being applied to elucidate potential molecular mechanisms involved in cardiotoxicity. Finally, we discuss combining systems biology approaches with iPSC technology to help discover molecular mechanisms associated with cardiotoxicity.

Clonal hematopoiesis is a precancerous state that is recognized as a new causal risk factor for cardiovascular disease. Therapy-related clonal hematopoiesis is a condition that is often found in cancer survivors. These clonal expansions are caused by mutations in DNA damage-response pathway genes that allow hematopoietic stem cells to undergo positive selection in response to the genotoxic stress. These mutant cells increasingly give rise to progeny leukocytes that display enhanced proinflammatory properties. Recent experimental studies suggest that therapy-related clonal hematopoiesis may contribute to the medium- to long-term risk of genotoxic therapies on the cardiovascular system.

Myocardial dysfunction in patients with cancer is a major cause of morbidity and mortality. Cancer therapy-related cardiotoxicities are an important contributor to the development of cardiomyopathy in this patient population. Furthermore, cardiac AL amyloidosis, cardiac malignancies/metastases, accelerated atherosclerosis, stress cardiomyopathy, systemic and pulmonary hypertension are also linked to the development of myocardial dysfunction. Herein, we summarize current knowledge on the mechanisms of myocardial dysfunction in the setting of cancer and cancer-related therapies. Additionally, we briefly outline key recommendations on the surveillance and management of cancer therapy-related myocardial dysfunction based on the consensus of experts in the field of cardio-oncology.

Over the last several decades, advancements in cancer screening and treatment have significantly improved cancer mortality and overall quality of life. Unfortunately, non–cancer-related side effects, including cardiovascular toxicities can impact the continued delivery of these treatments. Arrhythmias are an increasingly recognized class of cardiotoxicity that can occur as a direct consequence of the treatment or secondary to another type of toxicity such as heart failure, myocarditis, or ischemia. Atrial arrhythmias, particularly atrial fibrillation (AF) are most commonly encountered, however, ventricular- and bradyarrhythmias can also occur, albeit at lower rates. Treatment strategies tailored to patients with cancer are essential to allow for the safe delivery of the cancer treatment without affecting short- or long-term oncologic or cardiovascular outcomes.

Targeting cardioprotective strategies to patients at the highest risk for cardiac events can help maximize therapeutic benefits. Dexrazoxane, liposomal formulations, continuous infusions, and neurohormonal antagonists may be useful for cardioprotection for anthracycline-treated patients at the highest risk for heart failure. Prevalent cardiovascular disease is a risk factor for cardiac events with many cancer therapies, including anthracyclines, anti–human-epidermal growth factor receptor-2 therapy, radiation, and BCR-Abl tyrosine kinase inhibitors, and may be a risk factor for cardiac events with other therapies. Although evidence for cardioprotective strategies is sparse for nonanthracycline therapies, optimizing cardiac risk factors and prevalent cardiovascular disease may improve outcomes.

Radiation therapy (RT) is part of standard-of-care treatment of many thoracic cancers. More than 60% of patients receiving thoracic RT may eventually develop radiation-induced cardiac dysfunction (RICD) secondary to collateral heart dose. This article reviews factors contributing to a thoracic cancer patient's risk for RICD, including RT dose to the heart and/or cardiac substructures, other anticancer treatments, and a patient's cardiometabolic health. It is also discussed how automated tracking of these factors within electronic medical record environments may aid radiation oncologists and other treating physicians in their ability to prevent, detect, and/or treat RICD in this expanding patient population.

Cardiovascular events, ranging from arrhythmias to decompensated heart failure, are common during and after cancer therapy. Cardiovascular complications can be life-threatening, and from the oncologist's perspective, could limit the use of first-line cancer therapeutics. Moreover, an aging population increases the risk for comorbidities and medical complexity among patients who undergo cancer therapy. Many have established cardiovascular diagnoses or risk factors before starting these therapies. Therefore, it is essential to understand the molecular mechanisms that drive cardiovascular events in patients with cancer and to identify new therapeutic targets that may prevent and treat these two diseases. This review will discuss the metabolic interaction between cancer and the heart and will highlight current strategies of targeting metabolic pathways for cancer treatment. Finally, this review highlights opportunities and challenges in advancing our understanding of myocardial metabolism in the context of cancer and cancer treatment.

Tyrosine kinase inhibitors (TKIs) are used to treat several cancers; however, a myriad of adverse cardiotoxic effects remain a primary concern. Although hypertension (HTN) is the most common adverse effect reported with TKI therapy, incidents of arrhythmias (eg, QT prolongation, atrial fibrillation) and heart failure are also prevalent. These complications warrant further research toward understanding the mechanisms of TKI-induced cardiotoxicity. Recent literature has given some insight into the intracellular signaling pathways that may mediate TKI-induced cardiac dysfunction. In this article, we discuss the cardiotoxic effects of TKIs on cardiomyocyte function, signaling, and possible treatments.

Chimeric antigen receptor (CAR) T-cell and bispecific T-cell engager (BiTE) therapies have revolutionized the treatment of refractory or relapsed leukemia and lymphoma. Increased use of these therapies has revealed signals of significant cardiotoxicity, including cardiomyopathy/heart failure, arrhythmia, myocardial injury, hemodynamic instability, and cardiovascular death mainly in the context of a profound inflammatory response to CAR T-cell antitumor effects known as cytokine release syndrome (CRS). Preexisting cardiovascular risk factors and disease may increase the risk of such cardiotoxicity. High index of suspicion and close monitoring is required for prompt recognition. Supportive hemodynamic care and targeted anti-IL-6 therapy, as well as possibly broader immunosuppression with corticosteroids, are the cornerstones of the management.

Cardiovascular (CV) events are an increasingly common limitation of effective anticancer therapy. Over the last decade imaging has become essential to patients receiving contemporary cancer therapy. Herein we discuss the current state of CV imaging in cardio-oncology. We also provide a practical apparatus for the use of imaging in everyday cardiovascular care of oncology patients to improve outcomes for those at risk for cardiotoxicity, or with established cardiovascular disease. Finally, we consider future directions in the field given the wave of new anticancer therapies.

Amyloid deposits are defined by their tinctorial properties. Under the light microscope amyloid deposits are eosinophilic and amorphous when stained with hematoxylin and eosin. With Congo red staining the deposits are positive and under polarized light will exhibit green birefringence. Sixty years later electron microscopy demonstrated that all deposits were fibrillar. All amyloid deposits are protein derived. The clinical characteristics will be driven by the nature of the protein subunit. In cardiology, the 2 most common subunits accounting for well more than 90% of cardiac amyloidosis are either immunoglobulin light chain, amyloid light-chain (AL) amyloidosis, or transthyretin; transthyretin (TTR) amyloidosis. Although 70% of patients with systemic amyloidosis have cardiac involvement the diagnosis is made by cardiologists only 20% of the time, suggesting significant gaps in knowledge in how to establish a workflow to arrive at a diagnosis in everyday practice.

Consensus statements on recommended definitions and practice in cardio-oncology have been developed. There is recognition of the potential for anthracyclines, trastuzumab, pertuzumab, immune checkpoint inhibitors, tyrosine kinase inhibitors, cyclophosphamide, and radiotherapy to cause left ventricular dysfunction and heart failure with heterogeneous natural histories. Cardiac function should be evaluated by echocardiography before the initiation of these therapies. For the prevention of cardiotoxicity, there is evidence to support the use of dexrazoxane under specific circumstances; existing research does not support the use of angiotensin-converting enzyme inhibitors/angiotensin receptor blockers or β-blockers in unselected individuals but should be considered in specific instances.

Cardiovascular disease is a leading cause of death in cancer survivors, after recurrence of the primary tumor or occurrence of a secondary malignancy. Consequently, the interdisciplinary field of cardio-oncology has grown rapidly in recent years to address the cardiovascular care needs of this unique population through clinical care and research initiatives. Here, the authors discuss the ideal infrastructure for training and career development in cardio-oncology translational and implementation science and emphasize the importance of the multidisciplinary cardiovascular team for both research and patient care. Cardio-oncology training opportunities in general cardiology, hematology/oncology, and specialized cardio-oncology clinical and research fellowships are also considered.

Advances in cancer treatments have led to nearly 17 million survivors in the US today. Cardiovascular complications attributed to cancer treatments are the leading cause of morbidity and mortality in cancer survivors. In response, NCI and NHLBI held 2 workshops and issued funding opportunities to strengthen research on cardiotoxicity. A representative portfolio of NIH grants categorizing basic, interventional, and observational projects is presented. Compared with anthracyclines, research on radiation therapy and newer treatments is underrepresented. Multidisciplinary collaborative research that considers the cardiotoxicity stage and optimizes the balance between cardiovascular risk and cancer-treatment benefit might support continued improvements in cancer outcomes.

HEART FAILURE CLINICS

Preface

Translational Cardio-Oncology Research to Promote Better Outcomes for One and All

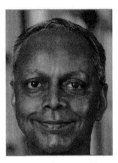

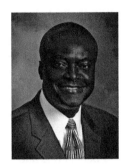

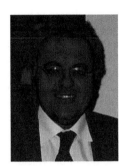

Ragavendra R. Baliga, MD, MBA, FACP, FRCP (Edin), FACC

George A. Mensah, MD, FACC, FAHA

Eduardo Bossone, MD, PhD, FCCP, FESC, FACC

Editors

Cardio-oncology is a vital, new discipline that has experienced exponential growth over the past decade. With the ever-increasing options for effective treatment of cancer, the burden of associated cardiovascular toxicity has continued to grow, making research in cardio-oncology a priority. This research needs to include the full spectrum of basic, clinical, and population science research (**Fig. 1**). Basic research, "conducted without thought of practical ends," results in "general knowledge and an understanding of nature and its laws."[1] Clinical research involves human

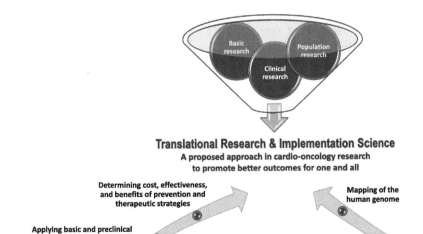

Translational Research & Implementation Science
A proposed approach in cardio-oncology research to promote better outcomes for one and all

Determining cost, effectiveness, and benefits of prevention and therapeutic strategies

Mapping of the human genome

Applying basic and preclinical research discoveries to the development of trials and studies in human subjects

Exploring implementation research and adopting best practices in the community

Advances in data science and computing power

Fundamental Discoveries

Fig. 1. Translational cardio-oncology research: key components and crucial tools.

Heart Failure Clin 18 (2022) xv–xvii
https://doi.org/10.1016/j.hfc.2022.04.001
1551-7136/22/© 2022 Published by Elsevier Inc.

heartfailure.theclinics.com

subjects, is patient-oriented, and includes research on mechanisms of human disease; behavioral studies; outcomes and health services research; preventive and therapeutic interventions; the development and testing of new health technologies; and clinical trials.[2] The National Institutes of Health has defined clinical trials as research studies in which "one or more human subjects are prospectively assigned to one or more interventions (which may include placebo or other control) to evaluate the effects of those interventions on health-related biomedical or behavioral outcomes."[2] Population research goes beyond individual patients to include cross-sectional and longitudinal epidemiological studies of cohorts, communities, or groups of people with known characteristics, such as age, sex/gender, race, and ethnicity, with or without a particular health condition.

Translational research and implementation science involve connecting the dots from basic, clinical, and population research to turn research discoveries into health impact in real-world settings. They include the application of fundamental discoveries to inform preclinical studies to the development of clinical trials and studies in humans, and research aimed at accelerating the adoption of best practices in the community. The latter includes research on the affordability, acceptability, reach, cost-effectiveness, and sustainability of prevention and therapeutic strategies. "It is the multi-disciplinary and multi-directional integration of basic research, patient-oriented research and population-based research."[3] Late-stage (T4) translation research and implementation science embrace the complexities of real-world settings—challenges in the "last mile on the long journey from fundamental discovery to population health impact."[4]

The scope of translational research is broad, and it is important that a focused effort be made to facilitate progress. Furthermore, the most meaningful patient-centered research requires attention to both quality and equity and collaborative efforts between basic scientists, clinical investigators, and implementation researchers. To ensure that the benefits of these efforts also reach populations that are often underserved and disproportionately impacted by cardiovascular diseases and cancer, systemic and structural inequities must be addressed.[5,6] The mapping of the human genome unleashed entirely new channels of exploration, including proteomics, transcriptomics, and gene-editing technology, which, in turn, have revolutionized translational research. These omics approaches are crucial tools for broadening the creativity, scope, and

innovativeness of cardio-oncology research. In addition, data science and computational advances have allowed analyses of big data of diverse communities facilitating community-engaged research. Sustained initiatives like these approaches applied in cardio-oncology will have a favorable impact on health care quality, including the amelioration of health inequities.

With these themes in mind, we invited the leaders of research in cardio-oncology to share with us their vision for the future. We are certain that these outstanding articles will provide additional seed for future research in the rapidly growing field of cardio-oncology research. The goal of this issue of *Heart Failure Clinics* is to ensure that a range of topics from bench to bedside and beyond, including implementation science, is discussed so that new models for promoting health and improving health care through translational cardio-oncology research develop to benefit one and all.

Ragavendra R. Baliga, MD, MBA,
FACP, FRCP
(Edin), FACC
Division of Cardiology
The Ohio State University Wexner Medical Center
Columbus, OH, USA

George A. Mensah, MD, FACC, FAHA
Center for Translation Research and
Implementation Science
National Heart, Lung, and Blood Institute
National Institutes of Health
Bethesda, MD, USA

Eduardo Bossone, MD, PhD,
FCCP, FESC, FACC
Division of Cardiology
AORN Antonio Cardarelli Hospital
Naples, Italy

E-mail addresses:
rrbaliga@gmail.com (R.R. Baliga)
george.mensah@nih.gov (G.A. Mensah)
ebossone@hotmail.com (E. Bossone)

REFERENCES

1. Bush V, editor. Science, the endless frontier: a report to the president by Vannevar Bush, Director of the Office of Scientific Research and Development. Washington, DC: United States Government Printing Office; 1945. Section 3 (The Importance of Basic Research), Chapter 3 (Science and the public welfare). Available at: http://www.nsf.gov/about/history/nsf50/vbush1945_content.jsp. Accessed March 20, 2022.

2. National Institutes of Health. NIH grants policy statement: definition of terms. 2021. Available at: https://grants.nih.gov/grants/policy/nihgps/HTML5/section_1/1.2_definition_of_terms.htm. Accessed March 20, 2022.

3. Rubio DM, Schoenbaum EE, Lee LS, et al. Defining translational research: implications for training. Acad Med 2010;85(3):470–5. https://doi.org/10.1097/ACM.0b013e3181ccd618.

4. Westfall JM, Mensah GA. T4 translational moonshot: making cardiovascular discoveries work for everyone. Circ Res 2018;122(2):210–2. https://doi.org/10.1161/circresaha.117.312273.

5. Mensah GA, Fuster V. Race, ethnicity, and cardiovascular disease: JACC focus seminar series. J Am Coll Cardiol 2021;78(24):2457–9. https://doi.org/10.1016/j.jacc.2021.11.001.

6. Churchwell K, Elkind MSV, Benjamin RM, et al. Call to action: structural racism as a fundamental driver of health disparities: a presidential advisory from the American Heart Association. Circulation 2020;142(24):e454–68.

Modeling Susceptibility to Cardiotoxicity in Cancer Therapy Using Human iPSC-Derived Cardiac Cells and Systems Biology

McKay Mullen, PhD[a], Wilson Lek Wen Tan, PhD[a], June-Wha Rhee, MD[b],*,
Joseph C. Wu, MD, PhD[a,c,d],*

KEYWORDS

• Cardiotoxicity • iPSC • Epigenetics • Genomics • Transcriptomics

KEY POINTS

- Cancer therapy-induced cardiotoxicity is an increasingly recognized problem in clinic; yet, its underlying mechanisms are poorly understood.
- Next generation sequencing combined with novel bioinformatic analysis has allowed researchers to identify genetic variants that may predispose patients to develop cardiotoxicity following the use of certain reagents.
- Advances in human genomics set the stage for the utilization of personalized medicine which caters cancer therapy to each individual's unique genome, maximizing anti-cancer effects while decreasing cardiotoxic adverse effects.

INTRODUCTION

During the past 2 decades, there have been remarkable advances in cancer therapies with newer agents of various categories being introduced in clinics every day. First, conventional chemotherapy refers to cancer treatment using chemicals with a specific toxic effect to destroy cancerous tissue.[1] Most available chemotherapeutic agents fall into various categories based on their mechanism of action, including but not limited to DNA-intercalating agents, antimetabolites, and tubulin-interactive agents. Chemotherapies are often used in conjunction with hormonal therapies, targeted therapies, and radiation therapies. Intercalators bind to DNA by inserting their chromophore moiety (ie, biological molecule that causes conformational change) between 2 consecutive base pairs, thus acting as a topoisomerase poison.[2,3] Hormonal therapies (ie, derivatives of synthetics of hormones, such as gonadotropin-releasing hormone [GnRH] modulators)[4] serve as a type of systemic therapy that, rather than being delivered directly to cancer cells, works by adding, blocking, or removing hormones from the body to slow or stop the growth of tumor cells.[5] Similarly, targeted therapy encompasses various direct and indirect approaches.[6] With targeted therapy, both direct and indirect methods rely on tumor antigens expressed on the cell surface as targets for ligands containing effector molecules (ie, monoclonal antibodies or small

a Stanford Cardiovascular Institute, Stanford University, 265 Campus Drive G1120B, Stanford, CA 94304, USA;
b Department of Medicine, City of Hope Comprehensive Cancer Center, 1500 E Duarte Rd, Duarte, CA 91010, USA; c Department of Medicine, Division of Cardiovascular Medicine, Stanford University; d Department of Radiology, Stanford University, 265 Campus Drive G1120B, Stanford, CA 94304, USA
* Co-corresponding authors. Department of Medicine, City of Hope Comprehensive Cancer Center, 1500 E Duarte Rd, Duarte, CA 91010 (J.R.); Stanford University, 265 Campus Drive, Room G1120B, Stanford, CA 94304 (J.C.W.).
E-mail addresses: jwrhee@stanford.edu (J.-W.R.); joewu@stanford.edu (J.C.W.)

Heart Failure Clin 18 (2022) 335–347
https://doi.org/10.1016/j.hfc.2022.02.009
1551-7136/22/© 2022 Elsevier Inc. All rights reserved.

molecule drugs that interfere with target proteins).[6] Finally, radiation therapy (ie, radiotherapy) involves the clinical use of ionizing radiation to kill cancer cells by inducing DNA damage.[7] One of the delivery modes is aiming the high-energy rays (ie, photons, protons, or particle radiation) at tumor site from outside the body.[8] Alternatively, internal radiation or brachytherapy is delivered from inside the body by radioactive sources, sealed in catheters into the tumor site.[8]

The development of cancer therapies into clinically useful agents has been based on their ability to selectively kill malignant cells.[9] As a result, modern treatment strategies have given patients a greater chance of surviving a cancer diagnosis; for example, the 5-year survival for early-stage breast cancer increased from 79% in 1990% to 90% in 2016.[10] However, on a global scale, cancer remains a significant burden that exacts a massive human cost, with 9.6 million deaths due to cancer in 2018.[10] In addition, cardiovascular disease (CVD) is one of the leading causes of long-term morbidity and mortality among cancer survivors.[5]

Patients who have a preexisting cardiovascular condition before their cancer diagnosis and then undergo treatments for their cancers are at a considerably increased risk of suffering worsening cardiovascular health.[11] Several current cancer therapies can increase cardiovascular risk in patients with cancer (eg, hypertension, cardiomyopathy, thrombosis, heart failure, and arrhythmias). For instance, in 2014, Herman and colleagues[12,13] reported that nilotinib (ie, a commonly used tyrosine kinase inhibitor) is associated with increased rates of arterial thrombosis, with 25% of patients experiencing an acute arterial event. In addition, recent studies show that CVD is the most common cause of death in patients with prostate cancer who have a survival rate longer than 10 years following a cancer diagnosis. Other epidemiologic studies have shown that an estimated 50% of patients are expected to undergo androgen deprivation therapy (ie, hormonal therapy) at some point in their treatment.[14] Of these patients, at least 20% to 30% will develop CVD, especially if they are taking GnRH agonists.[14]

Chemotherapeutic agents, targeted molecular therapies, and radiation therapy are all available cancer treatment options that can potentially harm the cardiovascular system.[15] Such damage can occur through the deterioration of the heart's function, peripherally by altering the hemodynamic flow, as well as through thrombotic events that often latently present in oncology patients.[15] Acute or subacute cardiotoxicity occurs when there are abnormalities in ventricular function, electrocardiographic QT-interval changes, arrhythmias, acute coronary syndromes, pericarditis, and myocarditis-like syndrome.[15] By comparison, chronic cardiotoxicity often occur in the form of asymptomatic systolic and/or diastolic left ventricular dysfunction that may progress to severe congestive cardiomyopathy and death.[15,16]

Thus far, it remains largely unknown how best to identify and treat those at risk for cardiotoxicity. Studies have shown that predictive markers (eg, natriuretic peptide) combined with pharmacologic intervention (eg, dexrazoxane) can help address chemotherapy-induced cardiotoxicity (**Table 1**).[11,17] Multiple clinical and epidemiologic studies have acknowledged that there may be underlying genetic suscpetibility to influence the severity of cardiotoxicity. However, conducting in vitro and in vivo studies has been challenging due to the lack of available clinically relevant models. More recently, innovative approaches using human-induced pluripotent stem cells (iPSCs), which can be produced from patients' somatic cells (eg, peripheral blood mononuclear cells or skin fibroblasts) and differentiated into relevant cardiovascular cell types, have proven valuable by providing a novel source of patient-specific genetic information, thus enabling personalized screening.[18] Moreover, remarkable advances in genetic sequencing technologies during the past decade have enabled more rapid discovery of new genes contributing to acute and chronic cardiotoxicity. In addition, advances in sequencing technologies (eg, next-generation sequencing [NGS], proteomics) and bioinformatics now allow researchers to investigate better mutations that result from chemotherapy (**Fig. 1**). This review will provide a detailed summary of various biomarkers and molecular mechanisms associated with cardiotoxicity discovered in genomics, transcriptomics, epitranscriptomics, and epigenetic studies.

GENOMICS

The human genome is made up of ∼3.2 billion base pairs of deoxyribonucleic acid (DNA) nucleotide, coiled and compressed into 23 pairs of chromosomes.[19] Human genetics has dramatically advanced during the past decades and deepened our understanding of the relationship between genetic diversity and disease predisposition, owing to the rapid development of novel sequencing technologies such as whole genome sequencing and whole exome sequencing.[20–24] These studies have identified millions of genetic variants, including short insertions and deletions, copy number variations, and other structural variations associated with complex traits and diseases.

Genome-wide association studies (GWAS) are among the more common population genetics

Table 1
Current imaging techniques and treatment approaches used to address chemotherapy-induced cardiotoxicity

Ref	Cancer Type	Approach	General Findings
Kavallaris [3] 2010	Breast cancer Non-Hodgkin lymphoma	Imaging	Newer technology is strain-echocardiography that allows for an improvement in the accuracy of calculating LVEF
Kavallaris [3] 2010	Breast cancer Non-Hodgkin lymphoma	Predictive biomarkers	Increased natriuretic peptide levels can detect chemotherapy-induced LVD
Leone-Bay et al, [4] 1996	Breast cancer acute leukemia	Predictive biomarkers	Negative troponin concentrations may identify patients with a very low risk of cardiomyopathy (negative predictive value, 99%)
Kavallaris [3] 2010, Baskar et al, [8] 2012	Metastatic breast cancer	Medication	Dexrazoxane significantly reduces anthracycline-related cardiotoxicity in adults with different solid tumors and in children with acute lymphoblastic leukemia and Ewing sarcoma
Kavallaris [3] 2010, Chandra et al, [7] 2021	Breast cancer	β-blockers	Carvedilol, a nonselective beta-blocker with antioxidant activity that is considered crucial in the treatment of patients with HF and LVD, is an effective cardioprotective agent during doxorubicin treatment

studies in which hundreds to millions of genetic variants across the genome of many individuals are tested to identify genotype–phenotype associations.[25] GWAS has successfully identified risk loci for a vast number of complex diseases and traits, including type 2 diabetes, heart failure, coronary artery disease, schizophrenia, and many types of cancers.[26–29] For predisposition to cardiotoxicity, multiple studies have reported genetic predisposition of individuals to anticancer therapy-induced cardiotoxicity.[30–35] Genetic polymorphisms for a handful of gene candidates, including *HER2*, *FCGR2*, and *FCGR3A*, have been reported to be associated with cardiotoxicity risk.[36] Aminkeng and colleagues[37] reported the association between a nonsynonymous genetic variant in the coding region of *RARG* genes with anthracycline-induced cardiotoxicity in childhood cancer. *RARG* has been shown to regulate the expression of topoisomerase II (*TOP2B*), which is also known to be involved in the progression of anthracycline-induced cardiotoxicity.[38,39] The identification of *RARG* genetic risk variant provides a clinical tool that may be used to predict genetic risk and improve cardiotoxicity risk stratification. In another study, Schneider and colleagues[31] reported no variants in a GWAS involving 845 patients with European-ancestry from a large adjuvant breast cancer clinical trial. Another promising variant, modestly replicated in 2 different cohorts, was found in a glucocorticoid receptor protein-binding site, which was hypothesized to play a crucial role in cardiac development.[40] In another genomic study involving a prespecified cardiomyopathy gene panel, rare truncating variants on *TTN* gene were associated with increased risk for cancer therapy-induced cardiomyopathy.[35] These studies highlight the potential of studying genetics as a risk factor for identifying patients with a higher risk for cancer-treatment-induced cardiomyopathy.

Although the genomic studies discussed above have provided a glimpse of genetic polymorphisms and aberrations associated with cancer therapy-induced cardiotoxicity, several considerations must be taken before applying genetic risk stratification for clinical practices. First, patients with cancer from diverse ancestries have to be included for future genomic studies.[41,42] Second, because most genomic studies recruited patients from specific cancer subtypes with personalized chemotherapy dosages and clinical practices,[35] the genetic loci reported from each genomic study may not be broadly relevant for the genotype-dependent cardiotoxicity risk stratification for all cancer types.[43] Nevertheless, current strategies to diagnose cancer therapy-induced cardiotoxicity and discontinue chemotherapy already have a decisive impact on the survival of patient with cancer. Therefore, the discovery of genetic risk factors may further help identify patient with cancer at high risk of cardiotoxicity and to tailor personalized cancer treatment regimens.

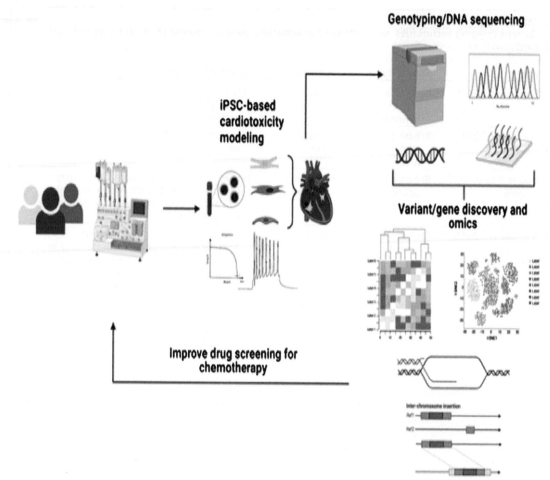

Fig. 1. *Application of iPSC-based cardiotoxicity screening and genomics to better understand the effects of* can-cer therapies *systemically.* PBMCs from patients are reprogrammed into iPSC and subsequently differentiated into various cardiac cell types, including cardiomyocytes, fibroblast, and endothelial cells using defined chemical methods. In addition, genomic DNA and transcriptome from the patient-specific iPSC lines can be analyzed using state-of-the-art multiomics sequencing technologies to identify genetic programs associated with cardiotoxicity risk. Genetic variants exerted their influence on cellular phenotype through transcriptomic and epigenetic regu-lations in a cell-type-specific manner. By understanding the interplay between genetics, epigenetics, and cardio-toxicity, personalized therapy can be designed for each patient to enhance the efficacy of cancer drugs and minimize the adverse impact on cardiovascular health. (Created with BioRender.com.)

TRANSCRIPTOMICS

Although nearly all cells in a multicellular organism share the same genetic blueprint, not every gene is expressed equally in every cell.[44] Different cells or tissues express a different set of genes that marks the particular cell's identity.[45] This variability in transcriptome underlies the wide range of phys-ical, biochemical, and developmental differences among diverse tissues, connecting genomic se-quences to gene function.[46] Therefore, the ability to determine the switching on and off of gene expression in response to challenges such as drug treatments, which form the basis to under-stand molecular pathways utilization in disease

causes, is a main objective of biomedical research.[47]

Recent decades have seen exponential growth in the sequencing technologies, resulting in ever more accessible and affordable genomics-related exper-iments. One of the earliest technologies in the 1980s for transcriptome profiling was the use of Sanger sequencing on expressed sequence tags.[48] Other low-throughput methods, including Northern blot-ting and reverse transcriptase quantitative PCR, were designed to study a limited number of genes.[49] Serial analysis of gene expression and DNA microarrays were developed in the 1990s for high-throughput transcriptome profiling.[50] DNA microarray, particularly, were widely used throughout 2000s due to their high throughput and lower cost.[50] However, DNA microarrays are limited to probing only known genes reported in the reference genome, and thus limiting their usage for novel transcript isoform discovery.[51] The massive research efforts in Human Genome Sequencing projects in the early 2000s has propelled the rapid development of high-throughput sequencing assays.[52] More specifically, RNA sequencing (RNA-seq) was invented for both the discovery and quantification of thousands of transcripts using a single high-throughput sequencing assay.[53] RNA-seq allows the quantification of RNAs over a broader dynamic range of 5 orders of magnitude, as compared with microarrays.[54] In addition to transcript quantification sensitivity, bioinformatics methods have also been developed to study the plethora of alternative RNA splicing events, a level of complexity that is captured by RNA-seq, but not by DNA microarray technology.[55]

Transcriptome-based toxicology analysis has been proposed to predict and risk-stratify patient-specific susceptibility to cardiotoxicity. Using tacrolimus and rosiglitazone, Matsa and colleagues[56] have performed RNA-seq to profile the gene expression responses on several human-induced pluripotent stem cell-derived cardiomyocyte (iPSC-CM) lines and showed that patient-specific iPSC-CM susceptibility to drug-induced cardiotoxicity could be computationally predicted, functionally validated, and rescued in vitro. Similarly, Burridge and colleagues[57] have observed a dose-dependent gene expression response from iPSC-CMs to doxorubicin exposure and identified several plausible molecular mechanisms governing doxorubicin-induced cardiotoxicity such as TGF-β signaling, p53 signaling, cardiac hypertrophy, G1/S checkpoint regulation, and retinoic acid receptor activation. Using clinically relevant doses of trastuzumab, Kitani and colleagues[58] performed RNA-seq on iPSC-CMs and functionally validated that metabolic pathway dysfunction, which was significantly enriched in trastuzumab-exposed iPSC-CMs, is the primary cause of cardiotoxic phenotype such as cardiomyocyte death and sarcomeric disorganization. The iPSC-CMs generated from patients who experienced severe cardiac dysfunction showed enhanced vulnerability to trastuzumab treatment. One of the study's highlights discovering that AMP-activated protein kinases activators (eg, metformin) can mitigate the adverse effects of trastuzumab-induced cardiotoxicity.[58] In another study, Sharma and colleagues[59] used both microarrays and RNA-seq to highlight the potential cardioprotective effect of insulin-mediated and IGF-mediated compensatory cardioprotection via VEGF/PDGFR-signaling during treatment with tyrosine kinase inhibitors (TKIs). Another study treated iPSC-CMs with various doxorubicin concentrations and identified a set of significantly downregulated genes with roles in DNA damage repair connected to p53.[60]

GWASs have uncovered genetic variants associated with cancer therapy-induced cardiotoxicity. However, the functional impact of these genetic variants remains elusive. Furthermore, many GWAS hits are found in intergenic regions, complicating the assignment of genes to these variants. Therefore, expression quantitative trait loci (eQTL), which measures the correlation between genotype and transcription of nearby genes, may provide a link between GWAS variant and cardiotoxicity phenotype. Scott and colleagues[22] performed an eQTL study to identify gene expression-related associations with anthracycline-induced cardiotoxicity (ACT) and revealed potential mechanisms underlying the development of this adverse reaction. The authors subsequently performed replication and functional validation analyses on the top association to further investigate its role in the development of ACT. In addition, using the gene expression profiles generated from transcriptome studies, the authors observed the downregulation of GDF5 across many tissues in ACT cases compared with controls, suggesting the involvement of GDF5 in protective mechanisms in cardiomyocytes against cardiotoxic agents at clinically relevant doses. In a separate study, Knowles and colleagues[33] used a panel of iPSC-CMs from 45 individuals exposed to 5 different drug concentrations to map the genetic basis of interindividual differences in doxorubicin-sensitivity. This study reported hundreds of genetic variants that modulated the spectrum of the transcriptomic response to doxorubicin treatment, many of which are predictive of ACT.[33]

Overall, transcriptome profiling has successfully dissected the molecular perturbation of anticancer therapy-induced cardiotoxicity, serving as a valuable tool for patient-specific cardiotoxicity prediction.

EPITRANSCRIPTOMICS

Although transcriptomic studies have revealed molecular responses to cardiotoxicities, there are other aspects of the transcript regulation that deserve equal attention. Epitranscriptomics, or "RNA-epigenetics," refers to chemical modifications on RNA that play essential roles in alternative splicing, nuclear export, transcript stability, and translations.[61] Various RNA modifications, including alternative splicing, adenosine-toinosine (A-to-I) modification, and RNA methylation, have been shown to regulate the mechanism of cancer drug resistance.[62] In particular, A-to-I editing, one of the most prevalent RNA modifications, is associated with cancer therapeutic resistance. A-to-I editing is catalyzed mainly by the adenosine deaminase acting on RNA (ADAR) family members, such as ADAR1, ADAR2, and ADAR3.[63] In multiple myeloma, ADAR1 was shown to enhance Alu-dependent editing of GLI1, a Hedgehog (Hh) signaling pathway transcriptional activator, leading to an R701 G amino acid change, which stabilized GL1 transcriptional activity by preventing the binding of a critical Hh signaling pathway inhibitor, resulting in resistance to immunotherapy.[64] Although the direct nexus between RNA modifications and cardiotoxicities remains elusive, cardiac-specific ablation of RNA-binding proteins such as ADAR1 and METTL3 in mice led to severe cardiac dysfunction, suggesting a potential role of RNA modifications in stress responses.[65,66]

EPIGENETICS

The term "epigenetics" was coined by Conrad Waddington in 1942, which he defined as alterations in phenotype without changes in the genotype to explain the concept of development for which there was little mechanistic understanding.[67] In other words, epigenetics represents the physiologic form of our genetic blueprint due to the regulation of gene expression levels without altering the underlying DNA sequence.[45]

Multiple epigenetic mechanisms have been studied, including methylation, acetylation, phosphorylation, ubiquitylation, and sumoylation.[68,69] DNA methylation, which happens predominantly on cytosine bases, involves the addition or removal of a methyl group on a nucleotide.[70] Methylation of cytosine, which involves the addition of methyl group, is catalyzed by DNA methyltransferases such DNMT1, DNMT3A, and DNMT3B.[71] Doxorubicin treatment in the animal model in vivo and in vitro has been associated with a global reduction in DNA methylation levels.[72–74] Nordgren and colleagues[73] performed a DNA methylation study on the heart tissues harvested from Sprague Dawley rats exposed to doxorubicin for 5 weeks. The study identified significant reduction in DNA methylation level on a handful of critical cardiac genes such as Rbm20, Scn5a, Nmnat2, and Cacna1c. In line with the animal model, Ferreira and colleagues[74] also observed global demethylation of the doxorubicin-treated rat cardiomyoblast H9C2 cell genome. Strikingly, one of the DNA methyltransferases, DNMT1, was also found to be repressed,

in line with the observation of global demethylation. DNMT1 plays an important role in the maintenance of DNA methylation of the mitochondrial genome.[71] Therefore, perturbation of DNMT1 and DNA methylation may affect the mitochondrial metabolism, thus affecting the toxicity induced by anthracycline treatment.

Another important epigenetic process is chromatin modification.[75–77] Chromatin is the complex of histone protein and DNA that is tightly bundled to fit into the nucleus.[78] Histone protein can be chemically modified by chromatin modifiers, such as histone deacetylases (HDAC) and histone acetyltransferase (KAT), by addition or removal of chemical groups, such as acetyl group, which have a direct impact on the gene regulation and chromatin folding.[79] High-throughput assays, such as chromatin immunoprecipitation followed by NGS (ChIP–seq), allows epigenome analysis at or near base-pair resolution, thus paving the way to epigenomic profiling for identifying genomic regions associated with chromatin modification alterations.[79] Anthracycline treatment has been associated with dysregulation of multiple chromatin modifiers such as HDAC2, HDAC6, and SIRT1.[80] In one study, doxorubicin treatment in rodents resulted in the upregulation of HDAC6, which led to deregulation of α-tubulin.[79] Genetic and pharmacologic inhibition of HDAC6 in mice was found to exhibit a cardioprotective effect by restoring autophagic flux.[79] Hanf and colleagues[81] reported the deregulation of SIRT1 and HDAC2 in rat cardiomyoblast cells on doxorubicin treatment. Downregulation of HDAC2 was also replicated in mouse heart tissues treated with doxorubicin.[82] Intriguingly, treatment of cells with antioxidants has been proposed to alleviate doxorubicin-induced cardiotoxicity.[83] One plausible mechanism was the recruitment of SIRT1, which may exert a cardioprotective effect against doxorubicin with an elevated deacetylation activity on antioxidant treatment.[84] In another study, Ma and colleagues[39] proposed a ROS-independent mechanism for doxorubicin-induced cardiotoxicity involving Rac1, a GTP-binding protein, and subunit of NADPH oxidase that resulted in the suppression of HDAC activity and upregulation of p53.

Apart from histone acetylation, doxorubicin treatment has also been reported to affect histone methylation.[85] Specifically, histone lysine demethylases, including KDM3A and LSD1, as well as histone lysine methyltransferases, including SET7 and SMYD1, have been shown to deregulate on doxorubicin treatment.[86,87] KDM3A was significantly upregulated on doxorubicin treatment of rat H9C2 cells.[81] In addition, long-term doxorubicin treatment also reduced the LSD1 expression level.[88,89]

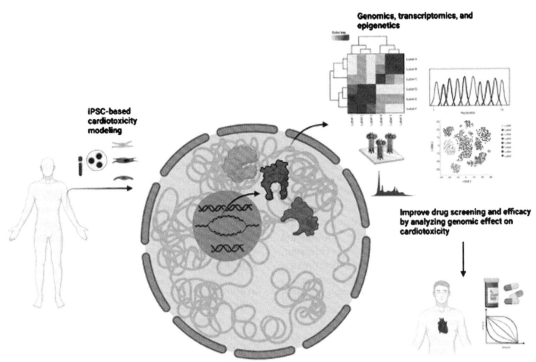

Fig. 2. *Application of system biology approaches and iPSC technology for future prediction of personalized cancer therapy-induced cardiotoxicity studies.* Patient-specific iPSC-derived cardiac cell can be used to perform functional genomics studies using high-throughput CRISPR screening to identify novel genetic biomarkers associated with cancer therapy-induced cardiotoxicity. Circulating cell-free DNA can also be used as a less invasive detection biomarker for patient-specific cardiotoxicity. Single-cell profiling can also be exploited to uncover cell-specific transcriptomics and epigenomics changes in response to cancer drug treatment at high resolution.

Similarly, significant overexpression of *SET7* and *SMYD1* was observed in long-term and high-dose doxorubicin treatment.[81] The molecular pathway for the concerted regulation of histone methyltransferases and demethylases may be due to the inhibition of *TOP2B* in the form of "eviction" of specific histones from chromatin, resulting in a potential shift of histone modification, and chromatin structure, around the promoter region of a gene.[90–92]

FUTURE OF FUNCTIONAL GENOMICS IN CARDIO-ONCOLOGY MODELING USING HUMAN-INDUCED PLURIPOTENT STEM CELLS

The application of iPSCs has been a valuable tool for recapitulating a clinically relevant readout in a high-throughput assay[93] (**Fig. 2**). In addition, the ability to differentiate iPSCs into a myriad of disease-relevant cell types, including cardiomyocytes,[94] fibroblast,[95] smooth muscle cells,[96] and endothelial cells,[97] allows researchers to apply chemical and functional genomics experiments to better elucidate and interpret disease pathways influencing chemotherapy-induced cardiotoxicity.[93,98]

Single-cell technologies have been widely adopted as a platform to study cell-type-specific

transcription programs.[99–101] In iPSC cultures, transcriptional heterogeneity, representing diverse cell states and differential gene responses has been described.[97] Therefore, the transcriptome and epigenome findings described earlier have mainly come from studies that average measurements over large populations of cells, many of which are functionally heterogeneous. These studies concealed or underestimated the actual variability among cells and therefore prevented us from determining the nature of heterogeneity at the molecular level as a basis for understanding biological complexity in response to drug treatments.[102] New approaches using single-cell profiling techniques such as single-cell RNA-seq, single-cell ChIP-seq, and single-cell assay for transposase accessible chromatin (ATAC)-seq now enable researchers to identify and uncover cell type-specific gene regulation on cancer therapy that has been masked by the averaging effect from older bulk sequencing technologies.[103,104]

The clustered regularly interspaced short palindromic repeats (CRISPR) system and other variants thereof have been widely adopted for genetic manipulation.[105] The high-throughput CRISPR screening technique can interrogate novel gene functions involved in various biological pathways, such as metastasis, synthetic lethal interactions, therapeutic resistance, immunotherapy response, cardiac pathologic condition, and tissue development, which are primarily performed in vitro.[106–109] CRISPR screening involves the delivery of hundreds or thousands of single-stranded guide RNAs targeting multiple genes.[106] Using quantifiable cellular and molecular readouts, CRISPR screens can identify key driver genes important for the fitness or survival of the cells in response to cancer drug treatment.[107] In a CRISPR screening study using iPSC-CM, 2 genes encoding for solute carrier organic anion transporters (SLCO1A2 and SLCO1B3) were reported to be the key transport mechanism underlying doxorubicin-induced cell death.[107] However, CRISPR screen is not without its shortcomings and blind spots.[106] Careful consideration has to be given in the interpretation of CRISPR screening results. In addition, Cas9 protein creates double-stranded DNA breaks, which might trigger a cellular response such as cell cycle arrest and apoptosis.[110–112] An alternative approach would be to use nuclease-dead mutants of Cas9 (dCas9) in the CRISPR screening experiments. dCas9, fused with transcriptional repressor domains such as Kruppel-associated box, blocks transcription of genes without creating DNA breaks.[113] Recently, CRISPR screening was coupled with single-cell transcriptome profiling (Perturb-seq) to elucidate detailed transcriptome changes in response to gene perturbation in a cell-type-specific manner.[114] Although the application of screening using CRISPR is still in its infancy for cardio-oncology, we thought this approach will help uncover many more molecular biomarkers for cardiotoxicity in an accelerated time frame.

Circulating cell-free DNA (cfDNA) is gaining traction in the oncology setting.[115–122] cfDNA released into the patient's blood circulation has been shown to distinguish early-stage cancers in an organ-specific manner without the need for invasive procedures to acquire biopsies from metastatic lesions.[116–120,122,123] Because of its stability in serum with a relatively short half-life of up to 3 hours, cfDNA serves as an attractive blood-based biomarker.[124] Genome sequencing of cfDNA in the patient's circulation has been applied to monitor metastasis, early detection of cancer progression, and drug resistance.[116,117,120,121,123] In the cardiovascular field, cfDNA has been used as a diagnostic marker to detect acute rejection after heart transplantation and to monitor cardiac pathologic conditions such as myocardial infarction.[124,125] Therefore, due to its specificity and sensitivity, cfDNA can serve as a potential alternative molecular readout for increased cardiac cell death in patients undergoing cancer therapy. The use of cfDNA for the detection of cardiotoxicity in patients with cancer has been assessed.[123] Also, the genomic sequence content encoded in the sequencing reads of iPSC-derived cfDNA might also provide information on disease-relevant genetic variants.[121] The prognostic value of these genetic polymorphisms encoded in cfDNA remains to be determined. Nonetheless, cfDNA remains relatively unexplored as a prognostic and diagnostic tool for cancer therapy-induced cardiotoxicity. Coupled with the versatility and scalability of iPSC technology, we thought cfDNA can be applied to design personalized cancer therapy regimes that will minimize the adverse effect of chemotherapy.

SUMMARY

In summary, iPSC technology, coupled with genomics and epigenomics approaches, has uncovered many molecular targets and biological mechanisms associated with cancer-therapy-induced cardiotoxicity. The future direction of research may involve using a large iPSC biobank looking into different CVD states related to cardio-oncology to investigate the influence of using genome-editing technologies (eg, CRISPR-cas9) to correct chemo-induced aberrant mutations. The implication of these results may lay the foundation for applying genetic profiling and genome editing as a novel approach to treating patients diagnosed with cancer.

CLINICS CARE POINTS

- Before starting cancer therapy, patients' cardiovascular history should be comprehensively assessed and well documented.
- Certain cancer therapy drugs (eg, doxorubicin) have been associated with significant cardiovascular complications. Close monitoring and optimization of cardiovascular health would be warranted when using these potentially cardiotoxic drugs, especially if patients have preexisting CVDs.
- It is important to continue to implement standard guideline-based therapies (eg, statins) to lower CVDs in patients with cancer.
- iPSC technology, genomics, and epigenomics approaches have provided insights into the biological mechanisms associated with cancer-therapy-induced cardiotoxicity and may uncover molecular targets for cardioprotective approaches.

ACKNOWLEDGMENTS

This study is supported by Stanford Propel Post-doctoral Scholar Award (M.M.); Stanford Postdoctoral Fellowship Award (W.L.W.T.); National Institutes of Health K08 HL148540 (J.W.R.); and American Heart Association SFRN 869015, R01 HL123968, R01 HL141851, R01 HL145676, and R01 HL150693 (J.C.W.).

REFERENCES

1. Johnstone RW, Ruefli AA, Lowe SW. Apoptosis. *Cell*. 2002;108(2):153–64.
2. Portugal J, Barceló F. Noncovalent binding to DNA: still a target in developing anticancer agents. Curr Med Chem 2016;23(36):4108–34.
3. Kavallaris M. Microtubules and resistance to tubulin-binding agents. Nat Rev Cancer 2010; 10(3):194–204.
4. Leone-Bay A, Ho K-K, Agarwal R, et al. *4-[4-[(2-Hydroxybenzoyl)Amino]Phenyl]*Butyric acid as a novel oral delivery agent for recombinant human growth hormone. J Med Chem 1996;39(13): 2571–8. https://pubs.acs.org/sharingguidelines.
5. Curigliano G, Cardinale D, Dent S, et al. Cardiotoxicity of anticancer treatments: epidemiology, detection, and management. CA Cancer J Clin 2016; 66(4):309–25.
6. Baudino T. Targeted cancer therapy: the next generation of cancer treatment. Curr Drug Discov Tech 2015;12(1):3–20.
7. Chandra RA, Keane FK, Voncken FEM, et al. Contemporary radiotherapy: present and future. Lancet 2021;398(10295):3–20.
8. Baskar R, Lee KA, Yeo R, et al. Cancer and radiation therapy: current advances and future directions. Int J Med Sci 2012;9(3):193–9.
9. Galluzzi L, Humeau J, Buqué A, et al. Immunostimulation with chemotherapy in the era of immune checkpoint inhibitors. Nat Rev Clin Oncol 2020; 17(12):725–41.
10. Siegel RL, Miller KD, Fuchs HE, et al. Cancer statistics, 2021. CA: A Cancer J Clinicians 2021;71(1): 7–33.
11. Gintant G, Burridge P, Gepstein L, et al. Use of human induced pluripotent stem cell-derived cardiomyocytes in preclinical cancer drug cardiotoxicity testing: a scientific statement from the American Heart Association. Circ Res 2019;125(10):e75–92.
12. Herrmann J, Lerman A. An update on cardio-oncology. Trends Cardiovasc Med 2014;24(7):285–95.
13. Cameron AC, Touyz RM, Lang NN. Vascular complications of cancer chemotherapy. Can J Cardiol 2016;32(7):852–62.
14. Muniyan S, Xi L, Datta K, et al. Cardiovascular risks and toxicity - the Achilles heel of androgen deprivation therapy in prostate cancer patients. Biochim Biophys Acta Rev Cancer 2020;1874(1): 188383.
15. Albini A, Pennesi G, Donatelli F, et al. Cardiotoxicity of anticancer drugs: The need for cardio-oncology and cardio-oncological prevention. J Natl Cancer Inst 2010;102(1):14–25.
16. Dolci A, Dominici R, Cardinale D, et al. Biochemical markers for prediction of chemotherapy-induced cardiotoxicity systematic review of the literature and recommendations for use. Am J Clin Pathol 2008;130(5):688–95.
17. Cheuk DK, Sieswerda E, van Dalen EC, et al. Medical interventions for treating anthracycline-induced symptomatic and asymptomatic cardiotoxicity during and after treatment for childhood cancer. Cochrane Database Syst Rev 2016;2016(8): CD008011.
18. Rhee J-W, Ky B, Armenian SH, et al. Primer on biomarker discovery in cardio-oncology. JACC: CardioOncology. 2020;2(3):379–84.
19. Craig Venter J, Adams MD, Myers EW, et al. The sequence of the human genome. Science 2001; 291(5507):1304–51.
20. Hirschhorn JN, Lohmueller K, Byrne E, et al. A comprehensive review of genetic association studies. Genet Med 2002;4(2):45–61.
21. Mitsuhashi S, Matsumoto N. Long-read sequencing for rare human genetic diseases. J Hum Genet 2020;65(1):11–9.
22. Scott EN, Wright GEB, Drögemöller BI, et al. Transcriptome-wide association study uncovers the role of essential genes in anthracycline-induced cardiotoxicity. NPJ Genomic Med 2021;6(1):35.
23. Van Hout CV, Tachmazidou I, Backman JD, et al. Exome sequencing and characterization of 49,960 individuals in the UK Biobank. Nature 2020;586(7831):749–56.
24. Sinnott-Armstrong N, Tanigawa Y, Amar D, et al. Genetics of 35 blood and urine biomarkers in the UK Biobank. Nat Genet 2021;53(2):185–94.
25. Tam V, Patel N, Turcotte M, et al. Benefits and limitations of genome-wide association studies. Nat Rev Genet 2019;20(8):467–84.
26. Mahajan A, Taliun D, Thurner M, et al. Fine-mapping type 2 diabetes loci to single-variant resolution using high-density imputation and islet-specific epigenome maps. Nat Genet 2018; 50(11):1505–13.
27. Shah S, Henry A, Roselli C, et al. Genome-wide association and Mendelian randomisation analysis provide insights into the pathogenesis of heart failure. Nat Commun 2020;11(1):1–12.
28. Nikpay M, Goel A, Won HH, et al. A comprehensive 1000 Genomes-based genome-wide association meta-analysis of coronary artery disease. Nat Genet 2015;47(10):1121–30.

29. Ripke S, Neale BM, Corvin A, et al. Biological insights from 108 schizophrenia-associated genetic loci. Nature 2014;511(7510):421–7.

30. Park B, Sim SH, Lee KS, et al. Genome-wide association study of genetic variants related to anthracycline-induced cardiotoxicity in early breast cancer. Cancer Sci 2020;111(7):2579–87.

31. Schneider BP, Shen F, Gardner L, et al. Genome-wide association study for anthracycline-induced congestive heart failure. Clin Cancer Res 2017;23(1):43–51.

32. Norton N, Crook JE, Wang L, et al. Association of genetic variants at TRPC6 With chemotherapy-related heart failure. Front Cardiovasc Med 2020;7(August):1–15.

33. Knowles DA, Burrows CK, Blischak JD, et al. Determining the genetic basis of anthracycline-cardiotoxicity by molecular response QTL mapping in induced cardiomyocytes. eLife 2018;7:1–25.

34. McOwan TN, Craig LA, Tripdayonis A, et al. Evaluating anthracycline cardiotoxicity associated single nucleotide polymorphisms in a paediatric cohort with early onset cardiomyopathy. Cardio-Oncology. 2020;6(1):4–9.

35. Garcia-Pavia P, Kim Y, Restrepo-Cordoba MA, et al. Genetic variants associated with cancer therapy-induced cardiomyopathy. Circulation 2019;140(1):31–41.

36. Gavin PG, Song N, Rim Kim S, et al. Association of polymorphisms in FCGR2A and FCGR3A with degree of trastuzumab benefit in the adjuvant treatment of ERBB2/HER2-positive breast cancer analysis of the NSABP B-31 trial. JAMA Oncol 2017;3(3):335–41.

37. Aminkeng F, Bhavsar AP, Visscher H, et al. A coding variant in RARG confers susceptibility to anthracycline-induced cardiotoxicity in childhood cancer. Nat Genet 2015;47(9):1079–84.

38. Yi LL, Kerrigan JE, Lin CP, et al. Topoisomerase IIβ-mediated DNA double-strand breaks: Implications in doxorubicin cardiotoxicity and prevention by dexrazoxane. Cancer Res 2007;67(18):8839–46.

39. Ma X, Zhu P, Ding Y, et al. Retinoid X receptor alpha is a spatiotemporally predominant therapeutic target for anthracycline-induced cardiotoxicity. Sci Adv 2020;6(5):1–15.

40. Rog-Zielinska EA, Thomson A, Kenyon CJ, et al. Glucocorticoid receptor is required for foetal heart maturation. Hum Mol Genet 2013;22(16):3269–82.

41. Sapkota Y. Harnessing genomics to predict and prevent anthracycline-associated cardiotoxicity. JACC: CardioOncology. 2020;2(5):707–9.

42. Litvak A, Batukbhai B, Russell SD, et al. Racial disparities in the rate of cardiotoxicity of HER2-targeted therapies among women with early breast cancer. Cancer 2018;124(9):1904–11.

43. Han X, Zhou Y, Liu W. Precision cardio-oncology: understanding the cardiotoxicity of cancer therapy. NPJ Precision Oncol 2017;1(1):31.

44. Karlsson M, Zhang C, Méar L, et al. A single–cell type transcriptomics map of human tissues. Sci Adv 2021;7(31):1–10.

45. Abascal F, Acosta R, Addleman NJ, et al. Expanded encyclopaedias of DNA elements in the human and mouse genomes. Nature 2020;583(7818):699–710.

46. Albert FW, Kruglyak L. The role of regulatory variation in complex traits and disease. Nat Rev Genet 2015;16(4):197–212.

47. Wang Z, Gerstein M, Snyder M. RNA-Seq: a revolutionary tool for transcriptomics. Nat Rev Genet 2009;10(January 2009):57–63.

48. Goodwin S, McPherson JD, McCombie WR. Coming of age: Ten years of next-generation sequencing technologies. Nat Rev Genet 2016;17(6):333–51.

49. Slatko BE, Gardner AF, Ausubel FM. Overview of next generation sequencing technologies (and bioinformatics) in cancer. Mol Biol 2018;122(1):1–15.

50. Lowe R, Shirley N, Bleackley M, et al. Transcriptomics technologies. PLoS Comput Biol 2017;13(5):1–23.

51. Zhao S, Fung-Leung WP, Bittner A, et al. Comparison of RNA-Seq and microarray in transcriptome profiling of activated T cells. PLoS One 2014;9(1):e78644.

52. Lander ES, Linton LM, Birren B, et al. Initial sequencing and analysis of the human genome. Nature 2001;412(6846):565–6.

53. Stark R, Grzelak M, Hadfield J. RNA sequencing: the teenage years. Nat Rev Genet 2019;20(11):631–56.

54. Wang B, Kumar V, Olson A, et al. Reviving the transcriptome studies: an insight into the emergence of single-molecule transcriptome sequencing. Front Genet 2019;10(APR):1–11.

55. Bonnal SC, López-Oreja I, Valcárcel J. Roles and mechanisms of alternative splicing in cancer — implications for care. Nat Rev Clin Oncol 2020;17(8):457–74.

56. Matsa E, Burridge PW, Yu KH, et al. Transcriptome profiling of patient-specific human iPSC-cardiomyocytes predicts individual drug safety and efficacy responses in vitro. Cell Stem Cell 2016;19(3):311–25.

57. Burridge PW, Li YF, Matsa E, et al. Human induced pluripotent stem cell-derived cardiomyocytes recapitulate the predilection of breast cancer patients to doxorubicin-induced cardiotoxicity. Nat Med 2016;22(5):547–56.

58. Kitani T, Ong SG, Lam CK, et al. Human-induced pluripotent stem cell model of trastuzumab-induced cardiac dysfunction in patients with breast cancer. Circulation 2019;139(21):2451–65.

59. Sharma A, Burridge PW, McKeithan WL, et al. High-throughput screening of tyrosine kinase inhibitor cardiotoxicity with human induced pluripotent stem cells. Sci Translational Med 2017;9(377): eaaf2584.

60. McSweeney KM, Bozza WP, Alterovitz WL, et al. Transcriptomic profiling reveals p53 as a key regulator of doxorubicin-induced cardiotoxicity. Cell Death Discov 2019;5(1):102.

61. Holoch D, Moazed D. RNA-mediated epigenetic regulation of gene expression. Nat Rev Genet 2015;16(2):71–84.

62. Song H, Liu D, Dong S, et al. Epitranscriptomics and epiproteomics in cancer drug resistance: therapeutic implications. Signal Transduction Targeted Ther 2020;5(1):193.

63. Nishikura K. A-to-I editing of coding and non-coding RNAs by ADARs. Nat Rev Mol Cell Biol 2016;17(2):83–96.

64. Lazzari E, Mondala PK, Santos ND, et al. Alu-dependent RNA editing of GLI1 promotes malignant regeneration in multiple myeloma. Nat Commun 2017;8(1):1–10.

65. Dorn LE, Lasman L, Chen J, et al. The N-methyladenosine mRNA methylase METTL3 controls cardiac homeostasis and hypertrophy. Circulation 2019;139(4):533–45.

66. el Azzouzi H, Vilaça AP, Feyen DAM, et al. Cardiomyocyte specific deletion of ADAR1 Causes severe cardiac dysfunction and increased lethality. Front Cardiovasc Med 2020;7(March):1–16.

67. Goldberg AD, Allis CD, Bernstein E. Epigenetics: a landscape takes shape. Cell 2007;128(4):635–8.

68. Handy DE, Castro R, Loscalzo J. Epigenetic modifications: basic mechanisms and role in cardiovascular disease. Circulation 2011;123(19):2145–56.

69. Allis CD, Jenuwein T. The molecular hallmarks of epigenetic control. Nat Rev Genet 2016;17(8): 487–500.

70. Greenberg MVC, Bourc'his D. The diverse roles of DNA methylation in mammalian development and disease. Nat Rev Mol Cell Biol 2019;20(10): 590–607.

71. Lyko F. The DNA methyltransferase family: a versatile toolkit for epigenetic regulation. Nat Rev Genet 2018;19(2):81–92.

72. Cheng Y, He C, Wang M, et al. Targeting epigenetic regulators for cancer therapy: mechanisms and advances in clinical trials. Signal Transduction Targeted Ther 2019;4(1):62.

73. Nordgren KKS, Hampton M, Wallace KB. The altered DNA methylome of chronic doxorubicin exposure in sprague dawley rats. Toxicol Sci 2017;159(2):470–9.

74. Ferreira LL, Cunha-Oliveira T, Veloso CD, et al. Single nanomolar doxorubicin exposure triggers compensatory mitochondrial responses in H9c2 cardiomyoblasts. Food Chem Toxicol 2019;124: 450–61.

75. Li E. Chromatin modification and epigenetic reprogramming in mammalian development. Nat Rev Genet 2002;3(9):662–73.

76. Bannister AJ, Kouzarides T. Regulation of chromatin by histone modifications. Cell Res 2011; 21(3):381–95.

77. Kouzarides T. Chromatin modifications and their function. Cell 2007;128(4):693–705.

78. Klemm SL, Shipony Z, Greenleaf WJ. Chromatin accessibility and the regulatory epigenome. Nat Rev Genet 2019;20(4):207–20.

79. Marmorstein R. Protein modules that manipulate histone tails for chromatin regulation. Nat Rev Mol Cell Biol 2001;2(6):422–32.

80. Kumari H, Huang W-H, Chan MWY. Review on the role of epigenetic modifications in doxorubicin-induced cardiotoxicity. Front Cardiovasc Med 2020;7(May):1–8.

81. Hanf A, Oelze M, Manea A, et al. The anti-cancer drug doxorubicin induces substantial epigenetic changes in cultured cardiomyocytes. Chemico-Biological Interactions 2019;313(September): 108834.

82. Piotrowska I, Isalan M, Mielcarek M. Early transcriptional alteration of histone deacetylases in a murine model of doxorubicin-induced cardiomyopathy. PLoS One 2017;12(6):1–12.

83. Vincent DT, Ibrahim YF, Espey MG, et al. The role of antioxidants in the era of cardio-oncology. Cancer Chemother Pharmacol 2013;72(6):1157–68.

84. Sin TK, Tam BT, Yung BY, et al. Resveratrol protects against doxorubicin-induced cardiotoxicity in aged hearts through the SIRT1-USP7 axis. J Physiol 2015;593(8):1887–99.

85. Greer EL, Shi Y. Histone methylation: A dynamic mark in health, disease and inheritance. Nat Rev Genet 2012;13(5):343–57.

86. Ohguchi H, Hideshima T, Bhasin MK, et al. The KDM3A-KLF2-IRF4 axis maintains myeloma cell survival. Nat Commun 2016;7:1–15.

87. Wallace KB, Sardão VA, Oliveira PJ. Mitochondrial determinants of doxorubicin- induced cardiomyopathy. Circ Res 2020;126:926–41.

88. Lin Y, Kang T, Zhou BP. Doxorubicin enhances Snail/LSD1-mediated PTEN suppression in a PARP1-dependent manner. Cell Cycle 2014; 13(11):1708–16.

89. Lee C, Rudneva VA, Erkek S, et al. Lsd1 as a therapeutic target in Gfi1-activated medulloblastoma. Nat Commun 2019;10(1):1–13.

90. Zhang S, Liu X, Bawa-Khalfe T, et al. Identification of the molecular basis of doxorubicin-induced cardiotoxicity. Nat Med 2012;18(11):1639–42.

91. Marinello J, Delcuratolo M, Capranico G. Anthracyclines as topoisomerase II poisons: from early

studies to new perspectives. Int J Mol Sci 2018; 19(11):3480.

92. Tewey KM, Rowe TC, Yang L, et al. Adriamycin-induced DNA damage mediated by mammalian DNA topoisomerase II. Science 1984;226(4673): 466–8.

93. Mullen M, Zhang A, Lui GK, et al. Race and genetics in congenital heart disease: application of iPSCs, omics, and machine learning technologies. Front Cardiovasc Med 2021;8:635280.

94. Burridge PW, Matsa E, Shukla P, et al. Chemically defined generation of human cardiomyocytes. Nat Methods 2014;11(8):855–60.

95. Zhang H, Tian L, Shen M, et al. Generation of quiescent cardiac fibroblasts from human induced pluripotent stem cells for in vitro modeling of cardiac fibrosis. Circ Res 2019;125(5):552–66.

96. Shen M, Quertermous T, Fischbein MP, et al. Generation of vascular smooth muscle cells From induced pluripotent stem cells. Circ Res 2021; 128(5):670–86.

97. Paik DT, Tian L, Lee J, et al. Large-scale single-cell RNA-Seq reveals molecular signatures of heterogeneous populations of human induced pluripotent stem cell-derived endothelial cells. Circ Res 2018; 123(4):443–50.

98. Rhee JW, Ky B, Armenian SH, et al. Primer on biomarker discovery in cardio-oncology: application of omics technologies. JACC: CardioOncology. 2020;2(3):379–84.

99. Yamada S, Nomura S. Review of single-cell RNA sequencing in the heart. Int J Mol Sci 2020; 21(21):1–15.

100. Butler A, Hoffman P, Smibert P, et al. Integrating single-cell transcriptomic data across different conditions, technologies, and species. Nat Biotechnol 2018;36(5):411–20.

101. Pierce SE, Kim SH, Greenleaf WJ. Finding needles in a haystack: dissecting tumor heterogeneity with single-cell transcriptomic and chromatin accessibility profiling. Curr Opin Genet Dev 2021;66:36–40.

102. Goldman SL, MacKay M, Afshinnekoo E, et al. The impact of heterogeneity on single-cell sequencing. Front Genet 2019;10:8.

103. Kashima Y, Sakamoto Y, Kaneko K, et al. Single-cell sequencing techniques from individual to multiomics analyses. Exp Mol Med 2020;52(9):1419–27.

104. Paik DT, Cho S, Tian L, et al. Single-cell RNA sequencing in cardiovascular development, disease and medicine. Nat Rev Cardiol 2020;17(8): 457–73.

105. Anzalone Av, Koblan LW, Liu DR. Genome editing with CRISPR–Cas nucleases, base editors, transposases and prime editors. Nat Biotechnol 2020; 38(7):824–44.

106. Doench JG. Am I ready for CRISPR? A user's guide to genetic screens. Nat Rev Genet 2018;19(2): 67–80.

107. Sapp V, Aguirre A, Mainkar G, et al. Genome-wide CRISPR/Cas9 screening in human iPS derived cardiomyocytes uncovers novel mediators of doxorubicin cardiotoxicity. Scientific Rep 2021;11(1): 13866.

108. Jaitin DA, Weiner A, Yofe I, et al. Dissecting immune circuits by linking CRISPR-pooled screens with single-cell RNA-seq. Cell 2016;167(7):1883–96.e15.

109. Tycko J, Wainberg M, Marinov GK, et al. Mitigation of off-target toxicity in CRISPR-Cas9 screens for essential non-coding elements. Nat Commun 2019;10(1):1–14.

110. van Overbeek M, Capurso D, Carter MM, et al. DNA Repair profiling reveals nonrandom outcomes at cas9-mediated breaks. Mol Cell 2016;63(4):633–46.

111. Wang T, Birsoy K, Hughes NW, et al. Identification and characterization of essential genes in the human genome. Science 2015;350(6264):1096–101.

112. Doench JG, Fusi N, Sullender M, et al. Optimized sgRNA design to maximize activity and minimize off-target effects of CRISPR-Cas9. Nat Biotechnol 2016;34(2):184–91.

113. Kampmann M. CRISPRi and CRISPRa screens in mammalian cells for precision biology and medicine. ACS Chem Biol 2018;13(2):406–41.

114. Dixit A, Parnas O, Li B, et al. Perturb-Seq: dissecting molecular circuits with scalable single-cell RNA profiling of pooled genetic screens. Cell 2016; 167(7):1853–66.e17.

115. Sadeh R, Sharkia I, Fialkoff G, et al. ChIP-seq of plasma cell-free nucleosomes identifies gene expression programs of the cells of origin. Nat Biotechnol 2021;39(5):586–98.

116. Snyder MW, Kircher M, Hill AJ, et al. Cell-free DNA comprises an in vivo nucleosome footprint that informs its tissues-Of-origin. Cell 2016;164(1–2): 57–68.

117. Zukowski A, Rao S, Ramachandran S. Phenotypes from cell-free DNA. Open Biol 2020;10(9):200119.

118. Lo YMD, Han DSC, Jiang P, et al. Epigenetics, fragmentomics, and topology of cell-free DNA in liquid biopsies. Science 2021;372(6538):eaaw3616.

119. Jiang P, Chan KCA, Lo YMD. Liver-derived cell-free nucleic acids in plasma: biology and applications in liquid biopsies. J Hepatol 2019;71(2):409–21. https://doi.org/10.1016/j.jhep.2019.04.003.

120. Gall TMH, Belete S, Khanderia E, et al. Circulating tumor cells and cell-free DNA in pancreatic ductal adenocarcinoma. Am J Pathol 2019;189(1):71–81.

121. Vietsch EE, Graham GT, McCutcheon JN, et al. Circulating cell-free DNA mutation patterns in early and late stage colon and pancreatic cancer. Cancer Genet 2017;218-219:39–50.

122. Lehmann-Werman R, Magenheim J, Moss J, et al. Monitoring liver damage using hepatocyte-specific methylation markers in cell-free circulating DNA. JCI Insight 2018;3(12):e120687.

123. Martinez Roth S, Vietsch EE, Barefoot ME, et al. Cardiomyocyte-specific circulating cell-free methylated DNA in esophageal cancer patients treated with chemoradiation. Gastrointest Disord 2021; 3(3). https://doi.org/10.3390/gidisord3030011.

124. de Vlaminck I, Valantine HA, Snyder TM, et al. Circulating cell-free DNA enables noninvasive diagnosis of heart transplant rejection. Sci Translational Med 2014;6(241):241ra77.

125. Zemmour H, Planer D, Magenheim J, et al. Noninvasive detection of human cardiomyocyte death using methylation patterns of circulating DNA. Nat Commun 2018;9(1). https://doi.org/10.1038/s41467-018-03961-y.

Therapy-Related Clonal Hematopoiesis
A New Link Between Cancer and Cardiovascular Disease

Yoshimitsu Yura, MD, PhD[a,b], Jesse D. Cochran, BS[a], Kenneth Walsh, PhD[a],*

KEYWORDS

- Clonal hematopoiesis • Cardio-oncology • Inflammation

KEY POINTS

- Clonal hematopoiesis is a new risk factor for cardiovascular disease.
- Both cardiovascular disease and clonal hematopoiesis are frequent in patients with cancer and cancer survivors who have been treated with genotoxic agents.
- Experimental studies have shown that cancer therapy-related clonal hematopoiesis contributes to worse cardiovascular disease outcome.

INTRODUCTION

The incidence of cancer and cardiovascular disease (CVD) increases with age, and there are a substantial number of individuals who suffer from both conditions.[1,2] Advances in cancer therapy over the past few decades have resulted in a large and growing population of long-term cancer survivors. Indeed, approximately half of patients diagnosed with cancer in high-income settings are now expected to survive for 10 years or longer.[3,4] This new aging population presents novel clinical challenges requiring further attention and investigation. Specifically, patients with cancer and cancer survivors display increased risks for CVD, including coronary artery disease (CAD) and heart failure (HF), owing in part to the side effects of genotoxic therapies.[3,5] To date, the acute effects of cancer drugs on cardiac myocytes have been extensively investigated.[6,7] However, it is difficult to reconcile how this mechanism can explain the medium- to long-term risk of cancer therapies on the cardiovascular system. Recently, clonal hematopoiesis (CH), a precancerous state in the hematopoietic system, has been recognized as a new causal risk factor for CVD.[8–13] This review introduces the concept of CH, summarizes recent epidemiologic and experimental studies linking CH to CVD, and discusses recent experimental studies demonstrating that cancer therapy-related CH (t-CH) can induce cardiac dysfunction. These studies suggest a new mechanism linking cancer therapy to cardiac toxicity.

WHAT IS CLONAL HEMATOPOIESIS?

Hematopoietic stem and progenitor cells (HSPC) typically reside in the bone marrow, produce multiple blood cell types, and replenish themselves through a self-renewal process.[14] The progeny immune cells of the HSPC fulfill critical roles in maintaining homeostasis and are also implicated in a myriad of disease states.[15] The rapid turnover of blood cells can contribute to the accumulation of mutant HSPC clones with age.[16] Although most mutations have little or no effect on cellular fitness, some mutations will occur in "driver" genes, such as oncogenes or tumor suppressor genes, that

[a] Hematovascular Biology Center, Robert M. Berne Cardiovascular Research Center, University of Virginia School of Medicine, 415 Lane Road, PO Box 801394, Suite 1010, Charlottesville, VA 22908, USA; [b] Department of Cardiology, Nagoya University Graduate School of Medicine, Nagoya, Japan.65 Tsurumai-cho, Showa-ku, Nagoya 466-8550, Japan
* Corresponding author.
E-mail address: kw9ar@virginia.edu

Heart Failure Clin 18 (2022) 349–359
https://doi.org/10.1016/j.hfc.2022.02.010

can enable the positive selection of mutant cells.[17–20] In this context, mutant cells can outcompete neighboring wild-type cells leading to their clonal expansion.[21] Notably, these mutant HSPC give rise to circulating immune cells that harbor the same mutant allele, and it has been shown that these mutations can alter the function of the progeny immune cells.[22] Clonal expansions in blood cells have been found to occur in relatively healthy individuals who lack overt signs of hematologic transformation. This condition has historically been referred to as CH and more recently as CH of indeterminate potential (CHIP) to distinguish it from the clonal expansions that occur in malignant blood cancers.[23]

CH can be detected by bulk DNA sequencing for driver gene mutations in the blood, bone marrow, or tissues infiltrated by blood cells.[24] Large-scale, next-generation sequencing (NGS) analyses of blood samples have identified somatic mutations in leukemia-associated genes of asymptomatic individuals who are void of any known hematologic disease.[18–20,25] These mutations are most prevalent in the epigenetic regulators DNA methyltransferase-3A (DNMT3A), ten-eleven translocation-2 (TET2), and additional sex combs like 1 (ASXL1). At lower frequencies, CH has also been associated with mutations in janus kinase 2 (JAK2), tumor protein 53(TP53), protein phosphatase, Mg^{2+}/Mn^{2+}-dependent 1D (PPM1D), BCL6 Corepressor (BCOR), guanine nucleotide binding protein, alpha stimulating complex locus (GNAS), Splicing Factor 3b Subunit 1 (SF3B1), and others.[23] In addition to single nucleotide variants (SNVs) and small insertions and deletions (Indels) in driver genes, CH can also be assessed cytogenetically by detecting the large mosaic chromosomal alterations in blood.[26,27]

Variant allele fraction (VAF) refers to the proportion of mutant allele copies relative to total copies sequenced, and it is directly proportional to the percentage of mutant clones within a cell population. Typical NGS has a sequence limitation of 1% to 2% owing to the intrinsic error rate of DNA sequencing. This sequencing shortcoming traditionally limited the threshold for CHIP to a VAF greater than 2% (meaning 2% of the sequenced alleles or 4% of cells assuming a heterozygous somatic mutation). Using this relatively insensitive VAF criteria, detectable mutations are rarely detected in the young individuals but highly prevalent in the elderly, with between 10% and 20% of people older than 70 years of age harboring a clones of appreciable size.[18–20,28,29] More recently, error-corrected DNA sequencing has been developed to detect clones with VAF values as low as 0.03% or below.[30,31] Using this

technology, smaller clones can be detected in the blood of younger individuals. These finding have led to the notion that relatively small clones are ubiquitous by middle age, and that these clones expand with age.

CLONAL HEMATOPOIESIS IS ASSOCIATED WITH CARDIOVASCULAR DISEASE

Many recent studies have linked CH with reduced survival.[18–20,27] Although CH increases the risk of a hematologic malignancy, as would be expected, blood cancer alone cannot account for the relatively large increase in mortality that is associated with this condition. Surprisingly, Jaiswal and colleagues[8,18] initially reported that individuals with CH displayed significantly increased incident coronary heart disease and ischemic stroke risks after adjusting for age and traditional risk factors. For these analyses, whole-exome sequencing of peripheral blood from 4726 individuals with coronary heart disease and 3529 control individuals was performed.[8] They reported that carriers of CH had an approximately 2-fold greater risk of coronary heart disease and a 4-fold greater incidence of early-onset myocardial infarction compared with noncarriers. In these analyses, mutations in DNMT3A, TET2, ASXL1, and JAK2 were each individually associated with coronary heart disease and CVD mortality. The risk ratio for CH is similar to or greater than that of conventional risk factors, underscoring the importance of CH in CVD.[32]

Other studies have confirmed and extended these findings. Bick and colleagues[9] analyzed whole-exome sequences from 35,416 individuals in the UK Biobank without prevalent CVD to identify participants with CH. They identified 1079 (3.0%) individuals with DNMT3A or TET2 CH and found that CH was associated with increased incident CVD event risk (hazard ratio [HR], 1.27) during a 6.9-year median follow-up. CVD risk was greater for larger clones compared with smaller clones (HR, 1.59). More recently, Nachun and colleagues[10] reported that a combination of CH and epigenetic aging has a strong predictive value in identifying patients with high risk of all-cause mortality and coronary heart disease. In this regard, epigenetic age acceleration manifests when the individual's estimated epigenetic age is older than that of his/her chronologic age. This study examined 5522 human samples from 4 cohorts within the Trans-omics for Precision Medicine program and found that ~40% of CHIP carriers exhibited epigenetic age acceleration. Individuals with both CH and aging acceleration displayed greater risks of all-cause mortality (HR, 2.90) and coronary heart disease (HR, 3.24) compared with individuals without CH and aging acceleration.[10] Notably, CH-positivity was not associated with mortality or CVD if it was independent of epigenetic age acceleration. Saiki and colleagues[11] performed a combination of targeted DNA sequencing for 23 CH-related genes and array-based copy number alterations (CNAs) detection in blood derived from 11,234 individuals from the BioBank Japan cohort. Driver gene SNVs and Indels or CNAs were detected in ~40% of individuals who were 60 years of age or greater. CH-related SNVs/indels and CNAs exhibited statistically significant cooccurrence within individuals. Notably, this study found that cooccurrence of CNAs and SNVs/indels in *DNMT3A*, *TET2*, *JAK2*, or *TP53* genes was associated with much higher cardiovascular mortality.[11] Collectively, these findings document a robust and frequent association between CH and CVD, and they are summarized in **Table 1**.

Because epidemiologic studies are correlative by nature, they generally cannot distinguish whether CH and CVD are causally linked or are simply an epiphenomenon of the aging process. Thus, potential mechanistic links between CH and CVD have been explored in model systems. Most of these studies have focused on the TET2 epigenetic regulator that is frequently mutated in CH. Two independent groups originally reported that *TET2*-mediated CH could be causal in the development of atherosclerosis using murine models.[8,33] In the study conducted by the authors' laboratory, a competitive bone marrow transplantation approach was performed to introduce a small number of *Tet2*-deficient HSPC to a recipient mouse, effectively mimicking the human scenario of individuals carrying a *TET2* somatic mutation that gradually expands over time.[33] *Tet2*-deficient HSPC displayed progressive expansion into all immune cell progeny with a bias toward cells of myeloid lineage. This model of *Tet2*-mediated clonal expansion led to a marked increase in plaque size in hyperlipidemic low-density lipoprotein receptor-deficient ($Ldlr^{-/-}$) mice.[33] Consistent with these observations, it was independently reported that the complete bone marrow transplantation of *Tet2*-deficient cells to hyperlipidemic mice also led to an increase in vascular plaque size.[8] Both studies showed that myeloid-specific ablation of *Tet2* was sufficient to promote atherosclerotic development.[8,33] Mechanistically, TET2 activates the NLR family pyrin domain containing 3 (NLRP3) inflammasome in immune cells to elevate proinflammatory cytokine release through an HDAC-dependent mechanism.[33] The NLRP3 inflammasome is a critical component of the innate immune system that controls the activation and

secretion of interleukin-1β(IL-1β) and IL-18.[34] Notably, it was shown that treatment with a small molecule NLRP3 inflammasome inhibitor reversed the accelerated atherosclerosis that was caused by the expansion of *Tet2*-deficient hematopoietic cells.[33] Subsequent experimental studies also found that *JAK2*-mediated CH may have a causal role in thrombosis, atherosclerosis, and pulmonary hypertension.[35–38] *JAK2* is a nonreceptor tyrosine kinase and associates with various receptors during signal transduction. $JAK2^{V617F}$ is a constitutively active mutant form that activates STAT (signal transducer and activator of transcription) transcription factors.

CLONAL HEMATOPOIESIS IS ASSOCIATED WITH HEART FAILURE

Recently, it was reported that CH, particularly sequence variations in *ASXL1*, *TET2*, and *JAK2*, represents a risk factor for incident HF.[12] In this study, CH status was determined from whole-exome or -genome sequence data of blood DNA in participants without prevalent HF or hematological malignancy from 5 large cohorts. Of the 56,597 individuals (41% men, mean age 58 years at baseline), CH could be detected in 3406 individuals (6%). During the follow-up period of up to 20 years, 4694 individuals developed HF (8.3%). After adjusting for demographic and clinical risk factors, CH was prospectively associated with a 25% increased risk of HF in the meta-analysis with consistent associations across all cohorts (HR, 1.25).[12] In addition, several studies have associated CH with poor outcomes in patients with preexisting HF. Dorsheimer and colleagues[39] analyzed 200 patients (median age 65 years) who had undergone autologous bone marrow treatment for acute myocardial infarction for mutations in candidate CH genes by deep-targeted amplicon sequencing. Using a VAF threshold of 2%, the prevalence of CH was 18.5% with *DNMT3A* and *TET2* being the most prevalent mutant genes. Patients with these forms of CH displayed significantly worse long-term clinical outcomes, including mortality and mortality combined with rehospitalization for HF.[39] Furthermore, when patients were grouped based on VAF, there was a dose-dependent relationship between clone size and clinical outcome, indicating that smaller clone sizes (between 1% and 2% VAF) were associated with worse prognoses.[39] Subsequently, Assmus and colleagues[40] analyzed CH in 419 patients with HF (stable HF symptoms, New York Heart Association ≥2, ischemic origin, and left ventricular dysfunction). Receiver operating characteristic (ROC) curve analysis of the data was used to

Table 1
Summary of studies showing associations between clonal hematopoiesis and cardiovascular disease

Source	Population	Sequencing Method	Findings
Jaiswal et al,[8] 2017	4726 patients with CHD 3529 controls	Whole-exome sequence	CHIP was associated with a greater risk of CHD (HR 2.0) and early-onset MI (HR 4.0)
Bick et al,[9] 2020	35,416 individuals without prevalent CVD	Whole-exome sequence	CHIP (*DNMT3A, TET2*) was associated with increased risk of incident CVD Genetically reduced IL-6 signaling was associated with an attenuated CVD risk in CHIP
Nachun et al,[10] 2021	5522 individuals	Whole-genome sequence DNA methylation array	CHIP and age acceleration were associated with increased risk of all-cause mortality (HR, 2.9) and CHD (HR, 3.2)
Saiki et al,[11] 2021	11,234 individuals	Targeted sequence of 23 CH genes Array-based CNAs detection	Cooccurrence of SNVs/indels and CNAs (*DNMT3A, TET2, JAK2, and TP53*) was associated with higher CVD mortality
Yu et al,[12] 2021	56,597 individuals without HF and hematological malignancy	Whole-exome sequence Whole-genome sequence	Mutations in *TET2, ASXL1,* and *JAK2* were prospectively associated with a 25% increased risk of HF
Bhattacharya et al,[13] 2021	7426 incident stroke cases 78,752 controls	Whole-exome sequence Whole-genome sequence	CHIP was associated with an increased risk of total stroke (HR, 1.14)
Dorsheimer et al,[39] 2019	200 patients undergoing autologous BMT for AMI	Error-corrected targeted exome sequencing	CH (*DNMT3A, TET2*) was associated with significantly worse long-term clinical outcomes, including mortality and mortality combined with rehospitalization for HF
Assmus et al,[40] 2021	419 patients with chronic HF	Error-corrected targeted exome sequencing	CH (*DNMT3A* and *TET2*) was an independent predictor of mortality in patients with HF Optimized VAF for *TET2* and *DNMT3A* were 0.73% and 1.13%, respectively

(*continued on next page*)

Table 1
(continued)

Source	Population	Sequencing Method	Findings
Cremer et al,[41] 2020	419 patients with chronic HF	Error-corrected targeted exome sequencing	CH (*DNMT3A, TET2, PHF6, SMC1A, PPM1D, EZH2, CEBPA, SRSF2, SETBP*) was an independent predictor of mortality in patients with chronic HF
Pascual-Figal et al,[43] 2021	62 patients with HF (EF < 45%)	Error collected targeted-exome sequencing for 54 genes	CHIP in either *DNMT3A* or *TET2* exhibited accelerated HF progression irrespective of ischemic/nonischemic cause

identify prognostic VAF cutoff values. Survival ROC analyses revealed optimized VAF cutoff values of 0.73% and 1.15% for *TET2* and *DNMT3A* clones, respectively. Using these respective cutoffs, 5-year mortality was increased in both *TET2* and *DNMT3A* carriers.[40] In the same cohort, Cremer and colleagues[41] reported that in addition to *TET2* and *DNMT3A*, clones with mutations in *PPM1D,* Serine and Arginine Rich Splicing Factor 2 (*SRSF2*), CCAAT Enhancer Binding Protein Alpha (*CEBPA*), PHD Finger Protein 6 (*PHF6*), Structural Maintenance of Chromosomes 1A (*SMC1A*), Enhancer of Zeste 2 Polycomb Repressive Complex 2 Subunit (*EZH2*), and SET Binding Protein (*SETBP*) were also associated with worse clinical outcomes.[42] Although the aforementioned studies focused on HF of ischemic origin, Pascual-Figal and colleagues recently reported that CH is associated with accelerated disease progression regardless of the HF cause.[43] In this study, blood samples from 62 patients with HF with left ventricular ejection fractions less than 45% underwent deep sequence analysis for 54 candidate CH genes. After adjusting for risk factors, patients with mutations in either *DNMT3A* or *TET2* exhibited accelerated HF progression as assessed through death (HR, 2.79), death or HF hospitalization (HR 3.84), and HF-related death or HF hospitalization (HR, 4.41). This association remained significant irrespective of ischemic/nonischemic cause.[43]

Experimental studies indicate that CH can causally contribute to HF. Various mouse models have been used to show that the CH models of *TET2*, *DNMT3A*, and *JAK2* genes promote adverse cardiac remodeling, and these findings are summarized in detail in recent reviews.[22,44] Briefly, in a model of *TET2* CH, mice were transplanted with *Tet2*-mutant HSPC and underwent left anterior descending artery (LAD) ligation or transverse aortic constriction (TAC) surgery. Mice transplanted with *Tet2*-mutant cells exhibited worse cardiac remodeling compared with mice transplanted with wild-type bone marrow.[45] As with the atherosclerosis model, inhibition of the NLRP3 inflammasome alleviated the adverse effects of CH in these HF models.[33] In another model, *Tet2*- or *Dnmt3a*-mutant HSPC were generated through lentivirus transfection of Cas9 protein and single guide RNA (sgRNA), and transplanted into recipient mice. Mice harboring *Tet2*- or *Dnmt3a*-mutant HSPC displayed worse cardiac remodeling following angiotensin II infusion compared with mice transplanted with wild-type HSPC.[46] It has also been shown that the adoptive transfer of *Tet2*-deficient HSPC to unconditioned mice (ie, no myeloablation to promote engraftment) leads to the development of age-related, spontaneous cardiomyopathy in the absence of surgical or pharmacologic stress.[47] Finally, it was found that lentivirus-mediated transduction of HSPC, leading to myeloid-specific expression of Jak2^{V617F}, promoted greater cardiac remodeling following TAC and LAD ligation.[48] These CVD features were observed in the absence of changes to hematocrit or blood cell counts that can occur when Jak2^{V617F} is expressed in hematopoietic cells (but is not a feature of CH). Collectively, multiple experimental findings illustrate that CH can contribute to the development of HF, and mechanistic features involving inflammatory cytokines have been defined.

THERAPY-ASSOCIATED CLONAL HEMATOPOIESIS IS PREVALENT IN PATIENTS WITH CANCER

Although CH spontaneously arises with aging, specific environmental perturbations can augment the fitness of mutant HSPC and contribute to clonal expansions in the hematopoietic system. Patients with cancers display higher prevalence of CH. Coombs and colleagues[49] analyzed candidate CH target genes in tumor and blood samples from 8810 individuals (median age of 58.3 years) and found a high prevalence of CH (25%). In addition to increasing age, CH was found to also be associated with tobacco use and prior radiation therapy or chemotherapy. Compared with the age-associated CH described previously, this population displayed an overlapping but distinct mutational landscape that is referred to as t-CH.[49] This form of CH occurs as a result of the selective pressure that the genotoxic stressors exert on HSPC. Mutations are found in the DNA damage-response pathway (DDR) genes, including Ataxia-telangiectasia-mutated (ATM), Checkpoint kinases 1, 2 (CHK1, CHK2), TP53, and PPM1D.[50,51] In the study of Coombs and colleagues,[49] although CH was found to be associated with increased incidence of hematologic cancers, the diminished survival could not be attributed to hematologic cancer alone, suggesting the presence of unknown contributors.

To expand upon these findings, Bolton and colleagues[52] reported an association between cancer treatments and CH mutations in 24,146 patients with cancer with variable primary tumor types (n = 56) and ages. CH mutations were identified in 7216 individuals, representing 30% of the patient cohort.[52] Of all treatment modalities, external beam radiation therapy, cytotoxic chemotherapy, and radionuclide therapy were most strongly associated with CH. Mutations in PPM1D were most strongly associated with previous exposure to platinum or radionuclide therapy.[52] There was also a strong enrichment in other DDR genes, including TP53 and CHK2.

Gibson and colleagues[53] performed targeted sequencing on cryopreserved aliquots of autologous stem cells from 401 patients with non-Hodgkin lymphoma (NHL). These patients underwent autologous stem cell transplantation (ASCT), an extreme hematopoietic stress in which autologous stem cells are harvested before the administration of myeloablative chemotherapy and then reinfused into the patient to repopulate the hematopoietic system. In this cohort, 120 patients (29.9%) had CH at the time of ASCT, and these patients had significantly lower overall survival compared with those without CH (10-year overall survival, 30.4% vs 60.9%).[53] The increase in death in this population resulted from therapy-related myeloid neoplasm and CVD.[53] A further investigation of this patient cohort by Kahn and colleagues[54] revealed that PPM1D mutations were 60 times more likely to be present in patients with chemotherapy-exposed lymphoma than in 28,418 individuals who were unselected for malignancy and adjusted for age.[18,19,54] Recently, Miller and colleagues[55] reported the effect of t-CH on clinical outcomes in patients with NHL and multiple myeloma (MM). In this study, 154 patients with NHL or MM receiving chimeric antigen receptor T cells (CAR T cells) were assessed by NGS of peripheral blood for mutations in known CH driver genes. It was found that CH was present in 48% of patients. Although CH was not associated with a difference in overall survival, it was associated with increased responsiveness to immune-targeting therapies and increased severity of cytokine release syndrome in patients younger than aged 60 years. These data suggest that CH can influence inflammatory pathways across numerous therapeutic contexts in patients with cancer and cancer survivors. These studies are summarized in **Table 2**.

Recent experimental studies have investigated the mechanisms that contribute to the clonal expansions induced by genotoxic agents. These studies have shown that the genotoxic stresses of chemotherapy or radiation therapy create selective pressures causing expansion of clones with mutations in DDR genes that confer resistance to these stressors.[54,56–58] PPM1D is a member of the PP2C family of serine-threonine phosphatases. PPM1D is induced by TP53 activation, which, in turn, dephosphorylates and inactivates TP53 through a negative feedback mechanism. In addition, several other proteins in the DDR pathway, including H2A Histone Family Member X (H2AX), ATM, and CHK2, are dephosphorylated by PPM1D. Therefore, PPM1D is a critical negative regulator of many components of the DDR pathway.[59] Most PPM1D mutations are truncating mutations in the terminal exon.[52,54,56] These exon 6 mutations are gain-of-function mutations that display elevated expression and activity owing to loss of a C-terminal degradation domain. The truncating PPM1D mutations confer a chemoresistance phenotype, resulting in the selective expansion of PPM1D-mutant HSPC in the presence of chemotherapeutic agents. The transcription factor TP53, which can be activated by DNA damage,[60] is also commonly mutated in t-CH.[52]

Table 2
Summary of the studies examining clonal hematopoiesis in patients with cancer

Source	Population	Sequencing Method	Findings
Coombs et al,[49] 2017	8810 individuals with nonhematologic cancers	Whole-exome sequence Paired (blood and cancer)	25% of patients had CH. 4.5% of patients had CH-PD CH was associated with increased age, prior radiation therapy, and tobacco use CH-PD was associated with diminished patient survival
Gibson et al,[53] 2017	12 patients with NHL before ASCT 401 patients with NHL after ASCT	Whole-exome sequence Targeted-NGS for 86 genes	29.9% of patients have CHIP CHIP was associated with inferior survival from tMN and CVD
Kahn et al,[54] 2018	401 patients with NHL 28,418 individuals unselected for cancer	Whole-exome sequence Targeted-NGS	PPM1D mutations were 60 times more prevalent in chemotherapy-exposed patients with NHL
Bolton et al,[52] 2020	24,146 patients with cancer (56 types of primary tumor)	Deep targeted amplicon sequence	30% of patients had CH Cancer treatment was associated with CH with enrichments in DDR genes (PPM1D, TP53, CHK2)
Miller et al,[55] 2021	154 NHL or MM patients receiving CAR T cells	NGS of the driver genes	48% of patients had CHIP CHIP was associated with increased CR rate and CRS severity

Abbreviations: CH-PD, clonal hematopoiesis of putative driver genes; CR, complete response; CRS, cytokine release syndrome; tMN, therapy-related myeloid neoplasms.

Most somatic *TP53* mutations are missense mutations in the DNA-binding domain of the TP53 protein, which leads to an inability to conduct DNA damage repair.[57,61] It has been reported that DNA damage by radiation triggers TP53-dependent cell competition in HSPC. This competition appears to be mediated by an induction of growth arrest and senescence-related genes in wild-type cells that become outcompeted by cells with mutations in *TP53*.[58] It has also been reported that mutant TP53 interacts with EZH2 to promote HSPC self-renewal and differentiation.[57] Collectively, these clinical and experimental studies reveal that chemotherapy and/or radiation therapy exert powerful selective pressure on mutant clones in the hematopoietic system, and this can lead to robust clonal expansions.

POSSIBLE LINKS BETWEEN THERAPY-ASSOCIATED CLONAL HEMATOPOIESIS AND CARDIOVASCULAR DISEASE

As noted previously, patients with cancer and cancer survivors display an increased risk of CVD development.[3,62] It is widely appreciated that radiation and/or chemotherapy contribute to the

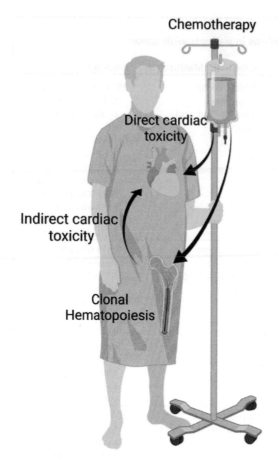

Chemotherapy

Direct cardiac toxicity

Indirect cardiac toxicity

Clonal Hematopoiesis

Fig. 1. The cardiac toxicity associated with genotoxic therapies may stem from both direct and indirect mechanisms. Patients with cancer treated with genotoxic therapies display a higher prevalence of CH, which may cause indirect cardiac toxicity. (Created with BioRender.com.)

development of nonischemic heart disease. For example, a recent large-scale electronic health record analysis of multiple databases examined CVD outcomes in 126,120 patients with cancer and 630,144 control individuals.[63] Increased risks of HF or cardiomyopathy were observed in patients with 10 of the 20 cancers examined, including hematological (HR, 1.94), esophageal (HR, 1.96), lung (HR, 1.82), kidney (HR, 1.73), and ovarian (HR, 1.59) cancer. Furthermore, it has been reported that mortality owing to CVD in cancer survivors is greater than that of the cancer itself after a 10-year follow-up.[3,62,63] Therefore, given the recent proliferation of new cancer therapies and the longer survival of patients with cancer, there is an increasing need to identify the molecular mechanisms that contribute to the CVD observed in these patients.

Given the mechanistic links between age-related CH and CVD, the authors speculated that the DDR genes commonly mutated in t-CH could contribute to the HF that is prevalent in patients with cancer and cancer survivors (**Fig. 1**). Thus, the authors tested whether causal relationships exist between t-CH and cardiac dysfunction by focusing on hematopoietic cell mutations in $PPM1D$[64] and $TP53$,[65] which represent the most enriched t-CH genes in patients receiving cancer therapy.[52,53] In one of these studies, the authors developed a mouse model using CRISPR-Cas9 technology to generate CH-associated mutations in exon 6 of $Ppm1d$, leading to its overactivation.[64] This model of t-CH was then used to examine whether somatic mutations of $PPM1D$ in hematopoietic cells can increase the heart's susceptibility to stress. This $Ppm1d$ mouse model of CH revealed worse cardiac remodeling as measured by echocardiography and greater cardiac fibrosis and myocyte hypertrophy following chronic infusion of angiotensin II.[64] Mechanistically, $Ppm1d$-mutant macrophages display impaired DDR pathway activation, greater DNA damage, higher reactive oxygen species production, and an augmented proinflammatory profile with elevations in IL-1β and IL-18.[64] It was further shown that the NLRP3 inflammasome inhibitor MCC950 effectively reverses the cardiac remodeling caused by transplantation of $Ppm1d$-mutant HSPC.[64] These data suggest that inflammasome activation and elevated cytokine production are critical for the enhanced pathologic cardiac phenotype associated with this form of t-CH.

In a second study, the authors examined a model of t-CH involving mutations in TP53.[65] This study used 3 distinct mouse strains to examine the relationship between t-CH of $TP53$ clones and cardiac function. The models included mice transplanted with Trp53 heterozygous-knockout bone marrow cells, myeloid-specific Trp53-deficient mice, and mice transplanted with bone marrow cells harboring a common $TP53$ missense mutation, $Trp53^{R270H}$. To establish a model of $TP53$-mediated t-CH, these mice were treated with a course of the chemotherapeutic agent doxorubicin (Dox). As expected, treatment of mice with Dox accelerated the expansion of hematopoietic TP53-mutant clones in the adoptive transfer model that avoids myeloablation. It was also found that mice transplanted with HSPC lacking TP53, or with mutant TP53, display worse Dox-induced cardiotoxicity compared with mice transplanted with wild-type HSPC. Mechanistically, treatment with Dox leads to exuberant and persistent neutrophil infiltration into the myocardium. In this context, the $Tp53$-mutant neutrophil produced greater ROS, leading to further damage of the myocardium and greater inflammatory cytokine production.[65]

Collectively, these findings provide precedence for the concept that t-CH can contribute to the development of CVD in patients with cancer and cancer survivors who have undergone therapy with genotoxic agents (see **Fig. 1**). Currently, there are no clinical studies to directly address this hypothesis; however, this possibility could be investigated through a prospective study of clinical outcomes in patients with cancer treated with genotoxic therapies. If validated by further studies, these data would suggest that t-CH is predictive of cardiac dysfunction in cancer survivors and that the pathological cardiac condition in these patients could be responsiveness to anti-inflammatory therapies. As mentioned above, t-CH owing to mutations in multiple DDR pathway genes, beyond *PPM1D* and *TP53*, is frequently observed in patients with cancer and cancer survivors, and these t-CH driver genes could potentially also affect the CVD outcomes. Thus, many future clinical and experimental studies are warranted.

SUMMARY AND FUTURE DIRECTIONS

In closing, CH is an emerging risk factor for both cancer and CVD. Patients with cancer and cancer survivors exhibit prevalent t-CH, a form of CH that is associated with DDR gene mutations in HSPC that enable clone expansion in response to genotoxic agent exposure. Given the growing appreciation of its role in CVD, an individual's t-CH status could become a critical consideration in assessing the risk and prognosis of the patient with cancer. Furthermore, recent experimental findings suggest that anti-inflammatory therapies have utility for treating the cardiac toxicities that develop in cancer survivors with t-CH. Thus, additional clinical and experimental studies are warranted to understand the mechanisms that give rise to t-CH and its effects on the cardiovascular system.

CLINICS CARE POINTS

- Although there are no existing guidelines on screening and treating patients with clonal hematopoiesis, it should be recognized that individuals with clonal hematopoiesis are at higher risk of cardiovascular disease.
- Currently, it is reasonable to suggest that modifiable conventional risk factors be

aggressively controlled in patients with clonal hematopoiesis. Also, additional cardiovascular disease screening could be considered in individuals with confirmed CH and a suspicion of cardiovascular disease based on age, symptoms, and prior treatment by anticancer therapies.

FUNDING

This work was funded by National Institutes of Health (Bethesda, MD) grants HL152174, AG073249, HL141256, and HL139819. The authors have no conflicts of interest or relationships with industry to disclose.

DISCLOSURE

The authors do not have anything to disclose.

REFERENCES

1. Handy CE, Quispe R, Pinto X, et al. Synergistic opportunities in the interplay between cancer screening and cardiovascular disease risk assessment: together we are stronger. Circulation 2018; 138:727–34.
2. Calvillo-Argüelles O, Jaiswal S, Shlush LI, et al. Connections between clonal hematopoiesis, cardiovascular disease, and cancer: a review. JAMA Cardiol 2019;4:380–7.
3. Zamorano JL, Gottfridsson C, Asteggiano R, et al. The cancer patient and cardiology. Eur J Heart Fail 2020;22:2290–309.
4. Arnold M, Rutherford MJ, Bardot A, et al. Progress in cancer survival, mortality, and incidence in seven high-income countries 1995-2014 (ICBP SURVMARK-2): a population-based study. Lancet Oncol 2019;20:1493–505.
5. Curigliano G, Lenihan D, Fradley M, et al. Management of cardiac disease in cancer patients throughout oncological treatment: ESMO consensus recommendations. Ann Oncol Off J Eur Soc Med Oncol 2020;31:171–90.
6. Moslehi JJ. Cardiovascular toxic effects of targeted cancer therapies. N Engl J Med 2016;375:1457–67.
7. Zhang S, Liu X, Bawa-Khalfe T, et al. Identification of the molecular basis of doxorubicin-induced cardiotoxicity. Nat Med 2012;18:1639–42.
8. Jaiswal S, Natarajan P, Silver AJ, et al. Clonal hematopoiesis and risk of atherosclerotic cardiovascular disease. N Engl J Med 2017;377:111–21.
9. Bick AG, Pirruccello JP, Griffin GK, et al. Genetic interleukin 6 signaling deficiency attenuates cardiovascular risk in clonal hematopoiesis. Circulation 2020;141:124–31.

10. Nachun D, Lu AT, Bick AG, et al. Clonal hematopoiesis associated with epigenetic aging and clinical outcomes. Aging Cell 2021;20:e13366.

11. Saiki R, Momozawa Y, Nannya Y, et al. Combined landscape of single-nucleotide variants and copy number alterations in clonal hematopoiesis. Nat Med 2021;27:1239–49.

12. Yu B, Roberts MB, Raffield LM, et al. Supplemental association of clonal hematopoiesis with incident heart failure. J Am Coll Cardiol 2021;78:42–52.

13. Bhattacharya R, Zekavat SM, Haessler J, et al. Clonal hematopoiesis is associated with higher risk of stroke. Stroke 2021;53:788–97.

14. Seita J, Weissman IL. Hematopoietic stem cell: self-renewal versus differentiation. Wiley Interdiscip Rev Syst Biol Med 2010;2:640–53.

15. Jaiswal S. Clonal hematopoiesis and nonhematologic disorders. Blood 2020;136:1606–14.

16. Welch JS, Ley TJ, Link DC, et al. The origin and evolution of mutations in acute myeloid leukemia. Cell 2012;150:264–78.

17. Busque L, Patel JP, Figueroa ME, et al. Recurrent somatic TET2 mutations in normal elderly individuals with clonal hematopoiesis. Nat Genet 2012;44:1179–81.

18. Jaiswal S, Fontanillas P, Flannick J, et al. Age-related clonal hematopoiesis associated with adverse outcomes. N Engl J Med 2014;371:2488–98.

19. Genovese G, Kahler AK, Handsaker RE, et al. Clonal hematopoiesis and blood-cancer risk inferred from blood DNA sequence. N Engl J Med 2014;371:2477–87.

20. Xie M, Lu C, Wang J, et al. Age-related mutations associated with clonal hematopoietic expansion and malignancies. Nat Med 2014;20:1472–8.

21. Shlush LI. Age-related clonal hematopoiesis. Blood 2018;131:496–504.

22. Yura Y, Sano S, Walsh K. Clonal hematopoiesis: a new step linking inflammation to heart failure. JACC Basic Transl Sci 2020;5:196–207.

23. Steensma DP, Bejar R, Jaiswal S, et al. Clonal hematopoiesis of indeterminate potential and its distinction from myelodysplastic syndromes. Blood 2015;126:9–16.

24. Shumilov E, Flach J, Pabst T, et al. Genetic alterations crossing the borders of distinct hematopoetic lineages and solid tumors: diagnostic challenges in the era of high-throughput sequencing in hemato-oncology. Crit Rev Oncol Hematol 2018;126:64–79.

25. McKerrell T, Vassiliou GS. Aging as a driver of leukemogenesis. Sci Transl Med 2015;7:306fs38.

26. Forsberg LA, Rasi C, Malmqvist N, et al. Mosaic loss of chromosome Y in peripheral blood is associated with shorter survival and higher risk of cancer. Nat Genet 2014;46:624–8.

27. Loh P-R, Genovese G, Handsaker RE, et al. Insights into clonal haematopoiesis from 8,342 mosaic chromosomal alterations. Nature 2018;559:350–5.

28. Jaiswal S, Ebert BL. Clonal hematopoiesis in human aging and disease. Science 2019;366.

29. Bick AG, Weinstock JS, Nandakumar SK, et al. Inherited causes of clonal haematopoiesis in 97,691 whole genomes. Nature 2020;586:763–8.

30. Young AL, Challen GA, Birmann BM, Druley TE. Clonal haematopoiesis harbouring AML-associated mutations is ubiquitous in healthy adults. Nat Commun 2016;7:12484.

31. Watson CJ, Papula AL, Poon GYP, et al. The evolutionary dynamics and fitness landscape of clonal hematopoiesis. Science 2020;367:1449–54.

32. Jaiswal S, Libby P. Clonal haematopoiesis: connecting ageing and inflammation in cardiovascular disease. Nat Rev Cardiol 2020;17:137–44.

33. Fuster JJ, MacLauchlan S, Zuriaga MA, et al. Clonal hematopoiesis associated with TET2 deficiency accelerates atherosclerosis development in mice. Science 2017;355:842–7.

34. Swanson KV, Deng M, Ting JP-Y. The NLRP3 inflammasome: molecular activation and regulation to therapeutics. Nat Rev Immunol 2019;19:477–89.

35. Wolach O, Sellar RS, Martinod K, et al. Increased neutrophil extracellular trap formation promotes thrombosis in myeloproliferative neoplasms. Sci Transl Med 2018;10.

36. Wang W, Liu W, Fidler T, et al. Macrophage inflammation, erythrophagocytosis, and accelerated atherosclerosis in Jak2 (V617F) mice. Circ Res 2018;123:e35–47.

37. Fidler TP, Xue C, Yalcinkaya M, et al. The AIM2 inflammasome exacerbates atherosclerosis in clonal haematopoiesis. Nature 2021;592:296–301.

38. Kimishima Y, Misaka T, Yokokawa T, et al. Clonal hematopoiesis with JAK2V617F promotes pulmonary hypertension with ALK1 upregulation in lung neutrophils. Nat Commun 2021;12:6177.

39. Dorsheimer L, Assmus B, Rasper T, et al. Association of mutations contributing to clonal hematopoiesis with prognosis in chronic ischemic heart failure. JAMA Cardiol 2019;4:25–33.

40. Assmus B, Cremer S, Kirschbaum K, et al. Clonal haematopoiesis in chronic ischaemic heart failure: prognostic role of clone size for DNMT3A- and TET2-driver gene mutations. Eur Heart J 2021;42:257–65.

41. Cremer S, Kirschbaum K, Berkowitsch A, et al. Multiple somatic mutations for clonal hematopoiesis are associated with increased mortality in patients with chronic heart failure. Circ Genomic Precis Med 2020;13:e003003.

42. Kiefer KC, Cremer S, Pardali E, et al. Full spectrum of clonal haematopoiesis-driver mutations in chronic heart failure and their associations with mortality. ESC Hear Fail 2021;8:1873–84.

43. Pascual-Figal DA, Bayes-Genis A, Díez-Díez M, et al. Clonal hematopoiesis and risk of progression

of heart failure with reduced left ventricular ejection fraction. J Am Coll Cardiol 2021;77:1747–59.

44. Wang Y, Sano S, Ogawa H, et al. Murine models of clonal hematopoiesis to assess mechanisms of cardiovascular disease. Cardiovasc Res 2021; cvab215.

45. Sano S, Oshima K, Wang Y, et al. Tet2-mediated clonal hematopoiesis accelerates heart failure through a mechanism involving the IL-1beta/NLRP3 inflammasome. J Am Coll Cardiol 2018;71:875–86.

46. Sano S, Oshima K, Wang Y, Katanasaka Y, Sano M, Walsh K. CRISPR-mediated gene editing to assess the roles of Tet2 and Dnmt3a in clonal hematopoiesis and cardiovascular disease. Circ Res 2018;123:335–41.

47. Wang Y, Sano S, Yura Y, et al. Tet2-mediated clonal hematopoiesis in nonconditioned mice accelerates age-associated cardiac dysfunction. JCI insight 2020;5.

48. Sano S, Wang Y, Yura Y, et al. JAK2 (V617F) -mediated clonal hematopoiesis accelerates pathological remodeling in murine heart failure. JACC Basic Transl Sci 2019;4:684–97.

49. Coombs CC, Zehir A, Devlin SM, et al. Therapy-related clonal hematopoiesis in patients with non-hematologic cancers is common and associated with adverse clinical outcomes. Cell Stem Cell 2017;21:374–82.e4.

50. Jackson SP, Bartek J. The DNA-damage response in human biology and disease. Nature 2009;461:1071–8.

51. Hakem R. DNA-damage repair; the good, the bad, and the ugly. EMBO J 2008;27:589–605.

52. Bolton KL, Ptashkin RN, Gao T, et al. Cancer therapy shapes the fitness landscape of clonal hematopoiesis. Nat Genet 2020;52:1219–26.

53. Gibson CJ, Lindsley RC, Tchekmedyian V, et al. Clonal hematopoiesis associated with adverse outcomes after autologous stem-cell transplantation for lymphoma. J Clin Oncol 2017;35:1598–605.

54. Kahn JD, Miller PG, Silver AJ, et al. PPM1D-truncating mutations confer resistance to chemotherapy and sensitivity to PPM1D inhibition in hematopoietic cells. Blood 2018;132:1095–105.

55. Miller PG, Sperling AS, Brea EJ, et al. Clonal hematopoiesis in patients receiving chimeric antigen receptor T-cell therapy. Blood Adv 2021;5:2982–6.

56. Hsu JI, Dayaram T, Tovy A, et al. PPM1D mutations drive clonal hematopoiesis in response to cytotoxic chemotherapy. Cell Stem Cell 2018;23:700–13.e6.

57. Chen S, Wang Q, Yu H, et al. Mutant p53 drives clonal hematopoiesis through modulating epigenetic pathway. Nat Commun 2019;10:5649.

58. Bondar T, Medzhitov R. p53-mediated hematopoietic stem and progenitor cell competition. Cell Stem Cell 2010;6:309–22.

59. Uyanik B, Grigorash BB, Goloudina AR, Demidov ON. DNA damage-induced phosphatase Wip1 in regulation of hematopoiesis, immune system and inflammation. Cell death Discov 2017;3:17018.

60. Brosh R, Rotter V. When mutants gain new powers: news from the mutant p53 field. Nat Rev Cancer 2009;9:701–13.

61. Boettcher S, Miller PG, Sharma R, et al. A dominant-negative effect drives selection of TP53 missense mutations in myeloid malignancies. Science 2019;365:599–604.

62. Stoltzfus KC, Zhang Y, Sturgeon K, et al. Fatal heart disease among cancer patients. Nat Commun 2020;11:2011.

63. Strongman H, Gadd S, Matthews A, et al. Medium and long-term risks of specific cardiovascular diseases in survivors of 20 adult cancers: a population-based cohort study using multiple linked UK electronic health records databases. Lancet (London, England) 2019;394:1041–54.

64. Yura Y, Miura-Yura E, Katanasaka Y, et al. The cancer therapy-related clonal hematopoiesis driver gene Ppm1d promotes inflammation and non-ischemic heart failure in Mice. Circ Res 2021;129:684–98.

65. Sano S, Wang Y, Ogawa H, et al. TP53-mediated therapy-related clonal hematopoiesis contributes to doxorubicin-induced cardiomyopathy by augmenting a neutrophil-mediated cytotoxic response. JCI insight 2021;6:e146076.

Myocardial Dysfunction in Patients with Cancer

Efstratios Koutroumpakis, MD[a], Nikhil Agrawal, MD[b], Nicolas L. Palaskas, MD[a],
Jun-ichi Abe, MD, PhD[a], Cezar Iliescu, MD[a], Syed Wamique Yusuf, MBBS[a],
Anita Deswal, MD, MPH[a],*

KEYWORDS

• Myocardial dysfunction • Cardiotoxicity • Cancer • Cancer therapy

KEY POINTS

- Cancer therapies, accelerated atherosclerosis, cancer-related stress, systemic arterial and pulmonary hypertension, cardiac amyloidosis and cardiac malignancies/metastases have all been linked to the development of myocardial dysfunction in the setting of cancer.
- Research over the last decades has increased our knowledge about the pathogenetic mechanisms that chemotherapy and cancer targeted therapy cause myocardial dysfunction.
- Surveillance protocols for patients treated with potentially cardiotoxic cancer therapies have been developed based on the consensus of experts in the field of cardio-oncology.

INTRODUCTION

The number of cancer survivors continues to increase in the United States, and may exceed 22 million by 2030.[1] Advances in cancer therapeutics have led to a significant improvement in longer-term survival for many types of cancer. The increased survival time has also resulted in increased recognition of cancer and cancer therapy-related cardiovascular (CV) disease, even more evident in survivors of childhood cancer. Myocardial dysfunction, which in a proportion of patients manifests as symptomatic heart failure (HF), represents the epitome of cancer-related cardiotoxicity.[2] In this article, we present current knowledge on the epidemiology and mechanisms of myocardial dysfunction related to cancer and cancer therapies. Cardiotoxicity related to CART-cell and radiation therapy and the detailed role of cardioprotective therapy are discussed in Upshaw and colleagues' article, "Cardioprotection of High-Risk Individuals," in this issue; Pedersen and colleagues' article, "Radiation-Induced Cardiac Dysfunction: Optimizing Radiation Delivery and Post-Radiation Care," in this issue; Stein-Merlob and colleagues' article, "T-cell Immunotherapy and Cardiovascular Disease: Chimeric Antigen Receptor T-Cell and Bispecific T-cell Engager Therapies" in this issue.

PREVALENCE OF MYOCARDIAL DYSFUNCTION IN PATIENTS WITH CANCER

The prevalence of myocardial dysfunction and HF in cancer survivors is substantially higher compared to individuals without malignancy. For example, new-onset HF was over three times more frequent among 900 survivors of breast cancer and lymphoma, when compared to 1550 control individuals in a study from Rochester MN.[3] The increased risk of HF was observed from the first year after diagnosis and persisted 20 years later.[3] Cancer and HF share common risk factors including older age, health behaviors (smoking and alcohol abuse), and comorbidities including diabetes mellitus and obesity, which partially

[a] Department of Cardiology, University of Texas MD Anderson Cancer Center, 1515 Holcombe Boulevard, Unit 1451, Houston, TX 77030, USA; [b] Division of Cardiology, Department of Internal Medicine, McGovern Medical School at The University of Texas Health Science Center at Houston, 6431 Fannin Street, Houston, TX 77030, USA
* Corresponding author. Department of Cardiology, University of Texas MD Anderson Cancer Center, Holcombe Boulevard, Houston, TX 77030.
E-mail address: adeswal@mdanderson.org

Heart Failure Clin 18 (2022) 361–374
https://doi.org/10.1016/j.hfc.2022.02.011
1551-7136/22/© 2022 Elsevier Inc. All rights reserved.

explains their frequent coexistence.[4] In addition, cancer and cancer therapies can cause myocardial dysfunction leading to the development of HF (**Box 1**; **Fig. 1**).

MYOCARDIAL DYSFUNCTION ASSOCIATED WITH CANCER

Certain malignancies can directly involve the heart and cause myocardial dysfunction and HF. One example is multiple myeloma and plasma cell dyscrasias, which can lead to the development of cardiac light chain (AL) amyloidosis. This leads to infiltrative, restrictive cardiomyopathy due to the extracellular deposition of amyloid fibrils[5] (see Morie Gertz's article "Cardiac Amyloidosis," in this issue).

Relatively infrequently, malignancies can directly affect the heart in the form of cardiac metastasis or as primary cardiac tumors. The frequency of cardiac metastases is between 0.7% and 3.5% in the general population and up to 9% in patients with known malignancies.[6] Primary cardiac tumors are rare (0.01%–0.1% on postmortem analysis).[6] Cardiac tumors or metastases are infrequently associated with localized myocardial dysfunction, but can also manifest with HF due to obstructive pathology.

Furthermore, malignancies can affect cardiac function indirectly. Malignancies have been associated with increased risk of venous thrombosis. Symptomatic venous thromboembolism is reported in up to 5% of hospitalized patients with cancer[7] and its prevalence is 4 to 7 times higher in patients with cancer compared with healthy individuals.[8] Extensive or recurrent pulmonary emboli can lead to pulmonary hypertension and right-sided myocardial dysfunction and HF. Additionally, myeloproliferative disorders, chronic anemia, and tumoral obstruction of the pulmonary arterial system have all been associated with

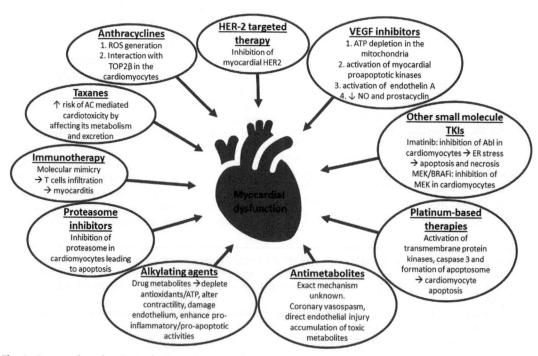

Fig. 1. Proposed mechanisms of cancer therapy-related myocardial dysfunction.

pulmonary hypertension (Group 5) and right-sided HF.[9] Furthermore, cancer-related chronic systemic inflammation, shared risk factors, and cancer therapies likely contribute to the process of accelerated atherosclerosis seen in cancer survivors, which can lead to ischemic cardiomyopathy.[10] The prevalence of stress (Takotsubo) cardiomyopathy in patients with cancer is increasingly recognized.[11] The physical and emotional stress of cancer, compounded by the external stress of treatments, and paraneoplastic syndromes, all likely contribute to the development of stress cardiomyopathy.[11]

Interestingly, not only has cancer been associated with myocardial dysfunction and HF, but HF has also been associated with the development of cancer.[12] Neurohormonal activation has been linked to cancer initiation, progression, and dissemination, a topic under active investigation.[12]

Definitions of Cancer Therapy-Related Cardiac Dysfunction

Definitions of cancer therapy-related cardiac dysfunction (CTRCD) have varied, but are usually focused on reduction in left ventricular ejection fraction (LVEF) with or without clinical HF. The lack of standardized definitions for CTRCD has hampered comparisons across studies and the generalizability of results. **Table 1** provides examples of definitions used. The LVEF cutoffs vary, and correlation with clinical outcomes is less clear. Furthermore, current LVEF-based definitions do not account for variability in measurements, changes in diastolic function, or HF with preserved LVEF (HFpEF).[13] Myocardial strain imaging and especially global longitudinal strain (GLS) is increasingly utilized as an early predictor of reduced cardiac function.[14] Although a reduction in GLS is a predictor of future overt LV systolic dysfunction, the clinical benefits of utilizing changes in strain to start cardioprotective therapy are not currently established.[15] Further, abnormal longitudinal trends in parameters such as LV volumes, LVEF, and diastolic function, even if individual values remain in the normal range, may predate the development of overt cardiomyopathy by a significant time period.[16] Integration of these trends into clinical practice with the help of information technology may provide earlier signals for initiating cardioprotective therapy.

Anthracycline- and HER-2 Targeted Therapy-associated Cardiotoxicity: the Origins and Evolution of the Field of Cardio-Oncology

Anthracyclines (ACs), introduced in the early 1970s, represent a mainstay of chemotherapeutic regimens for several solid and hematologic cancers. Human epidermal growth factor receptor 2 (HER2)-targeted agents include the monoclonal antibodies trastuzumab and pertuzumab, as well as the tyrosine kinase inhibitor (TKI), lapatinib, and have been used for the treatment of HER2 overexpressing breast and gastric tumors.[17,18]

Mechanisms of cardiotoxicity

Anthracycline and trastuzumab-induced cardiotoxicity have been critical components of cardio-oncology research, based on which Ewer and Lippman introduced the concept of two types of cardiotoxicity: irreversible injury (type 1) and reversible dysfunction (type 2),[19] a concept that is now debated.[20]

Anthracyclines cause dose-dependent cardiotoxicity, which was classically thought to represent irreversible cardiac damage. One of the critical mechanisms of cardiotoxicity is reactive oxygen species (ROS) generation. The high affinity of AC to metal ions elicits the reduction of the quinone moiety-Fe3+ complex and subsequently induces the Fenton reaction and ROS production.[21] Lipid peroxidation caused by ROS promotes cellular membrane and DNA damage.[22] Dexrazoxane, an intercellular iron chelator, which inhibits iron-assisted ROS production, has shown to decrease the risk of HF after AC treatment.[23]

Another proposed mechanism is the interaction of AC with topoisomerase 2β (TOP2β). Topoisomerase-2 has two isoforms. TOP2α is expressed in proliferating cells such as cancer cells, while TOP2β is the predominant isoform in adult cardiomyocytes. AC bind both DNA and TOP2 and form a DNA cleavage complex. This complex prevents DNA replication and dsDNA break religation, leading to cell death. The depletion of TOP2β from the heart inhibits AC-induced DNA damage response, induces ROS generation, and leads to cardiomyocyte death. Our group recently reported that the depletion of TOP2β promotes diastolic dysfunction via activation of p53 and inhibition of Akt (protein kinase B) signaling.[24] Of note, AC do not directly inhibit TOP2 topoisomerase activity. Instead, AC capture TOP2 in the DNA-TOP2-AC complex and inhibit TOP2 function as a mediator of DNA replication, a process referred to as TOP2 poisoning.[25] Therefore, the cardiomyocyte-specific TOP2β knock-out mice do not show any cardiac dysfunction at the basal level. Furthermore, depletion of TOP2β can prevent AC-induced cardiac dysfunction because of the loss of AC's binding partner in the inhibition of DNA replication.[26]

In contrast to AC, trastuzumab-induced cardiotoxicity is dose-independent and reversible in

Table 1
Examples of the varied definitions of CTRCD

Organization or Study Group	Definition of CTRCD
National Cancer Institute CTCAE v 5.0[98]	Classifies HF or LVD separately as events based on Grades 1 through 5. Grade 1: asymptomatic elevations in biomarkers or abnormalities on imaging. Grades 2 and 3: symptoms with mild and moderate exertion. Grade 4: severe, life-threatening symptoms requiring hemodynamic support Grade 5: death.
US Food and Drug Administration[99]	For anthracyclines: ≥10% decline in LVEF to below the lower limit of normal or an absolute LVEF of 45%, or a ≥ 20% decline in LVEF at any level.
Cardiac Review and Evaluation Committee[100]	1. Cardiomyopathy is characterized by a decrease in LVEF globally or more severe in the septum. 2. Signs and symptoms of HF. 3. Decline of EF ≥ 5% to final LVEF < 55% with symptoms of HF. 4. Asymptomatic decline of LVEF ≥ 10% to final LVEF < 55%.
Herceptin Adjuvant (HERA) trial[18]	LVEF decrease by ≥ 10% from baseline to an LVEF <50% with or without HF symptoms.
Breast Cancer International Research Group (BCIRG)[101]	Symptomatic LVD: >10% reduction from baseline LVEF without HF symptoms
American Society of Echocardiography and European Association of Cardiovascular Imaging[102]	≥10% decline in LVEF to final LVEF < 53% (confirmed by repeat imaging). Also suggested relative decrease from baseline in LV GLS by ≥ 15%.
Schwartz RG, et al. 1987[103]	Decline in LVEF > 10% to final LVEF < 50%.

Abbreviation: CTCAE, common terminology criteria for adverse events; GLS, global longitudinal strain; LVD, left ventricular dysfunction; LVEF, left ventricular ejection fraction.

many cases.[27] Trastuzumab targets HER2/Erb2, a receptor tyrosine kinase that is overexpressed in 15% to 20% of breast cancers.[28] HER2 is also expressed in myocytes and might have a protective role against myocardial stress.[29] Neuregulin, an EGF-family ligand, ErbB2, and ErbB4 receptor tyrosine kinases are involved in cell–cell crosstalk and mediate cellular responses to cardiac stress.[30] Inhibition of myocardial HER2 by the HER2-targeted agents is likely responsible for their cardiotoxicity.[31]

The toxic effects of AC and trastuzumab on the vasculature have been recently recognized and may also contribute to their cardiotoxic phenotype.[32] Doxorubicin-induced excess mitochondrial ROS decreased eNOS expression and phosphorylation in endothelial cells.[33] Likewise, the trastuzumab-induced M1-like macrophage phenotype and endothelial dysfunction may lead to vascular dysfunction and subsequent atherosclerosis.[34,35]

Although the categorization of AC- and trastuzumab-induced cardiotoxicity into types 1 and 2 was initially justified, it is now known that AC-induced cardiotoxicity is not always permanent,[22] and trastuzumab-induced cardiotoxicity is not always reversible.[36] Furthermore, there is probably overlap in the pathogenetic mechanisms of AC- and trastuzumab-induced cardiotoxicity. Both AC and trastuzumab can inhibit TOP2β expression in cardiomyocytes, and concurrent or sequential treatment with doxorubicin and trastuzumab significantly enhanced apoptosis and induced ROS production in human cardiomyocytes as compared to either agent alone.[37] Thus, the differentiation between type 1 and type 2 cardiotoxicity is less clear.

Clinical considerations

Transient LV dysfunction shortly after anthracycline infusion occurs rarely. More commonly, the subacute (within 1 year of therapy) and chronic (late onset > 1 year after therapy) changes are more clinically relevant.[13] AC-induced cardiac dysfunction is dependent on the cumulative dose and has been reported as 3% to 5% after 400 mg/m^2, 7% to 26% after 550 mg/m^2, and 18% to 48% after 700 mg/m^2 of doxorubicin.[38] *Large variations in the frequency of asymptomatic LVEF decrease and clinical HF across studies are likely due to differing definitions and heterogeneity in patient risk factors* (**Box 2**). In a large study of 2625 patients who received AC therapy and underwent frequent monitoring of LVEF, almost all cases (98%) of CTRCD were identified within the first year after therapy completion.[22] Additionally, after early treatment with renin–angiotensin system (RAS) inhibitors, improvement of LVEF occurred in 82% cases, although recovery of LVEF to pretherapy values occurred in a minority (11%).[22]

Concomitant administration of trastuzumab with ACs in the initial trials was associated with higher rates of cardiotoxicity. In a large breast cancer trial, development of NYHA class III or IV HF was observed in 27% of patients treated with the combination of trastuzumab, AC and cyclophosphamide compared to 8% of those treated with chemotherapy alone without trastuzumab.[28] The risk of cardiotoxicity has subsequently been reduced by trastuzumab being administered

---

Box 2
Patients at high risk for myocardial dysfunction related to cancer therapies

Increasing age (>60–65 years) or very young (children)

Prior anthracycline therapy

Prior mediastinal or chest radiation therapy

History of smoking

Comorbidities:

- Hypertension
- Diabetes mellitus
- Obesity
- Chronic Kidney Disease

Pre-existing heart disease, including coronary artery disease and borderline and reduced LVEF less than 55%

Elevated cardiac biomarkers (cardiac troponin or natriuretic peptides) at baseline

Single-nucleotide polymorphisms (SNPs) identified as risk factors in childhood cancer survivors.

Data from Refs[94,96,104,105]

---

sequentially after instead of concurrently with AC.[36] In a recent meta-analysis of large breast cancer trials, the incidence of trastuzumab associated HF was 2.5% compared to 0.4% in the control group (pooled relative risk for HF, 5.1, and for LVEF decline, 1.8).[39] When trastuzumab was used in patients with gastric cancer concomitantly with antimetabolites and alkylating agents, the reported rates of reduction in LVEF and HF were in the range of 5% and 1%, respectively.[40] In the Herceptin Adjuvant trial, among 1693 patients, trastuzumab-induced cardiac dysfunction improved in 80% after treatment with RAS inhibitors or digoxin,[41] even though cardiac function has been reported to recover after trastuzumab withdrawal, even without cardioprotective HF therapy.[27]

The cardiotoxic effects of pertuzumab and lapatinib are similar and not more frequent when used with trastuzumab.[42,43] The incidence of cardiotoxicity with HER2 targeted therapies is slightly higher in registries and retrospective studies compared to clinical trials, likely due to the younger age and lack of cardiac comorbidities in many clinical trials.[44]

Tyrosine Kinase Inhibitors

There are over 500 kinases encoded in the human genome, responsible for cell signal transduction that occurs via phosphorylation. Aberrant activation of different tyrosine kinases plays a critical role in cancer pathogenesis, which has led to the development of several TKIs as effective targeted cancer therapies.[29,45] Tyrosine kinase inhibition can be achieved at different levels. Monoclonal antibodies or soluble decoy receptors work by binding the receptor kinase or its ligand. Alternatively, small-molecule inhibitors work intracellularly by interfering with the binding of kinases to ATP or substrates.[45] A major focus of kinase-directed therapy is the vascular endothelial growth factor (VEGF) signaling pathway.

Vascular endothelial growth factor pathway inhibition

VEGF plays a central role in angiogenesis, promoting endothelial proliferation, migration and invasion.[46] VEGF inhibitors (VEGFi) including VEGF signaling pathway small molecule TKIs halt angiogenesis and starve tumor cells of necessary oxygen and nutrients.[46] They are approved for the treatment of solid tumors such as metastatic renal cell, hepatocellular, colorectal, and lung cancer. There are several proposed mechanisms leading to hypertension and direct cardiotoxicity with VEGFi, including endothelial cell dysfunction and death and microvascular dysfunction due to adenosine triphosphate (ATP) depletion in the mitochondria, activation of myocardial proapoptotic kinases, profound vasoconstriction by the activation of endothelin A, decrease of nitric oxide and prostacyclin, and capillary rarefaction.[47,48] Although exact TKI cardiac toxicity mechanisms remain unclear, mitochondrial dysfunction appears at the center of many adverse CV effects.

Clinically, CV toxicities manifest as hypertension, hypertension-induced HF, myocardial ischemia, and LV dysfunction.[49] For example, the incidence of hypertension has been reported as 15%-47% with sunitinib and 17%-42% with sorafenib.[50] The incidence may be higher in patients with comorbidities. In addition to direct cardiac effects, the commonly observed effect of hypertension with VEGFi may contribute to myocardial dysfunction and HF, including HFpEF. In a multicenter prospective study of 90 patients with metastatic renal cell carcinoma treated with sunitinib the predicted risk for ≥10% decline in LVEF to a value of less than 50% was 9.7%.[51] The majority of events happened after the first treatment cycle, and LVEF recovered to normal in all patients after careful management.[51] In another retrospective study of patients treated with sunitinib, 28% had an absolute LVEF reduction of at least 10%, while 8% developed symptomatic HF.[52] A meta-analysis found that 4.1% of 6935 patients developed HF on treatment with sunitinib versus 1.8% treated with placebo.[53] An approximately 5-fold increase in HF risk has also been reported with the VEGF-binding monoclonal antibody, bevacizumab.[54]

Other small molecule TKIs

Small molecule multitargeted TKIs, such as the BCR-ABL kinase inhibitors, are used in a wide array of malignancies.[55] Imatinib was the first of such TKIs, still widely used for the treatment of chronic myeloid leukemia (CML), Philadelphia chromosome-positive acute lymphocytic leukemia (ALL), and gastrointestinal stromal tumors.[56] Imatinib has been associated with a decline of LVEF and HF, although uncommonly.[57] In cultured cardiomyocytes, imatinib led to cell death with features of both apoptosis and necrosis.[58] Imatinib targets Abl, ARG (Abl-related gene), PDGFRα/β, and c-Kit. Lentivirus-mediated expression of an imatinib-resistant mutant of Abl prevented imatinib toxicity in cardiomyocytes.[58] Therefore, inhibition of Abl is believed to cause imatinib's cardiotoxicity. Inhibition of Abl in cardiomyocytes induces endoplasmic reticulum stress through a buildup of misfolded proteins leading to cellular apoptosis.[57]

Dasatinib, nilotinib, and ponatinib were subsequently developed for the treatment of CML. These newer multitargeted TKIs have also been associated with cardiopulmonary adverse effects, including pulmonary hypertension with dasatinib, and vascular atherosclerotic and thrombotic events with nilotinib and ponatinib.[59] Pulmonary hypertension and coronary events can lead to the development of myocardial dysfunction. In a pooled analysis of 911 patients from single-arm trials examining dasatinib's safety, 4% developed HF.[60] Asymptomatic decline in LVEF has also been reported with pazopanib (7%-11%).[50]

The use of combination of MEK (mitogen-activated protein kinase)/BRAF (v-raf murine sarcoma viral oncogene homolog B) inhibitors can also be associated with cardiotoxicity.[61] The cardiac effects are based on the key role of MEK for cardiomyocyte maintenance, repair, and survival under basal and stress situations. In phase 3 clinical trials, reduction in LVEF was reported in 5.7% to 11.7% of the patients treated with BRAF inhibitor/MEK inhibitors.[61] In a recent meta-analysis of randomized trials (>2300 patients), combined therapy with inhibitors of BRAF/MEK was associated with a higher relative risk of LVEF decrease as compared to monotherapy with BRAF inhibitors.[62] More significant reduction in LVEF (LVEF <40% or LVEF reduction >20% compared to baseline) was found in 8% of the patients treated with a BRAF/MEK inhibitor combination, with patients younger than 55 years being at significantly higher risk. Of note, MEK-induced cardiotoxicity is asymptomatic in most cases and is usually noted during a follow-up echocardiogram. The reduction in LVEF is usually reversible after treatment interruption.

Immunotherapy

Over the last decade, indications for the use of immune checkpoint inhibitors (ICI) in the treatment of cancer have rapidly expanded.[63] Currently, 8 FDA approved ICI target cytotoxic T-lymphocyte–associated protein 4 (CTLA-4), programmed cell death receptor 1 (PD-1), and programmed cell death ligand 1 (PD-L1). Despite their success in cancer treatment, ICI can cause immune-related adverse events (irAE) involving almost any organ. The most rare irAE is myocarditis (0.5%–1%, now being increasingly recognized), but is highly fatal (25%–50%).[64,65] ICI-associated myocarditis ranges from asymptomatic rises in troponin to life-threatening conditions presenting with cardiogenic shock and/or advanced atrioventricular block.[66]

The exact pathophysiology of myocarditis is unclear. Proposed mechanisms include a process of molecular mimicry in which T cells recognize the same or similar epitopes in the tumor and the myocardium.[67] Autopsy studies of patients with ICI-associated myocarditis have shown that the same T cell clones are present in the tumor, myocardium, and skeletal muscle further supporting this mechanism.[67] Early mouse models with genetic deletion of PD-1 demonstrated the development of cardiomyopathy; however, this was due to autoantibodies against troponin I, and lacked the T cell infiltration seen in humans.[68] More recently, a mouse model with heterozygous alleles for CTLA-4 and homozygous PD-1 deletion $(ctla4^{+/-}pdcd1^{-/-})$ recapitulated the pathology seen in humans with predominant myocardial CD8+ T cell infiltration, arrhythmias, and decreased cardiac function.[69] In another study, cynomolgus monkeys given combined CTLA-4 (ipilimumab) and PD-1 (nivolumab) inhibition developed cardiomyopathy with myocardial CD8+ and CD4+ T cell infiltration.[70] The predominant endomyocardial biopsy findings described with ICI-associated myocarditis resemble acute cellular rejection in transplanted hearts, with the predominant inflammatory infiltrate being CD8+ T cells followed by CD4+ T cells and rare macrophages.[66,67] In addition to the predominant T cell myocardial infiltration, ICI-associated myocarditis may also have an antibody-mediated component with endomyocardial biopsy samples showing pericapillary C4d staining on immunohistochemistry.[71] HF is a common clinical presentation of ICI-associated myocarditis. Most of the patients maintain a preserved LVEF even though those with normal LVEF have similar adverse CV event rates compared to those with depressed LVEF.[72,73]

Other Conventional Chemotherapeutic Agents

Alkylating agents
Especially at higher doses, cyclophosphamide has been associated with hemorrhagic myocarditis and cardiomyopathy. Metabolites of cyclophosphamide are responsible for the depletion of antioxidants/ATP level, altered contractility, damaged endothelium, and enhanced proinflammatory/proapoptotic activities leading to myocarditis, cardiomyopathy, myocardial infarction, and HF.[74] Although doses greater than 270 mg/kg for 1 to 4 days or ≥ 1.55 g/m^2 are associated with a higher risk, lower doses can also be cardiotoxic. These effects are rare and usually occur within days after the initiation of treatment. The reported mortality in patients with cyclophosphamide-related cardiomyopathy and HF has ranged from 2% to 17%.[2,75]

Platinum-based chemotherapy agents
The proposed mechanism of cisplatin cardiotoxicity involves the activation of several transmembrane protein kinases, caspase 3, and formation of apoptosome leading to apoptosis of the cardiomyocytes.[76] Cisplatin-induced cardiotoxic effects have been reported to manifest through hypertension, life-threatening arrythmias, myopericarditis, coronary vasospasm, and myocardial infarction.[77] A recent analysis of CV outcomes in more than 15,000 patients treated with cisplatin suggested that there is a 5-fold increased risk of CV death in the first year after treatment.[78]

Taxanes
Anti-microtubule agents are commonly used in the treatment of solid tumors such as breast adenocarcinoma, ovarian cancer, and head and neck tumors.[79] Taxanes do not directly impact the myocardium, but increase the risk of AC mediated LV dysfunction by affecting its metabolism and excretion.[80] There is low incidence of LV dysfunction (0.7%), although there is higher incidence of brady- and tachyarrhythmias.[81]

Antimetabolites
The exact mechanism of 5-FU capecitabine-mediated cardiac toxicity is poorly understood although it is likely driven by coronary vasospasm as evidenced by in vitro vasoconstriction of vascular smooth muscle cells.[82] Other proposed mechanisms include direct endothelial injury and accumulation of toxic metabolites.[83] Cardiotoxicities include arrhythmias, HF, stress (Takotsubo) cardiomyopathy, myocardial infarction, cardiogenic shock and sudden death.[84] A meta-analysis reported the incidence of symptomatic cardiotoxicity with 5-FU to be 0% to 20%, and with capecitabine 3% to 35%.[85]

Proteasome inhibitors
Malignant plasma cells have high rates of proteasome activity and protein turnover and make excellent targets for proteasome inhibitors such as bortezomib (reversible) and carfilzomib (irreversible), which are approved for the treatment of mantle cell lymphoma and multiple myeloma. The proposed mechanism of cardiotoxicity and myocardial dysfunction is through apoptosis of cardiomyocytes which, have high rates of proteasome activity similar to malignant plasma cells.[86] Cardiomyocytes are particularly susceptible to proteotoxicity due to the high protein turnover of contractile proteins in the sarcomere. There is,

Table 2
Baseline evaluation, surveillance, and management of myocardial dysfunction in patients with cancer treated with chemotherapy or targeted cancer therapies; Key recommendations based on the American Society of Clinical Oncology (ASCO), American Society of Echocardiography (ASE), European Society for Medical Oncology (ESMO) and the European Society of Cardiology (ESC) guidelines

	Baseline Evaluation	Surveillance	Treatment
General principles applicable to all cardiotoxic cancer therapies	• Baseline cardiac assessment including clinical history, physical exam, a 2D/3D echocardiogram, GLS, and cardiac enzymes including troponin ± BNP/NT-proBNP is recommended, especially in those considered to be at high risk for the development of CTRCD. • Baseline risk assessment and identification of CV risk factors.	• Routine surveillance with history, physical exam, and imaging with echocardiography (preferably 3D and including GLS) is recommended during cardiotoxic therapy, in patients at increased risk of developing cardiac dysfunction. • Frequency of surveillance with cardiac imaging during cardio-toxic therapy is as specified below or otherwise based on the discretion of the treating clinician. • Troponin levels ± BNP/NTpro-BNP before and/or 24 h after each chemotherapy cycle may be considered in high-risk patients. • Cardiac MRI or MUGA may be offered if an echocardiogram is not available or technically feasible, with preference given to cardiac MRI. • After treatment conclusion, repeat cardiac imaging at 6–12 mo, at 2 y, and possibly periodically thereafter.	• Treatment of LV systolic dysfunction with or without HF symptoms with RAS blockers.
Anthracyclines	• See general principles above. No specific recommendations.	• Surveillance with quantitative 2D/3D echocardiography or CMR i) within 6–12 mo of completion of therapy or ii) once a cumulative dose of 250 mg/m2 of doxorubicin or its	• Discuss risk-benefit of continued anthracycline use. • Use of dexrazoxane and/or liposomal doxorubicin could be considered for the prevention of cardiotoxicity in high-risk

patients or high dose of anthracyclines.

equivalent anthracycline has been administered and iii) after each additional 100 mg/m2.

HER-2 targeted therapy	• See general principles above. No specific recommendations.	• Surveillance with quantitative 2D/3D echocardiography or CMR every 3 mo while on therapy	• If trastuzumab is stopped, repeat LVEF within 3–6 wk, and resume trastuzumab therapy if LVEF has normalized to >50%. RAS inhibitors of LV systolic dysfunction ± HF
VEGF inhibitors	• Establishment of a baseline BP.	• Close monitoring of blood pressure and surveillance echocardiography at 1 mo and every 3–6 mo while on therapy with VEGF or VEGF receptor inhibitors.	• BP control. • Discussion and assessment to determine whether reinstituting therapy is appropriate • RAS inhibitors for LV systolic dysfunction
ICIs	• See general principles above. No specific recommendations.	• See general principles above. No specific recommendations.	• Withhold further therapy with ICIs • Start high-dose corticosteroids • For steroid-refractory or high-grade myocarditis with hemodynamic instability, other immunosuppressive therapies, for example, anti-thymocyte globulin, infliximab (not in patients with HF), mycophenolate mofetil, or abatacept considered.

Abbreviations: BP, blood pressure; CV, cardiovascular; GLS, global longitudinal strain, BB, beta blockers; HF, heart failure; ICI, immune checkpoint inhibitors; RAS, renin–angiotensin system.

Data from Refs.[94–97]

however, conflicting data on whether there are an increased risk of clinical cardiotoxicity with bortezomib. One meta-analysis (5718 patients) suggested no significant increase in the risk of cardiotoxicity compared to control patients, whereas multiple case reports suggest otherwise.[87,88] In the ASPIRE trial, LV dysfunction was significantly higher with carfilzomib therapy (3.8%) as compared to the control group (1.8%) and was associated with a higher rate of uncontrolled hypertension (4.7% vs 1.8%).[89] Carfilzomib-associated CV toxicity was confirmed to occur at a higher incidence compared to bortezomib in the ENDEAVOR trial.[90]

Chronochemotherapy and cardiotoxicity

As we try to understand mechanisms of action and toxicity of individual drug classes, research over the last two decades has also revealed a complex association between clock genes, circadian rhythm interruption, and carcinogenesis.[91] In extension to this, it has been hypothesized that delivery of chemotherapy at the appropriate phase of the circadian rhythm might have optimal efficacy. The rationale of this hypothesis is based on the following three concepts: a) efficacy of an agent may vary with time of day administered depending on its mechanism of action[92] b) pharmacokinetics and metabolism of agents may vary with circadian phase that they were delivered[93] c) toxicity of agents may also vary with time of day that they were administered.[93] The idea that cancer therapy administration at specific times of the day (chronochemotherapy) can achieve better outcomes with less toxicity, including cardiotoxicity, is very appealing. However, empiric use of chronochemotherapy has shown conflicting outcomes in the first clinical studies conducted.[91] A cancer-specific, individualized, mechanism-based chronochemotherapy regimen that combines optimal circadian timing of specific agent administration, drug availability and metabolism, and drug toxicity is required to evaluate the potential of this approach in treating cancer and eliminating associated cardiotoxicity.

MONITORING FOR AND MANAGEMENT OF CTRCD

The American Society of Clinical Oncology (ASCO), American Society of Echocardiography (ASE), European Society for Medical Oncology (ESMO), and European Society of Cardiology (ESC) have published guidelines for the screening, monitoring as well as the management of cardiotoxicities in cancer survivors.[94–97] Some of the key recommendations are summarized in **Table 2**.

SUMMARY

Cancer itself, as a systemic disease, as well as cancer-targeted therapies can lead to myocardial dysfunction and subsequently clinical HF. Increased knowledge on the pathogenetic mechanisms leading to myocardial dysfunction has allowed the development of surveillance protocols and establishment of interventions that ameliorate the cardiotoxic potential of cancer and its treatments. Continued research is necessary for further improvement in the prevention and management of cancer-related myocardial dysfunction.

CLINICS CARE POINTS

- Myocardial dysfunction is increasingly recognized as a major cause of therapy interruptions, and morbidity and mortality in patients with cancer.
- Cancer itself, as a systemic disease, as well as chemotherapy and cancer targeted therapies can lead to myocardial dysfunction and subsequently clinical heart failure (HF).
- Increased knowledge about the pathogenetic mechanisms leading to myocardial dysfunction has allowed the development of surveillance protocols and establishment of preventive and therapeutic interventions that ameliorate the cardiotoxic potential of cancer and its treatments.
- Continued research is necessary for further improvement in the management of cancer-related myocardial dysfunction.

DISCLOSURE STATEMENT

Dr. Deswal is supported in part by the Ting Tsung and Wei Fong Chao Distinguished Chair. Dr. Palaskas is supported by the Cancer Prevention & Research Institute of Texas and the Andrew Sabin Family Foundation. Other authors have no conflicts of interest to disclose.

REFERENCES

1. Miller KD, Nogueira L, Mariotto AB, et al. Cancer treatment and survivorship statistics, 2019. CA Cancer J Clin 2019;69(5):363–85.
2. Herrmann J. Adverse cardiac effects of cancer therapies: cardiotoxicity and arrhythmia. Nat Rev Cardiol 2020;17(8):474–502.
3. Larsen C, Dasari H, Calle MCA, et al. Short and long term risk of congestive heart failure in breast cancer and lymphoma patients compared to

controls: an epidemiologic study. J Am Coll Cardiol 2018;71(11_Supplement):A695.

4. Koene RJ, Prizment AE, Blaes A, et al. Shared risk factors in cardiovascular disease and cancer. Circulation 2016;133(11):1104–14.

5. Falk RH, Alexander KM, Liao R, et al. AL (Light-Chain) cardiac amyloidosis: a review of diagnosis and therapy. J Am Coll Cardiol 2016;68(12):1323–41.

6. Goldberg AD, Blankstein R, Padera RF. Tumors metastatic to the heart. Circulation 2013;128(16):1790–4.

7. Piazza G, Rao AF, Nguyen TN, et al. Venous thromboembolism in hospitalized patients with active cancer. Clin Appl Thromb Hemost 2013;19(5):469–75.

8. Mukai M, Oka T. Mechanism and management of cancer-associated thrombosis. J Cardiol 2018;72(2):89–93.

9. Simonneau G, Gatzoulis MA, Adatia I, et al. Updated clinical classification of pulmonary hypertension. J Am Coll Cardiol 2013;62(25 Suppl):D34–41.

10. Ridker PM. Clinician's guide to reducing inflammation to reduce atherothrombotic risk: JACC review topic of the week. J Am Coll Cardiol 2018;72(25):3320–31.

11. Javaid AI, Monlezun DJ, Iliescu G, et al. Stress cardiomyopathy in hospitalized patients with cancer: machine learning analysis by primary malignancy type. ESC Heart Fail 2021;8(6):4626–34.

12. Bertero E, Canepa M, Maack C, et al. Linking heart failure to cancer: background evidence and research perspectives. Circulation 2018;138(7):735–42.

13. Bloom MW, Hamo CE, Cardinale D, et al. Cancer therapy-related cardiac dysfunction and heart failure: part 1: definitions, pathophysiology, risk factors, and imaging. Circ Heart Fail 2016;9(1):e002661.

14. Oikonomou EK, Kokkinidis DG, Kampaktsis PN, et al. Assessment of prognostic value of left ventricular global longitudinal strain for early prediction of chemotherapy-induced cardiotoxicity: a systematic review and meta-analysis. JAMA Cardiol 2019;4(10):1007–18.

15. Thavendiranathan P, Negishi T, Somerset E, et al. Strain-guided management of potentially cardiotoxic cancer therapy. J Am Coll Cardiol 2021;77(4):392–401.

16. Border WL, Sachdeva R, Stratton KL, et al. Longitudinal changes in echocardiographic parameters of cardiac function in pediatric cancer survivors. JACC CardioOncol 2020;2(1):26–37.

17. Goldenberg MM. Trastuzumab, a recombinant DNA-derived humanized monoclonal antibody, a novel agent for the treatment of metastatic breast cancer. Clin Ther 1999;21(2):309–18.

18. Piccart-Gebhart MJ, Procter M, Leyland-Jones B, et al. Trastuzumab after adjuvant chemotherapy in HER2-positive breast cancer. N Engl J Med 2005;353(16):1659–72.

19. Ewer MS, Lippman SM. Type II chemotherapy-related cardiac dysfunction: time to recognize a new entity. J Clin Oncol 2005;23(13):2900–2.

20. Riccio G, Coppola C, Piscopo G, et al. Trastuzumab and target-therapy side effects: Is still valid to differentiate anthracycline type I from type II cardiomyopathies? Hum Vaccin Immunother 2016;12(5):1124–31.

21. Gammella E, Maccarinelli F, Buratti P, et al. The role of iron in anthracycline cardiotoxicity. Front Pharmacol 2014;5:25.

22. Cardinale D, Colombo A, Bacchiani G, et al. Early detection of anthracycline cardiotoxicity and improvement with heart failure therapy. Circulation 2015;131(22):1981–8.

23. Abdel-Qadir H, Ong G, Fazelzad R, et al. Interventions for preventing cardiomyopathy due to anthracyclines: a Bayesian network meta-analysis. Ann Oncol 2017;28(3):628–33.

24. Moudgil R, Samra G, Ko KA, et al. Topoisomerase 2B decrease results in diastolic dysfunction via p53 and Akt: a novel pathway. Front Cardiovasc Med 2020;7:594123.

25. Pommier Y, Leo E, Zhang H, et al. DNA topoisomerases and their poisoning by anticancer and antibacterial drugs. Chem Biol 2010;17(5):421–33.

26. Zhang S, Liu X, Bawa-Khalfe T, et al. Identification of the molecular basis of doxorubicin-induced cardiotoxicity. Nat Med 2012;18(11):1639–42.

27. Ewer MS, Vooletich MT, Durand JB, et al. Reversibility of trastuzumab-related cardiotoxicity: new insights based on clinical course and response to medical treatment. J Clin Oncol 2005;23(31):7820–6.

28. Slamon DJ, Leyland-Jones B, Shak S, et al. Use of chemotherapy plus a monoclonal antibody against HER2 for metastatic breast cancer that overexpresses HER2. N Engl J Med 2001;344(11):783–92.

29. Perez IE, Taveras Alam S, Hernandez GA, et al. Cancer therapy-related cardiac dysfunction: an overview for the clinician. Clin Med Insights Cardiol 2019;13. 1179546819866445.

30. Odiete O, Hill MF, Sawyer DB. Neuregulin in cardiovascular development and disease. Circ Res 2012;111(10):1376–85.

31. Monsuez JJ, Charniot JC, Vignat N, et al. Cardiac side-effects of cancer chemotherapy. Int J Cardiol 2010;144(1):3–15.

32. Herrmann J. Vascular toxic effects of cancer therapies. Nat Rev Cardiol 2020;17(8):503–22.

33. He H, Wang L, Qiao Y, et al. Doxorubicin induces endotheliotoxicity and mitochondrial dysfunction

via ROS/eNOS/NO pathway. Front Pharmacol 2019;10:1531.

34. Bloom MJ, Jarrett AM, Triplett TA, et al. Anti-HER2 induced myeloid cell alterations correspond with increasing vascular maturation in a murine model of HER2+ breast cancer. BMC Cancer 2020; 20(1):359.

35. Sandoo A, Kitas GD, Carmichael AR. Endothelial dysfunction as a determinant of trastuzumab-mediated cardiotoxicity in patients with breast cancer. Anticancer Res 2014;34(3):1147–51.

36. de Azambuja E, Procter MJ, van Veldhuisen DJ, et al. Trastuzumab-associated cardiac events at 8 years of median follow-up in the Herceptin Adjuvant trial (BIG 1-01). J Clin Oncol 2014;32(20): 2159–65.

37. Jiang J, Mohan N, Endo Y, et al. Type IIB DNA topoisomerase is downregulated by trastuzumab and doxorubicin to synergize cardiotoxicity. Oncotarget 2018;9(5):6095–108.

38. Curigliano G, Cardinale D, Dent S, et al. Cardiotoxicity of anticancer treatments: Epidemiology, detection, and management. CA Cancer J Clin 2016;66(4):309–25.

39. Moja L, Tagliabue L, Balduzzi S, et al. Trastuzumab containing regimens for early breast cancer. Cochrane Database Syst Rev 2012;2012(4): Cd006243.

40. Shah MA. Update on metastatic gastric and esophageal cancers. J Clin Oncol 2015;33(16):1760–9.

41. Suter TM, Procter M, van Veldhuisen DJ, et al. Trastuzumab-associated cardiac adverse effects in the herceptin adjuvant trial. J Clin Oncol 2007;25(25): 3859–65.

42. Lenihan D, Suter T, Brammer M, et al. Pooled analysis of cardiac safety in patients with cancer treated with pertuzumab. Ann Oncol 2012;23(3): 791–800.

43. Piccart-Gebhart M, Holmes E, Baselga J, et al. Adjuvant lapatinib and trastuzumab for early human epidermal growth factor receptor 2-positive breast cancer: results from the randomized phase III Adjuvant Lapatinib and/or Trastuzumab treatment optimization trial. J Clin Oncol 2016;34(10): 1034–42.

44. Bowles EJ, Wellman R, Feigelson HS, et al. Risk of heart failure in breast cancer patients after anthracycline and trastuzumab treatment: a retrospective cohort study. J Natl Cancer Inst 2012;104(17): 1293–305.

45. Moslehi JJ. Cardiovascular toxic effects of targeted cancer therapies. N Engl J Med 2016;375(15): 1457–67.

46. Ellis LM, Hicklin DJ. VEGF-targeted therapy: mechanisms of anti-tumour activity. Nat Rev Cancer 2008;8(8):579–91.

47. Ferrara N. Role of vascular endothelial growth factor in regulation of physiological angiogenesis. Am J Physiol Cell Physiol 2001;280(6):C1358–66.

48. Lankhorst S, Saleh L, Danser AJ, et al. Etiology of angiogenesis inhibition-related hypertension. Curr Opin Pharmacol 2015;21:7–13.

49. Groarke JD, Choueiri TK, Slosky D, et al. Recognizing and managing left ventricular dysfunction associated with therapeutic inhibition of the vascular endothelial growth factor signaling pathway. Curr Treat Options Cardiovasc Med 2014;16(9):335.

50. Lee W-S, Kim J. Cardiotoxicity associated with tyrosine kinase-targeted anticancer therapy. Mol Cell Toxicol 2018;14(3):247–54.

51. Narayan V, Keefe S, Haas N, et al. Prospective evaluation of sunitinib-induced cardiotoxicity in patients with metastatic renal cell carcinoma. Clin Cancer Res 2017;23(14):3601–9.

52. Chu TF, Rupnick MA, Kerkela R, et al. Cardiotoxicity associated with tyrosine kinase inhibitor sunitinib. Lancet 2007;370(9604):2011–9.

53. Richards CJ, Je Y, Schutz FA, et al. Incidence and risk of congestive heart failure in patients with renal and nonrenal cell carcinoma treated with sunitinib. J Clin Oncol 2011;29(25):3450–6.

54. Choueiri TK, Mayer EL, Je Y, et al. Congestive heart failure risk in patients with breast cancer treated with bevacizumab. J Clin Oncol 2011;29(6):632–8.

55. Chaar M, Kamta J, Ait-Oudhia S. Mechanisms, monitoring, and management of tyrosine kinase inhibitors-associated cardiovascular toxicities. Onco Targets Ther 2018;11:6227–37.

56. Zhong L, Li Y, Xiong L, et al. Small molecules in targeted cancer therapy: advances, challenges, and future perspectives. Signal Transduct Target Ther 2021;6(1):201.

57. Chen MH, Kerkelä R, Force T. Mechanisms of cardiac dysfunction associated with tyrosine kinase inhibitor cancer therapeutics. Circulation 2008; 118(1):84–95.

58. Kerkelä R, Grazette L, Yacobi R, et al. Cardiotoxicity of the cancer therapeutic agent imatinib mesylate. Nat Med 2006;12(8):908–16.

59. Moslehi JJ, Deininger M. Tyrosine Kinase Inhibitor-Associated Cardiovascular Toxicity in Chronic Myeloid Leukemia. J Clin Oncol 2015;33(35): 4210–8.

60. Brave M, Goodman V, Kaminskas E, et al. Sprycel for chronic myeloid leukemia and Philadelphia chromosome-positive acute lymphoblastic leukemia resistant to or intolerant of imatinib mesylate. Clin Cancer Res 2008;14(2):352–9.

61. Arangalage D, Degrauwe N, Michielin O, et al. Pathophysiology, diagnosis and management of cardiac toxicity induced by immune checkpoint

inhibitors and BRAF and MEK inhibitors. Cancer Treat Rev 2021;100:102282.

62. Mincu RI, Mahabadi AA, Michel L, et al. Cardiovascular adverse events associated with BRAF and MEK inhibitors: A systematic review and meta-analysis. JAMA Netw Open 2019;2(8):e198890.

63. Robert C. A decade of immune-checkpoint inhibitors in cancer therapy. Nat Commun 2020;11(1): 3801.

64. Wang DY, Salem J-E, Cohen JV, et al. Fatal toxic effects associated with immune checkpoint inhibitors: a systematic review and meta-analysisfatal toxic effects associated with immune checkpoint inhibitorsfatal toxic effects associated with immune checkpoint inhibitors. JAMA Oncol 2018;4(12): 1721–8.

65. Salem JE, Manouchehri A, Moey M, et al. Cardiovascular toxicities associated with immune checkpoint inhibitors: an observational, retrospective, pharmacovigilance study. Lancet Oncol 2018; 19(12):1579–89.

66. Palaskas NL, Segura A, Lelenwa L, et al. Immune checkpoint inhibitor myocarditis: elucidating the spectrum of disease through endomyocardial biopsy. Eur J Heart Fail 2021;23(10):1725–35.

67. Johnson DB, Balko JM, Compton ML, et al. Fulminant myocarditis with combination immune checkpoint blockade. N Engl J Med 2016;375(18): 1749–55.

68. Okazaki T, Tanaka Y, Nishio R, et al. Autoantibodies against cardiac troponin I are responsible for dilated cardiomyopathy in PD-1-deficient mice. Nat Med 2003;9(12):1477–83.

69. Wei SC, Meijers WC, Axelrod ML, et al. A genetic mouse model recapitulates immune checkpoint inhibitor-associated myocarditis and supports a mechanism-based therapeutic intervention. Cancer Discov 2021;11(3):614–25.

70. Ji C, Roy MD, Golas J, et al. Myocarditis in cynomolgus monkeys following treatment with immune checkpoint inhibitors. Clin Cancer Res 2019; 25(15):4735–48.

71. Balanescu DV, Donisan T, Palaskas N, et al. Immunomodulatory treatment of immune checkpoint inhibitor-induced myocarditis: pathway toward precision-based therapy. Cardiovasc Pathol 2020; 47:107211.

72. Mahmood SS, Fradley MG, Cohen JV, et al. Myocarditis in patients treated with immune checkpoint inhibitors. J Am Coll Cardiol 2018;71(16): 1755–64.

73. Awadalla M, Mahmood SS, Groarke JD, et al. Global longitudinal strain and cardiac events in patients with immune checkpoint inhibitor-related myocarditis. J Am Coll Cardiol 2020;75(5):467–78.

74. Iqubal A, Iqubal MK, Sharma S, et al. Molecular mechanism involved in cyclophosphamide-induced cardiotoxicity: old drug with a new vision. Life Sci 2019;218:112–31.

75. Dhesi S, Chu MP, Blevins G, et al. Cyclophosphamide-induced cardiomyopathy: a case report, review, and recommendations for management. J Investig Med High Impact Case Rep 2013;1(1). 2324709613480346.

76. Ma H, Jones KR, Guo R, et al. Cisplatin compromises myocardial contractile function and mitochondrial ultrastructure: role of endoplasmic reticulum stress. Clin Exp Pharmacol Physiol 2010;37(4):460–5.

77. Dugbartey GJ, Peppone LJ, de Graaf IA. An integrative view of cisplatin-induced renal and cardiac toxicities: Molecular mechanisms, current treatment challenges and potential protective measures. Toxicology 2016;371:58–66.

78. Fung C, Fossa SD, Milano MT, et al. Cardiovascular disease mortality after chemotherapy or surgery for testicular nonseminoma: a population-based study. J Clin Oncol 2015;33(28):3105–15.

79. Field JJ, Kanakkanthara A, Miller JH. Microtubule-targeting agents are clinically successful due to both mitotic and interphase impairment of microtubule function. Bioorg Med Chem 2014;22(18): 5050–9.

80. Colombo T, Parisi I, Zucchetti M, et al. Pharmacokinetic interactions of paclitaxel, docetaxel and their vehicles with doxorubicin. Ann Oncol 1999;10(4): 391–5.

81. Sawaya H, Sebag IA, Plana JC, et al. Assessment of echocardiography and biomarkers for the extended prediction of cardiotoxicity in patients treated with anthracyclines, taxanes, and trastuzumab. Circ Cardiovasc Imaging 2012;5(5): 596–603.

82. Mosseri M, Fingert HJ, Varticovski L, et al. In vitro evidence that myocardial ischemia resulting from 5-fluorouracil chemotherapy is due to protein kinase C-mediated vasoconstriction of vascular smooth muscle. Cancer Res 1993;53(13):3028–33.

83. Peng J, Dong C, Wang C, et al. Cardiotoxicity of 5-fluorouracil and capecitabine in Chinese patients: a prospective study. Cancer Commun (Lond) 2018;38(1):22.

84. Kosmas C, Kallistratos MS, Kopterides P, et al. Cardiotoxicity of fluoropyrimidines in different schedules of administration: a prospective study. J Cancer Res Clin Oncol 2008;134(1):75–82.

85. Polk A, Vaage-Nilsen M, Vistisen K, et al. Cardiotoxicity in cancer patients treated with 5-fluorouracil or capecitabine: a systematic review of incidence, manifestations and predisposing factors. Cancer Treat Rev 2013;39(8):974–84.

86. Cole DC, Frishman WH. Cardiovascular complications of proteasome inhibitors used in multiple myeloma. Cardiol Rev 2018;26(3):122–9.

87. Xiao Y, Yin J, Wei J, et al. Incidence and risk of cardiotoxicity associated with bortezomib in the treatment of cancer: a systematic review and meta-analysis. PLoS One 2014;9(1):e87671.

88. Meseeha MG, Kolade VO, Attia MN. Partially reversible bortezomib-induced cardiotoxicity: an unusual cause of acute cardiomyopathy. J Community Hosp Intern Med Perspect 2015; 5(6):28982.

89. Stewart AK, Rajkumar SV, Dimopoulos MA, et al. Carfilzomib, lenalidomide, and dexamethasone for relapsed multiple myeloma. N Engl J Med 2015;372(2):142–52.

90. Dimopoulos MA, Moreau P, Palumbo A, et al. Carfilzomib and dexamethasone versus bortezomib and dexamethasone for patients with relapsed or refractory multiple myeloma (ENDEAVOR): a randomised, phase 3, open-label, multicentre study. Lancet Oncol 2016;17(1):27–38.

91. Sancar A, Van Gelder RN. Clocks, cancer, and chronochemotherapy. Science 2021;371(6524): eabb0738.

92. Ozturk N, Ozturk D, Kavakli IH, et al. Molecular aspects of circadian pharmacology and relevance for cancer chronotherapy. Int J Mol Sci 2017;18(10).

93. Dallmann R, Okyar A, Lévi F. Dosing-time makes the poison: circadian regulation and pharmacotherapy. Trends Mol Med 2016;22(5):430–45.

94. Curigliano G, Lenihan D, Fradley M, et al. Management of cardiac disease in cancer patients throughout oncological treatment: ESMO consensus recommendations. Ann Oncol 2020; 31(2):171–90.

95. Armenian SH, Lacchetti C, Barac A, et al. Prevention and monitoring of cardiac dysfunction in survivors of adult cancers: american society of clinical oncology clinical practice guideline. J Clin Oncol 2017;35(8):893–911.

96. Zamorano JL, Lancellotti P, Rodriguez Muñoz D, et al. 2016 ESC position paper on cancer treatments and cardiovascular toxicity developed under the auspices of the ESC committee for practice guidelines: the task force for cancer treatments and cardiovascular toxicity of the European society of cardiology (ESC). Eur Heart J 2016; 37(36):2768–801.

97. Brahmer JR, Lacchetti C, Schneider BJ, et al. Management of immune-related adverse events in patients treated with immune checkpoint inhibitor therapy: american society of clinical oncology clinical practice guideline. J Clin Oncol 2018;36(17): 1714–68.

98. U.S Department of Health and Human Services. Common terminology criteria for adverse events (CTCAE) version 5.0. 2017. Available at. https://ctep.cancer.gov/protocoldevelopment/electronic_applications/docs/ctcae_v5_quick_reference_5x7.pdf. Accessed on: 10/7/2021.

99. U.S. Food and Drug Administration. Definition. Available at: https://www.accessdata.fda.gov/drugsatfda_docs/label/2012/062921s022lbl.pdf. Accessed on: 10/7/2021.

100. Seidman A, Hudis C, Pierri MK, et al. Cardiac dysfunction in the trastuzumab clinical trials experience. J Clin Oncol 2002;20(5):1215–21.

101. Slamon D, Eiermann W, Robert N, et al. Adjuvant trastuzumab in HER2-positive breast cancer. N Engl J Med 2011;365(14):1273–83.

102. Plana JC, Galderisi M, Barac A, et al. Expert consensus for multimodality imaging evaluation of adult patients during and after cancer therapy: a report from the American society of echocardiography and the European association of cardiovascular imaging. J Am Soc Echocardiogr 2014;27(9): 911–39.

103. Schwartz RG, McKenzie WB, Alexander J, et al. Congestive heart failure and left ventricular dysfunction complicating doxorubicin therapy. Seven-year experience using serial radionuclide angiocardiography. Am J Med 1987;82(6): 1109–18.

104. Ezaz G, Long JB, Gross CP, et al. Risk prediction model for heart failure and cardiomyopathy after adjuvant trastuzumab therapy for breast cancer. J Am Heart Assoc 2014;3(1):e000472.

105. Alexandre J, Cautela J, Ederhy S, et al. Cardiovascular toxicity related to cancer treatment: a pragmatic approach to the american and european cardio-oncology guidelines. J Am Heart Assoc 2020;9(18):e018403.

Arrhythmic Complications Associated with Cancer Therapies

Naga Venkata K. Pothineni, MD[a], Herman Van Besien, MD[b],
Michael G. Fradley, MD[c],*

KEYWORDS

- Cardiovascular toxicities • Arrhythmias • Myocarditis • Heart failure • Cardio-oncology
- Cardiotoxicity

KEY POINTS

- Arrhythmias are a common complication of cancer therapy and can be either a direct consequence of the treatment or secondary to another type of toxicity such as heart failure, myocarditis, or ischemia.
- Atrial arrhythmias, particularly atrial fibrillation (AF) are most commonly encountered, while ventricular- and bradyarrhythmias occur at lower rates.
- At present, the management of cancer-treatment associated AF is the same as that for the patients with noncancer with AF.
- QT interval prolongation is common in patients with cancer though associated adverse arrhythmic events are rare
- Autonomic dysfunction (AD) frequently affects patients with cancer and survivors and can impact both morbidity and mortality.

INTRODUCTION

Over the last several decades, improved screening and detection have led to a significant increase in cancer survivorship. Moreover, the development of targeted and immunotherapies has also substantially improved cancer mortality, with some advanced malignancies now being managed as chronic diseases. Despite this improvement in cancer outcomes, there is increased recognition of treatment-related cardiovascular complications which can impact morbidity and mortality. Cardio-oncology is collaborative discipline aimed at the prevention of management of cardiovascular disease in patients with cancer. Beyond left ventricular dysfunction and heart failure, cancer treatments can have either direct or indirect electrophysiologic effects ranging from both tachy- and bradyarrhythmias (**Table 1**). Cardio-oncologists must be familiar with the myriad of arrhythmic complications, working closely with medical oncologists and electrophysiologists to provide the optimal electrophysiology and cancer care to these complex patients.

ATRIAL FIBRILLATION AND OTHER ATRIAL ARRHYTHMIAS

Atrial fibrillation (AF) is a commonly encountered arrhythmia in patients with cancer. Incident AF has been associated with the development of heart failure and stroke in patients with cancer.[1] While natural atrial remodeling with age contributes to AF, additional cancer-specific factors

[a] Kansas City Heart Rhythm Institute, Overland Park, KS, USA; [b] Department of Medicine, Hospital of the University of Pennsylvania, Perelman School of Medicine at the University of Pennsylvania, Philadelphia, PA, USA; [c] Division of Cardiology, Department of Medicine, Cardio-Oncology Center of Excellence, Perelman School of Medicine at the University of Pennsylvania, Philadelphia, PA, USA
* Corresponding author. 3400 Civic Center Boulevard PCAM 2-355S, Philadelphia, PA 19104.
E-mail address: Michael.fradley@pennmedicine.upenn.edu

Heart Failure Clin 18 (2022) 375–383
https://doi.org/10.1016/j.hfc.2022.02.006

Table 1
Arrhythmias associated with cancer treatments

Drug Class	Specific Agents	Associated Arrhythmias
Alkylating Agents	Melphalan	Atrial Arrhythmias
Anthracyclines	Doxorubicin	Atrial Arrhythmias Ventricular Arrhythmias
Antimetabolites	5-Fluorouracil	Ventricular Arrhythmias
Arsenic		QT Prolongation
Cyclin-Dependent Kinase 4/6 Inhibitors	Ribociclib	QT Prolongation
Immunotherapy	Checkpoint Inhibitors (ie, pembrolizumab)	Atrial Arrhythmias Ventricular Arrhythmias Bradyarrhythmias
Proteasome Inhibitors	Carfilzomib	Atrial Arrhythmias
Radiation Therapy (photon, proton)	Mediastinal; Head and Neck	Autonomic Dysfunction
Taxanes	Paclitaxel	Bradyarrhythmias
Tyrosine Kinase Inhibitors	Ibrutinib (BTK Inhibitor) Nilotinib, Dasatinib, Vandetanib ALK Inhibitors	Atrial Arrhythmias; Ventricular Arrhythmias; Bradyarrhythmias (rare) QT Prolongation Bradyarrhythmias

such as systemic inflammation, cancer-related metabolic stress (hypoxia, anemia), direct cytotoxic effect of chemotherapeutic agents, and on- and off-target effects on intracellular signaling pathways also play a role in AF development.[2]

A variety of anticancer drugs are known to increase the risk of AF. Doxorubicin and other anthracyclines are well-known causes of LV dysfunction. Multiple prior studies have also shown a higher incidence of AF even in patients with normal LV function receiving anthracyclines. Kilickap and colleagues reported a 10.3% incidence of AF following one infusion of doxorubicin using continuous rhythm monitoring.[3] In addition, the occurrence of LV dysfunction as a result of anthracyclines is also associated with a high rate of AF similar to other nonischemic cardiomyopathies.[4] Hematopoietic stem cell transplantation performed for various hematological malignancies is a well-recognized risk factor for atrial arrhythmias.[5] Sureddi and colleagues reported a 27% incidence of AF in patients with multiple myeloma undergoing stem cell transplantation.[6] In another retrospective analysis of patients undergoing hematopoietic stem cell transplantation, Chang and colleagues reported a 10.6% cumulative incidence of AF.[7] Interestingly, baseline left atrial function was a significant predictor of incident AF in this cohort. While metabolic factors such as renal failure, hypertension, and amyloid were associated with increased AF incidence, effect of anticancer agents such as melphalan and carfilzomib are also contributory. Importantly, posttransplant atrial arrhythmias are associated with worse long-term outcomes.[8] Immune checkpoint inhibitors are well associated with myocarditis and can be quite arrhythmogenic including an increased risk of atrial arrhythmias.[9,10] Finally, chimeric antigen receptor T(CAR-T) cell therapy has emerged as a novel therapeutic modality for various hematological malignancies with increasing use. CART-T therapy has been associated with a 5% to 7.5% risk of AAs.[11,12] Whether this represents a direct cytotoxic effect or a reflection of systemic inflammatory response is not well known.

Tyrosine kinase inhibitors (TKIs) such as sorafenib are another class of drugs linked with an increased risk of atrial arrhythmias. One proposed mechanism for increased arrhythmic risk is the inhibition of the phosphoinositide 3-kinase (PI3K) signaling pathway, leading to prolonged cardiac repolarization.[13] Vascular endothelial growth factor receptor (VEGFR) inhibitors block angiogenesis and can contribute to hypertension, LV dysfunction and incident atrial arrhythmias.[14] Other TKIs such as ponatinib and bosutinib have also been shown to have a modest association with incident AF in various studies.[15] Multiple studies have also shown that ibrutinib, a Bruton's tyrosine kinase

(BTK) inhibitor used for the treatment of hematological malignancies is associated with increased AF risk.[16] Yun and colleagues conducted a meta-analysis of 4 randomized trials and reported an 8-fold higher risk of AF with use of ibrutinib compared with other anticancer regimens.[17] Another recent review of 8 randomized clinical trials comprising 2580 patients showed an approximately 5-fold increased risk of AF with use of ibrutinib.[18] The mechanism of ibrutinib-induced AF remains unclear. Studies using animal models demonstrated that the use of ibrutinib leads to the prolongation of atrial refractory periods along with atrial dilation and fibrosis and subsequently increased AF inducibility. Importantly this increase in AF inducibility was evident even in mice that were not treated with ibrutinib, implying the mechanism of AF may be unrelated to BTK inhibition. A more recent study by Xiao and colleagues suggested off-target inhibition of C-terminal Src kinase may be the primary mechanism of increased AF susceptibility with ibrutinib, especially as acalabrutinib, a second-generation BTK inhibitor does not impact this kinase and has been associated with significantly lower rates of AF.[19] However, a recent randomized trial of acalabrutinib versus ibrutinib showed a 9.6% of incident AF in the acalabrutinib group compared with 16% in the ibrutinib group, suggesting that the mechanisms of AF may be multifactorial in this population and continues to be elusive.[20]

Atrial Fibrillation Management in Patients with Cancer

Management of AF in patients with active cancer presents a frequent clinical challenge (**Fig. 1**). While rate and rhythm control were considered equally efficacious for AF management,[21] more recent studies such as the EAST AF-NET have clearly demonstrated a clinical benefit of early rhythm control, especially with catheter ablation.[22] However, patients with active cancer were excluded from almost all clinical trials of AF management, leading to an individualized risk-benefit decision making by the treating clinician. Symptom status, effect on LV function, and expected long-term prognosis remains the main determinants of an optimal treatment approach, which include rate control and rhythm control, either with pharmacologic agents or catheter ablation.

Beta-blockers and calcium channel blockers remain the cornerstone for rate control in patients with AF. In patient with cancer, however, nondihydropyridine calcium channel blockers and digoxin should be used with caution due to frequent, specific drug–drug interactions that impact cytochrome P450 3A4 and p-glycoprotein metabolism.[23,24] Additional metabolic factors such as anemia and dehydration can lead to compensatory rapid ventricular rates should be adequately addressed.

Symptoms of AF and the presence of LV dysfunction and/or heart failure are the main drivers of choosing a rhythm control strategy. Pharmacologic options for rhythm control in patients with cancer are often limited, either due to similar drug interactions or the presence of underlying comorbidities. Class 1c agents such as flecainide are contraindication in patients with ischemic heart disease, LV dysfunction, and significant LV hypertrophy, which are often seen in patients with cancer and those with chemotherapy-induced cardiomyopathy. Other agents such as dronedarone have significant interactions with chemotherapeutic agents through both the CYP3A4 and P glycoprotein systems.[25] Class III agents such as sotalol and dofetilide have QT-prolonging effects which can be exacerbated by multiple anticancer drugs. In addition, underlying renal dysfunction can also limit their use. Amiodarone is the most frequently chosen anti-arrhythmic drug in patients with cancer owing given that it is relatively well-tolerated in most cases; however, the long-term deleterious effects of amiodarone should be carefully weighed against the benefits.[26]

Catheter ablation has emerged as the preferred rhythm control strategy in most patients with AF. Several randomized trials have shown increased AF-free survival with catheter ablation. Specifically, catheter ablation has been shown to improve heart failure outcomes in patients with AF and heart failure.[27] A recent substudy of EAST AF-NET also showed that instituting catheter ablation within 1 year of diagnosis of AF is associated with overall improved outcomes in patients with either heart failure with reduced or preserved ejection fraction.[28] However, several aspects of ablative therapy must be addressed in patients with cancer. First, pulmonary vein isolation is the cornerstone of AF ablation as the pulmonary veins are the source of AF triggers in greater than 90% of patients with AF.[29] Whether the same pathophysiology applies to AF induced by anticancer drugs is unknown. Contribution of nonpulmonary vein triggers, atrial scarring/fibrosis, and systemic inflammation can all influence the occurrence of AF and alter ablation outcomes. Second, while AF ablation has been shown to be safe, rates of bleeding complications are higher in patients with cancer and survivors, particularly those with hematological disorders.[30] Third, active malignancy is associated with hypercoagulability

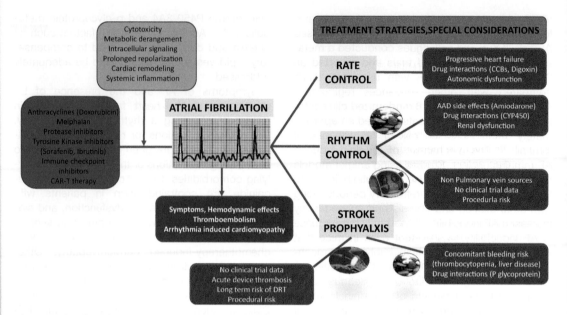

Fig. 1. Pathophysiology and management of atrial fibrillation in patients with cancer.

that can potentially increase the risk of thrombo-embolic complications with left atrial instrumentation. Finally, performing AF ablation dictates the use of uninterrupted anticoagulation at least for 4 to 6 weeks which may be challenging in some patients. While these considerations are valid, an individualized approach can help identify specific patients on anticancer therapy that may benefit from catheter ablation of AF.[24]

Stroke Prophylaxis

Oral anticoagulation remains the mainstay of stroke prophylaxis in patients with AF. However, anticoagulation decisions in patients with cancer are further complicated by an increased risk of bleeding due to hematological side effects of chemotherapy, hepatic/renal dysfunction, and presence of metastatic deposits in high-risk anatomic regions such as the brain. In addition, commonly used chemotherapeutic agents often use the same metabolic pathways such as the cytochrome and P-glycoprotein systems that are used by various direct oral anticoagulants (DOACs) such as apixaban, dabigatran and rivaroxaban.[24] Nevertheless, there are data to support the efficacy and safety of DOACs for stroke prophylaxis in patients with cancer with AF.[31] Based on current evidence and consensus, patients with cancer with elevated CHADS-VASc score and no elevated bleeding risk are candidates for OAC.[24] Despite this general recommendation, a significant number of patients with cancer may not be receiving adequate anticoagulation when AF is identified particularly in the setting of recent chemotherapy exposure.[32] Nevertheless, there is increasing evidence that the CHADS-VASc score may not be adequate to assess risk in patients with cancer emphasizing the need to develop cancer-specific algorithms.[33] While left atrial appendage occlusion (LAAO) has emerged as an effective alternative therapy for patients with AF unable to tolerate OAC, the pivotal trials of LAAO excluded patients with active cancer. Hence, thromboembolic prophylaxis decisions are largely based on expert consensus and multidisciplinary team evaluations. Although there is the paucity of trial data, observational data on the use of LAAO in patients with cancer have been reported. In a study of 364 patients with active cancer undergoing LAAO from the National Readmission Database, those with active cancer had a higher risk of in-hospital stroke/TIA after LAAO compared with those without cancer which may reflect an increased hypercoagulability with cancer.[34] In patients with elevated bleeding risk (thrombocytopenia, liver dysfunction and so forth), consideration can be given to LAAO if a short-term course of OAC can be tolerated. In patients who cannot tolerate even a short course of OAC, enrollment in an ongoing multicenter registry may offer the option of being on an antiplatelet agent instead in the short term.[35] Even after successful LAAO, the long-term risk of device-related thrombosis specifically in patients with active cancer who have a hypercoagulable state has not been systematically evaluated though a recent multicenter registry study identified hypercoagulability as an independent risk factor for long-term device-related thrombosis.[36]

VENTRICULAR ARRHYTHMIAS
QTc Prolongation and Torsade's de Pointes

The vast majority of iatrogenic QTc prolongation occurs through a drug's effect on the IKr potassium channel, responsible for the rapid repolarization of the myocyte membrane during phase 3 of the cardiac action potential.[24] This holds true for most anticancer agents as well, with a few exceptions. Notably, oxaliplatin has been shown to act via gain of function of inward Na + -channels, and arsenic trioxide (ATO) has an inhibitory effect on both IKr and IKs channels.[37,38]

Of the conventional chemotherapies, ATO has the most QT-prolonging potential, with some studies showing that a QTc greater than 500 ms can occur in more than 40% of patients.[39] Anthracyclines and most other cytotoxic chemotherapies have relatively little impact on the QTc despite the presence of various other cardiotoxicities.[24] Conversely, various targeted cancer therapies, particularly TKIs have demonstrated a significant QT-prolonging effect. A retrospective cohort study showed more than 13 years, one-third of TKIs administered resulted in QTc greater than 60 ms from baseline, with nearly 5% of those cases associated with life-threatening complications.[40] In that study, nilotinib and dasatinib were shown to have the highest rates of QTc prolongation. A meta-analysis demonstrated that vandetanib has a dose-dependent effect on the QTc interval affecting 15 to 20% of patients.[41] Approximately 3% of patients treated with the CDK4/6 inhibitor ribociclib demonstrated significant QT prolongation (>60 ms from baseline) in clinical trials.[42] The HDAC inhibitors romidepsin, panobinostat, and vorinostat are also associated with substantial QT prolongation.[41] Finally, hormonal therapies, such as selective estrogen receptor modifying (SERM) agents and androgen deprivation therapy, have been shown to have QT-prolonging effects.[43]

The clinical relevance of QTc prolongation has yet to be specifically determined for many cancer therapeutics. In one retrospective study of 113 patients treated with ATO, only 1 patient developed torsade's de pointes (in the setting of marked hypokalemia and hypomagnesemia) despite 65% having a Bazett corrected QT interval of greater than 500 ms.[39] Nevertheless, there is still need for caution when initiating these medications or adjusting their dose. Frequent ECG monitoring is a mainstay of safe administration, along with careful monitoring and repletion of electrolytes. During induction chemotherapy, many patients require

the use of antiemetics and antibiotics, and careful attention should be made in selecting agents that do not further lengthen the QT interval. There is a largely additive, if not synergistic effect, of combining QT-prolonging agents as part of a chemotherapy regimen.[24,44] Adjustment and or cessation of noncancer agents with QT-prolonging potential should be prioritized over altering the cancer treatment. Should TdP develop, prompt administration of magnesium sulfate is essential. In addition, the heart rate should be maintained at greater than 100 bpm with either isoproterenol or transvenous pacing.[45]

Ventricular Arrhythmias

Most cases of VT/VF in cancer are directly attributed to the physiologic burden of the disease itself, as VT/VF are more common in patients with widely metastatic disease. Metastasis to the heart itself, although rare, has also been implicated in the development of VAs.[46] Ventricular arrhythmias in the setting of cancer treatment are most commonly due to QT-prolonging effects as discussed above, or secondary to another primary cardiotoxicity (such as ischemia or LV dysfunction), though the BTK inhibitor ibrutinib likely has a direct arrhythmogenic effect with ventricular arrhythmias identified rare yet lethal side effect of this class of drugs.[47-49] The arrhythmogenic complications of antimetabolites such as 5-fluorouracil can be readily ascribed to ischemia from vasospasm,[50,51] while anthracyclines and anti-HER2-targeted therapies such as trastuzumab are known to induce cardiomyopathies from which ventricular arrhythmias can sometimes arise. Myocarditis is estimated to occur in 1.14% of all patients receiving immune checkpoint inhibitor therapy, with greater prevalence among anti-CTLA4 therapies over anti-PD1/PDL1. Ventricular arrhythmias frequently occur in the setting of fulminant disease.[52]

There are few studies that have specifically addressed the management of ventricular arrhythmias due to chemotherapy. Current guidelines are more general, recommending implantable cardioverter-defibrillator in patients with LVEF less than 35% refractory to guideline-directed medical therapy, NYHA class II–III symptoms, and life expectancy greater than 1 year. A population study from Denmark Primary Prevention of 3500 patients with an ICD and cancer showed no significant difference in mortality among those with and without cancer and implantation of a primary preventions ICD (4-year cumulative risk – 26.9% and 19.7%, respectively). In those patients with a secondary prevention ICD, there was significantly higher mortality in patients with cancer (4-year cumulative risk – 43.5% for patients with cancer and 18.1% for patients with non-cancer). Nevertheless, 2/3 of these patients were alive at 3-year follow-up and almost 60% received life-saving appropriate therapy from the device.[53] This emphasizes the need to develop a patient-oriented shared decision-making approach specifically for patients with cancer.

In patients with a wide QRS interval, the landmark MADIT-CHIC trial in 2019 provides evidence of the benefit of cardiac resynchronization therapy (CRT) in patients with chemotherapy-induced cardiomyopathy. This prospective study enrolled 30 patients with chemotherapy-induced cardiomyopathy (73% with breast cancer, most patients with anthracyclines exposure) from 12 different medical centers demonstrating improvement in LVEF of an average of 10.6% (95% confidence interval (CI): 8.0%–13.3%) with a concomitant reduction in LVESV and LVEDV and improvement of heart failure symptoms in 83% of patients assessed by New York Heart Association class.[54] Although this study was limited by its small sample size and lack of a control group, it represents an important first step in studying the specific impact of implantable devices in chemotherapy-induced cardiomyopathy.

BRADYARRHYTHMIAS AND AUTONOMIC DYSFUNCTION

Bradyarrhythmias due to cancer therapeutics are uncommon and rarely require intervention though symptomatic bradycardia and advanced atrioventricular block have been reported.[24] Paclitaxel is associated with reversible asymptomatic sinus bradycardia in up to 30% of patients, likely due to off-target effects on the histamine receptor.[55] In contrast, sinus bradycardia has been reported in up to 40% of patients treated with thalidomide with some requiring pacemaker implantation; however, this has not been demonstrated with other immunomodulatory drugs (IMiDs) such as lenalidomide.[56] While initial reports suggested elevated rates of symptomatic bradycardia with 5-fluorouracil (5-FU), a systematic review demonstrated a low incidence of clinically significant bradycardia.[50,57]

Targeted and immunotherapies can also cause bradycardia. The anaplastic lymphoma kinase (ALK) inhibitors, crizotinib, and ceritinib, which are used to treat nonsmall cell lung cancer, are well known to cause sinus bradycardia; episodes are generally asymptomatic and do not require intervention.[58] Ibrutinib can also lead to bradyarrhythmias—one large analysis reported a 2.3%

occurrence of conduction defects, 42% of which were high grade or complete atrioventricular block, with an 18% fatality rate.[48] High-degree atrioventricular block can be the first manifestation of ICI-related myocarditis with an analysis of adverse drug event data from the World Health Organization reporting a 0.12% risk of conduction abnormalities with immune checkpoint inhibitor.[59] While definitive prevention strategies have not been established, patients taking AV nodal blocking drugs may need closer monitoring and potentially dose reduction. In general, an alternative to nondihydropyridine calcium channel blockers should be considered due to the frequency of drug-drug interactions.

AUTONOMIC DYSFUNCTION IN CANCER

Autonomic dysfunction (AD) or dysregulation of the parasympathetic (PNS) and sympathetic nervous systems (SNS) is manifested by elevated heart rates/inappropriate sinus tachycardia, decreased heart rate variability or heart rate recovery after exercise and exaggerated blood pressure responses/orthostasis and is more prevalent in patients with cancer and cancer survivors compared with healthy controls.[60,61] Multiple aspects of cancer treatment contribute to AD: cancer therapy, psychological stress, sleep disturbances, weight gain, and loss of cardiometabolic fitness.[62] Anthracyclines, taxanes, vinca-alkaloids, platinum-based agents, head and neck irradiation, chest and mantle radiation and stem cell transplantation have all been associated with AD.[63] The presence of abnormal heart rate recovery was associated with increased mortality in survivors of Hodgkin lymphoma treated with mediastinal radiation.[64] Similarly, in survivors of bone marrow transplantation, decreased heart rate variability was associated with decreased functional capacity and increased mortality.[65] Management of AD requires a nuanced approach with increasing attention paid to exercise training and physical therapy to improve outcomes.[66]

SUMMARY

Arrhythmias are a common but often underappreciated toxicity of cancer therapies ranging from traditional cytotoxic chemotherapy to target and immunotherapies. While AF and other atrial arrhythmias are the most commonly encountered rhythm disturbances, both ventricular and bradyarrhythmias are important complications with the potential for adverse outcomes. There is a clear need for rigorous studies to better define the scope of the problem and understand the mechanism of arrhythmogenesis to tailor treatment to this unique population. Regardless of the type of arrhythmia, a collaborative and nuanced approach tailored to patients with cancer must be established so as to minimize arrhythmic risk while ensuring the continued delivery of optimal cancer therapy.

CLINICS CARE POINTS

- Atrial fibrillation (AF) is a common cardiovascular toxicity associated with BTK inhibitors, immunotherapy, and stem cell transplantation.
- When treating patients with AF and other arrhythmias, be mindful of interactions with cytochrome P450 3A4 and 2D6 system as well as p-glycoprotein
- Focus on fixing nononcologic contributors to QT prolongation (like electrolyte abnormalities and the use of concomitant QT-prolonging drugs) before altering cancer treatments.
- Implantable cardiac devices, particularly cardiac resynchronization therapy (CRT) can be effective in treating patients with cancer treatment associated cardiac dysfunction
- Bradyarrhythmias due to cancer therapeutics rarely require treatment or intervention

FINANCIAL DISCLOSURES

M.G. Fradley – Consulting/Advisory Board: AstraZeneca, Abbott, Myovant, Takeda; Research Grant: Medtronic. The remaining authors have nothing to disclose.

REFERENCES

1. Hu YF, Liu CJ, Chang PM, et al. Incident thromboembolism and heart failure associated with new-onset atrial fibrillation in cancer patients. Int J Cardiol 2013;165:355–7.
2. Farmakis D, Parissis J, Filippatos G. Insights into onco-cardiology: atrial fibrillation in cancer. J Am Coll Cardiol 2014;63:945–53.
3. Kilickap S, Barista I, Akgul E, et al. Early and late arrhythmogenic effects of doxorubicin. South Med J 2007;100:262–5.
4. Fradley MG, Viganego F, Kip K, et al. Rates and risk of arrhythmias in cancer survivors with chemotherapy-induced cardiomyopathy compared with patients with other cardiomyopathies. Open Heart 2017;4:e000701.
5. Shah N, Rochlani Y, Pothineni NV, et al. Burden of arrhythmias in patients with multiple myeloma. Int J Cardiol 2016;203:305–6.
6. Sureddi RK, Amani F, Hebbar P, et al. Atrial fibrillation following autologous stem cell transplantation in patients with multiple myeloma: incidence and risk factors. Ther Adv Cardiovasc Dis 2012;6: 229–36.
7. Chang EK, Chanson D, Teh JB, et al. Atrial Fibrillation in Patients Undergoing Allogeneic Hematopoietic Cell Transplantation. J Clin Oncol 2021;39: 902–10.
8. Tonorezos ES, Stillwell EE, Calloway JJ, et al. Arrhythmias in the setting of hematopoietic cell transplants. Bone Marrow Transpl 2015;50:1212–6.
9. Chitturi KR, Xu J, Araujo-Gutierrez R, et al. Immune Checkpoint Inhibitor-Related Adverse Cardiovascular Events in Patients With Lung Cancer. JACC: CardioOncology 2019;1:182–92.
10. Power JR, Alexandre J, Choudhary A, et al. Electrocardiographic Manifestations of Immune Checkpoint Inhibitor Myocarditis. Circulation 2021;144:1521–3.
11. Lefebvre B, Kang Y, Smith AM, et al. Cardiovascular Effects of CAR T Cell Therapy: A Retrospective Study. J Am Coll Cardiol Cardioonc 2020;2:193–203.
12. Alvi RM, Frigault MJ, Fradley MG, et al. Cardiovascular Events Among Adults Treated With Chimeric Antigen Receptor T-Cells (CAR-T). J Am Coll Cardiol 2019;74:3099–108.
13. Fradley MG, Moslehi J. QT Prolongation and Oncology Drug Development. Card Electrophysiol Clin 2015;7:341–55.
14. Mego M, Reckova M, Obertova J, et al. Increased cardiotoxicity of sorafenib in sunitinib-pretreated patients with metastatic renal cell carcinoma. Ann Oncol 2007;18:1906–7.
15. Lipton JH, Chuah C, Guerci-Bresler A, et al. Ponatinib versus imatinib for newly diagnosed chronic myeloid leukaemia: an international, randomised, open-label, phase 3 trial. Lancet Oncol 2016;17: 612–21.
16. Fradley MG, Gliksman M, Emole J, et al. Rates and Risk of Atrial Arrhythmias in Patients Treated With Ibrutinib Compared With Cytotoxic Chemotherapy. Am J Cardiol 2019;124:539–44.
17. Yun S, Vincelette ND, Acharya U, et al. Risk of Atrial Fibrillation and Bleeding Diathesis Associated With Ibrutinib Treatment: A Systematic Review and Pooled Analysis of Four Randomized Controlled Trials. Clin Lymphoma Myeloma Leuk 2017;17:31–37 e13.
18. Caldeira D, Alves D, Costa J, et al. Ibrutinib increases the risk of hypertension and atrial fibrillation: Systematic review and meta-analysis. PLoS One 2019;14:e0211228.
19. Xiao L, Salem JE, Clauss S, et al. Ibrutinib-Mediated Atrial Fibrillation Attributable to Inhibition of C-Terminal Src Kinase. Circulation 2020;142:2443–55.

20. Byrd JC, Hillmen P, Ghia P, et al. Acalabrutinib Versus Ibrutinib in Previously Treated Chronic Lymphocytic Leukemia: Results of the First Randomized Phase III Trial. J Clin Oncol 2021;JCO2101210.

21. Wyse DG, Waldo AL, DiMarco JP, et al. A comparison of rate control and rhythm control in patients with atrial fibrillation. N Engl J Med 2002; 347:1825–33.

22. Kirchhof P, Camm AJ, Goette A, et al. Early Rhythm-Control Therapy in Patients with Atrial Fibrillation. N Engl J Med 2020 Oct 1;383(14).

23. Ganatra S, Sharma A, Shah S, et al. Ibrutinib-Associated Atrial Fibrillation. JACC Clin Electrophysiol 2018;4:1491–500.

24. Fradley MG, Beckie TM, Brown SA, et al. Recognition, Prevention, and Management of Arrhythmias and Autonomic Disorders in Cardio-Oncology: A Scientific Statement From the American Heart Association. Circulation 2021;144:e41–55.

25. Yamreudeewong W, DeBisschop M, Martin LG, et al. Potentially significant drug interactions of class III antiarrhythmic drugs. Drug Saf 2003;26:421–38.

26. Santangeli P, Di Biase L, Burkhardt JD, et al. Examining the safety of amiodarone. Expert Opin Drug Saf 2012;11:191–214.

27. Marrouche NF, Brachmann J, Andresen D, et al. Catheter Ablation for Atrial Fibrillation with Heart Failure. N Engl J Med 2018;378:417–27.

28. Rillig A, Magnussen C, Ozga AK, et al. Early Rhythm Control Therapy in Patients With Atrial Fibrillation and Heart Failure. Circulation 2021;144:845–58.

29. January CT, Wann LS, Calkins H, et al. AHA/ACC/HRS Focused Update of the 2014 AHA/ACC/HRS Guideline for the Management of Patients With Atrial Fibrillation: A Report of the American College of Cardiology/American Heart Association Task Force on Clinical Practice Guidelines and the Heart Rhythm Society. J Am Coll Cardiol 2019;74:104–32.

30. Giustozzi M, Ali H, Reboldi G, et al. Safety of catheter ablation of atrial fibrillation in cancer survivors. J Interv Card Electrophysiol 2021 Apr;60(3):419–26.

31. Deitelzweig S, Keshishian AV, Zhang Y, et al. Effectiveness and Safety of Oral Anticoagulants Among Nonvalvular Atrial Fibrillation Patients With Active Cancer. JACC CardioOncol 2021;3:411–24.

32. Fradley MG, Ellenberg K, Alomar M, et al. Patterns of Anticoagulation Use in Patients With Cancer With Atrial Fibrillation and/or Atrial Flutter. JACC CardinoOncol 2020;2:747–54.

33. D'Souza M, Carlson N, Fosbol E, et al. CHA2DS2-VASc score and risk of thromboembolism and bleeding in patients with atrial fibrillation and recent cancer. Eur J Prev Cardiol 2018;25:651–8.

34. Isogai T, Saad AM, Abushouk AI, et al. Procedural and Short-Term Outcomes of Percutaneous Left Atrial Appendage Closure in Patients With Cancer. Am J Cardiol 2021;141:154–7.

35. Holmes DR, Reddy VY, Buchbinder M, et al. The Assessment of the Watchman Device in Patients Unsuitable for Oral Anticoagulation (ASAP-TOO) trial. Am Heart J 2017;189:68–74.

36. Simard T, Jung RG, Lehenbauer K, et al. Predictors of Device-Related Thrombus Following Percutaneous Left Atrial Appendage Occlusion. J Am Coll Cardiol 2021;78:297–313.

37. Adelsberger H, Quasthoff S, Grosskreutz J, et al. The chemotherapeutic oxaliplatin alters voltage-gated Na(+) channel kinetics on rat sensory neurons. Eur J Pharmacol 2000;406:25–32.

38. Drolet B, Simard C, Roden DM. Unusual effects of a QT-prolonging drug, arsenic trioxide, on cardiac potassium currents. Circulation 2004;109:26–9.

39. Roboz GJ, Ritchie EK, Carlin RF, et al. Prevalence, management, and clinical consequences of QT interval prolongation during treatment with arsenic trioxide. J Clin Oncol 2014;32:3723–8.

40. Abu Rmilah AA, Lin G, Begna KH, et al. Risk of QTc prolongation among cancer patients treated with tyrosine kinase inhibitors. Int J Cancer 2020 Dec 1; 147(11):3160–7.

41. Porta-Sanchez A, Gilbert C, Spears D, et al. Incidence, Diagnosis, and Management of QT Prolongation Induced by Cancer Therapies: A Systematic Review. J Am Heart Assoc 2017;6.

42. Hortobagyi GN, Stemmer SM, Burris HA, et al. Updated results from MONALEESA-2, a phase III trial of first-line ribociclib plus letrozole versus placebo plus letrozole in hormone receptor-positive, HER2-negative advanced breast cancer. Ann Oncol 2018;29:1541–7.

43. Barber M, Nguyen LS, Wassermann J, et al. Cardiac arrhythmia considerations of hormone cancer therapies. Cardiovasc Res 2019;115:878–94.

44. Kim PY, Irizarry-Caro JA, Ramesh T, et al. How to Diagnose and Manage QT Prolongation in Cancer Patients. JACC CardioOncol 2021;3:145–9.

45. Badri M, Patel A, Patel C, et al. Mexiletine Prevents Recurrent Torsades de Pointes in Acquired Long QT Syndrome Refractory to Conventional Measures. JACC Clin Electrophysiol 2015;1:315–22.

46. Enriquez A, Biagi J, Redfearn D, et al. Increased Incidence of Ventricular Arrhythmias in Patients With Advanced Cancer and Implantable Cardioverter-Defibrillators. JACC Clin Electrophysiol 2017;3:50–6.

47. Guha A, Derbala MH, Zhao Q, et al. Ventricular Arrhythmias Following Ibrutinib Initiation for Lymphoid Malignancies. J Am Coll Cardiol 2018;72:697–8.

48. Salem J-E, Manouchehri A, Bretagne M, et al. Cardiovascular Toxicities Associated With Ibrutinib. J Am Coll Cardiol 2019;74:1667–78.

49. Salem JE, Nguyen LS, Moslehi JJ, et al. Anticancer drug-induced life-threatening ventricular arrhythmias: a World Health Organization pharmacovigilance study. Eur Heart J 2021;42:3915–28.

50. Polk A, Vaage-Nilsen M, Vistisen K, et al. Cardiotoxicity in cancer patients treated with 5-fluorouracil or capecitabine: A systematic review of incidence, manifestations and predisposing factors. Cancer Treat Rev 2013;39:974–84.

51. Yilmaz U, Oztop I, Ciloglu A, et al. 5-fluorouracil increases the number and complexity of premature complexes in the heart: a prospective study using ambulatory ECG monitoring. Int J Clin Pract 2007; 61:795–801.

52. Mahmood SS, Fradley MG, Cohen JV, et al. Myocarditis in Patients Treated With Immune Checkpoint Inhibitors. J Am Coll Cardiol 2018;71:1755–64.

53. Christensen AM, Bjerre J, Schou M, et al. Clinical outcome in patients with implantable cardioverter-defibrillator and cancer: a nationwide study. Europace 2019;21:465–74.

54. Singh JP, Solomon SD, Fradley MG, et al. Association of Cardiac Resynchronization Therapy With Change in Left Ventricular Ejection Fraction in Patients With Chemotherapy-Induced Cardiomyopathy. JAMA 2019;322:1799–805.

55. Arbuck SG, Strauss H, Rowinsky E, et al. A reassessment of cardiac toxicity associated with Taxol. J Natl Cancer Inst Monogr 1993;117–30.

56. Minoia C, Giannoccaro M, Iacobazzi A, et al. Antineoplastic drug-induced bradyarrhythmias. Expert Opin Drug Saf 2012;11:739–51.

57. Khan MA, Masood N, Husain N, et al. A retrospective study of cardiotoxicities induced by 5-fluouracil (5-FU) and 5-FU based chemotherapy regimens in Pakistani adult cancer patients at Shaukat Khanum Memorial Cancer Hospital & Research Center. J Pakistan Med Assoc 2012;62: 430–4.

58. Ou SH, Tang Y, Polli A, et al. Factors associated with sinus bradycardia during crizotinib treatment: a retrospective analysis of two large-scale multinational trials (PROFILE 1005 and 1007). Cancer Med 2016;5:617–22.

59. Salem JE, Manouchehri A, Moey M, et al. Cardiovascular toxicities associated with immune checkpoint inhibitors: an observational, retrospective, pharmacovigilance study. Lancet Oncol 2018;19:1579–89.

60. Martin R, Delgado JM, Molto JM, et al. Cardiovascular reflexes in patients with malignant disease. Ital J Neurol Sci 1992;13:125–9.

61. Noor B, Akhavan S, Leuchter M, et al. Quantitative assessment of cardiovascular autonomic impairment in cancer survivors: a single center case series. Cardiooncology 2020;6:11.

62. Lakoski SG, Jones LW, Krone RJ, et al. Autonomic dysfunction in early breast cancer: Incidence, clinical importance, and underlying mechanisms. Am Heart J 2015;170:231–41.

63. Coumbe BGT, Groarke JD. Cardiovascular Autonomic Dysfunction in Patients with Cancer. Curr Cardiol Rep 2018;20:69.

64. Groarke JD, Tanguturi VK, Hainer J, et al. Abnormal exercise response in long-term survivors of hodgkin lymphoma treated with thoracic irradiation: evidence of cardiac autonomic dysfunction and impact on outcomes. J Am Coll Cardiol 2015;65:573–83.

65. Deuring G, Kiss A, Halter JP, et al. Cardiac autonomic functioning is impaired among allogeneic hematopoietic stem cell transplantation survivors: a controlled study. Bone Marrow Transpl 2017;52: 66–72.

66. Gilchrist SC, Barac A, Ades PA, et al. Cardio-Oncology Rehabilitation to Manage Cardiovascular Outcomes in Cancer Patients and Survivors: A Scientific Statement From the American Heart Association. Circulation 2019;139:e997–1012.

Cardioprotection of High-Risk Individuals

Jenica N. Upshaw, MD, MS*, Sharanya Mohanty, MD, Akash Rastogi, BA

KEYWORDS

- Cardio-oncology • Heart failure • Chemotherapy • Anthracyclines • Radiation
- Cardiovascular disease

KEY POINTS

- Comorbid cardiovascular disease or cardiac risk factors are associated with an increased risk of cardiovascular events during cancer treatment
- The risk for heart failure, atherosclerotic cardiovascular events, myocarditis, hypertension, and arrhythmias varies based on the specific cancer therapy(ies) and comorbid cardiovascular disease.
- Prevalent cardiovascular disease should be managed according to standard cardiovascular guidelines.
- Modest evidence exists for cardioprotective strategies for anthracycline and trastuzumab treated patients at the highest risk for heart failure.
- Further research is needed to explore cardioprotective strategies for other cancer therapies.

INTRODUCTION

Advances in screening and treatment have improved survival for patients with many types of cancer[1]; however, cardiovascular (CV) disease is a major cause of long-term non–cancer-related morbidity and mortality that threatens to limit gains in life expectancy made over the past decades.[2,3] In the general population, CV disease is the leading cause of death in both women and men.[4] Cancer survivors face even higher rates of CV disease compared with age-matched controls without cancer.[2,5,6] This review describes the evidence for CV risk stratification and cardioprotective strategies in a range of cancer types and treatments.

RISK STRATIFICATION

Targeting cardioprotective strategies to patients at the highest risk for cardiac events can help to maximize the benefits of these therapies. Risk stratification can be accomplished in several complementary ways including considerations of (1) specific cancer therapies, (2) preexisting CV disease, (3) CV imaging or biomarkers, and (4) multivariable clinical prediction models (**Fig. 1**).

Risk Stratification by Cancer Therapy

One of the most common applications of risk stratification is the recognition of specific chemotherapy agents or regimens that are associated with greater risk of CV events. For anthracyclines, this is accomplished in 2 main ways—(1) cumulative lifetime dose and (2) combination cardiotoxic exposures such as anthracyclines in combination with chest radiation, anti–human-epidermal growth factor receptor-2 (HER2) therapy, or anti-vascular endothelial growth factor (VEGF) therapy. Multiple studies have demonstrated the association between lifetime cumulative dose of anthracyclines and increased risk of cardiomyopathy or congestive heart failure. The risk of cardiomyopathy and heart failure increases exponentially with

Funding: This study is supported in part by National Institutes of Health grant K08HL146959 (Dr. Upshaw)
Division of Cardiology, Tufts Medical Center, 800 Washington St, Boston, MA 02111, USA
* Corresponding author. 800 Washington Street, Box 5931, Boston, MA 02111.
E-mail address: jupshaw@tuftsmedicalcenter.org

heartfailure.theclinics.com

Risk Stratification

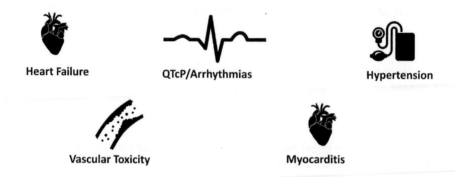

Specific Cancer Agent | Cardiac Risk Factors including Age | Comorbid CV disease | Biomarkers and Imaging | Prediction Model if Available

Heart Failure   **QTcP/Arrhythmias**   **Hypertension**

Vascular Toxicity   **Myocarditis**

❖ Management of Cardiac Comorbidities According to Standard Guidelines
❖ Cardioprotective Medications for High risk Individuals
❖ Monitoring
❖ Referral to Cardiology/CardioOncology

Fig. 1. CV risk stratification for patients with cancer should factor in the specific CV risks associated with the cancer therapy, the patient's cardiac risk factors, and any prevalent CV disease. In some cases, biomarkers, imaging, and prediction models may be of benefit. Existing CV disease should be managed according to standard guidelines. In those with prevalent CV disease or very high risk owing to cancer therapy, cardioprotective strategies, monitoring, and referral to cardiology or cardio-oncology should be considered.

cumulative anthracycline dose.[7,8] In a pooled analysis in the metastatic cancer setting, reductions in left ventricular ejection fraction (LVEF) to less than normal or clinical heart failure occurred in 6%, 14%, 33%, 59%, and 76% of patients at a cumulative doxorubicin dose of 250, 300, 400, 500, and 600 mg/m, respectively.[7] Even at lower cumulative doses of doxorubicin of 240 mg/m^2, commonly used in breast cancer, cardiomyopathy can occur in 10% to 15% of patients and heart failure in more than 5%.[9,10] The combination of anthracycline therapy with chest radiation is associated with an increased risk of heart failure, even at low cumulative anthracycline doses.[11,12] Similarly, sequential treatment with anthracyclines followed by anti-HER2 therapy is associated with the higher risk of LVEF declines compared with anthracyclines only or anti-HER2 therapy without prior anthracycline therapy.[13,14] Finally, sequential anthracyclines followed by the anti-VEGF agent, bevacizumab, leads to higher rates of LVEF decreases compared with anthracyclines without anti-VEGF therapy.[15]

For radiation therapy (RT), higher dose estimates to the heart and cardiac substructures are associated with a higher risk for ischemic heart disease and heart failure in a range of patient populations, cancer types, and radiation doses.[16–19] As discussed elsewhere in this article,

anthracyclines and chest radiation have synergistic effects on CV toxicity. Vascular toxicity with the BCR-Abl kinase inhibitor, ponatinib, has been shown to be dose dependent.[20] The myocarditis risk is greater with 2 immune checkpoint inhibitors (ICIs) compared with one.[21] As the number of targeted therapies and immunotherapies continue to increase, it will be important to understand the specific CV risks, such as heart failure, myocardial infarction, hypertension, and arrhythmias, seen with new therapies and any synergistic effects when cancer therapies are used in combination.

Risk Stratification by Prevalent Cardiovascular Disease or Cardiac Risk Factors

Individuals with CV risk factors or preexisting coronary artery disease, valvular heart disease or cardiomyopathy have been shown to be at increased risk for heart failure with anthracyclines and anti-HER2 therapy.[22–27] In addition, traditional cardiac risk factors such as hypertension, diabetes, tobacco use, hyperlipidemia, obesity, and advancing age have been associated with an increased risk of cardiotoxicity with anthracyclines, trastuzumab, or radiation.[5,10,22–28] In childhood cancer survivors treated with anthracyclines or chest radiation, the interval development of cardiac risk factors, particularly hypertension, is associated with an increased risk of subsequent cardiac events, including coronary artery disease and heart failure.[29] Similarly, cardiac risk factors, particularly hypertension and diabetes, are associated with an increased risk for heart failure and atherosclerotic CV events in those undergoing hematopoietic cell transplantation.[30–32] In older individuals with colorectal cancer, a significant interaction between the presence of hypertension and chemotherapy was seen for an increased risk of atherosclerotic CV events and a significant interaction between diabetes and chemotherapy for heart failure.[33]

Risk Stratification Using Biomarkers and Imaging

Serum biomarkers

Troponin (Tn) assays have been applied during and after anthracycline treatment for risk stratification and the early detection of cardiotoxicity. The largest study to date showed that a Tn inhibitor threshold of 0.08 ng/mL was predictive of subsequent cardiac events, defined as CV death, heart failure, life-threatening arrhythmia, or an asymptomatic LVEF decrease of 25% or more in a population treated with high-dose chemotherapy with autologous stem cell rescue.[34] Several smaller studies have also shown a correlation between early elevations in serum Tn and LVEF changes or cardiac events in cohorts of adults treated with the current standard of care anthracycline regimens for breast cancer and hematologic malignancies, although with variable predictive performance.[35–39] Tn has also been shown to be predictive of cardiotoxicity in pediatric populations treated with anthracyclines.[40–42] In a single-center study of 111 patients treated with anthracyclines, both baseline brain natriuretic peptide and post-treatment brain natriuretic peptide were significantly higher in patients who developed a cardiac event (defined as significant asymptomatic LVEF decreases, symptomatic heart failure, significant arrhythmia, sudden death, or acute coronary syndrome).[43] Although a moderate level of evidence suggests that cardiac Tn and natriuretic peptides can help with risk stratification and the early identification of anthracycline cardiotoxicity, further research is needed to understand the predictive performance of these biomarkers for the detection of cardiotoxicity during nonanthracycline regimens and to understand whether routine monitoring improves outcomes when used during modern-day cancer treatment regimens.

Global longitudinal strain

Global longitudinal strain (GLS) using echocardiographic speckle tracking has emerged as a sensitive early marker of anthracycline-induced cardiotoxicity.[9,35,44] Multiple studies have suggested that relative GLS decrements between 10% and 15% or absolute changes of 2% to 3% have good sensitivity and specificity for the prediction of subsequent decreases in LVEF.[44] Importantly, significant changes in GLS can be detected when the LVEF remains preserved, but predict subsequent reductions in LVEF at 6 to 12 months after the completion of chemotherapy.[44] The SUCCOUR trial compared GLS-guided cardioprotective medication use with LVEF-guided cardioprotective medication use strategy in a randomized trial of 330 anthracycline-treated participants (91% breast cancer, 9% lymphoma, 80% sequential anthracycline and trastuzumab).[45] Although there was no difference between the 2 groups in the primary end point of change in the LVEF from baseline to 1 year, there were more individuals started on cardioprotective therapies in the GLS arm and fewer individuals had an LVEF reduction of more than 10% to less than 55%. Given the negative primary end point, longer term monitoring of this population and/or future studies are needed before the widespread implementation of routine cardioprotection based on decrement in GLS alone, although this strategy is promising for early detection and intervention.

Risk Stratification Using Clinical Prediction Models

Prediction models use multiple variables in combination to estimate an individual patient's absolute risk for a given event. Using data from the Childhood Cancer Survivor Study, separate prediction models for (1) heart failure or (2) the composite of ischemic heart disease or stroke have been developed and validated externally with an online calculator available for personalized risk estimates for heart failure and stroke risk up to the age of 50.[12,46] There are 2 prediction models for trastuzumab associated cardiotoxicity in HER2–positive breast cancer and 1 model for anthracycline cardiotoxicity in HER2–negative breast cancer, although none of these models have been validated in external populations and are thus are not used routinely in clinical practice.[22,23,47] A prediction model for the composite of hospitalization for acute myocardial infarction, unstable angina, transient ischemic attack, stroke, peripheral vascular disease, heart failure, or CV death was derived in a large population-based cohort of early breast cancer cohort.[48] This model includes age, hypertension, diabetes, ischemic heart disease, atrial fibrillation, heart failure, cerebrovascular disease, peripheral vascular disease, chronic obstructive pulmonary disease, and chronic renal failure with excellent discrimination in the development and split-sample internal validation cohort, but has not yet been validated in an external population.

CARDIOPROTECTIVE STRATEGIES OF ANTHRACYCLINES
Anthracycline Cardiotoxicity

Anthracycline chemotherapeutic agents can cause heart failure owing to cardiac and vascular oxidative and nitrosative stress, mitochondrial dysfunction, and apoptosis.[14,49,50] Several cardioprotective strategies have emerged, including (1) using a nonanthracycline regimen if noninferior for cancer treatment, (2) administration of cardioprotective agents such as dexrazoxane or neurohormonal antagonist therapy, and (3) a continuous infusion or liposomal formulation of anthracyclines to decrease the anthracycline dose to the heart.

Dexrazoxane

Dexrazoxane remains the only US Food and Drug Association (FDA)-approved therapy for the prevention of anthracycline cardiotoxicity.[51] Dexrazoxane inhibits DNA topoisomerase IIb-anthracycline-mediated double-stranded DNA breaks and decreases oxygen free radical formation in cardiomyocytes. Dexrazoxane was approved initially by the US FDA in 1995 for patients with metastatic breast cancer who have already received more than 300 mg/m^2 of doxorubicin and who would benefit from ongoing doxorubicin therapy.[51–53] Although there were initial concerns about the loss of oncologic efficacy or an increased risk of secondary malignancies in children and adolescents treated with dexrazoxane,[54] more recent studies have demonstrated less echocardiographic evidence of cardiotoxicity with no difference in cancer recurrence, early mortality, or secondary malignancies with dexrazoxane in the pediatric and adolescent/young adult populations.[55–58] A recent meta-analysis of randomized and observational studies in breast cancer showed significant decreases in the risk of heart failure or cardiac events with no significant difference in oncologic outcomes.[59] In adults with advanced soft tissue sarcomas, the combination of doxorubicin with dexrazoxane allowed patients to receive high doses of doxorubicin (up to 600 mg/m^2) with a relatively low incidence of cardiac adverse events.[60] Further research is needed to understand the efficacy of dexrazoxane in other populations (eg, older patients with multiple cardiac risk factors who require anthracyclines) and

to understand the effect of dexrazoxane on long-term clinical CV events in the pediatric and adolescent and young adult populations.[51,61]

Liposomal Anthracycline Formulations

Liposomal anthracycline formulations decrease drug delivery to tissues with tight capillary junctions, including the heart. Pegylated liposomal doxorubicin (Doxil/CAELYX) was the first liposomal formulation to be FDA approved in 1995 after studies showed benefit in ovarian cancer and AIDS-related Kaposi sarcoma, and an indication for multiple myeloma was subsequently added.[62] A nonpegylated liposomal formulation of doxorubicin (Myocet) has been compared with conventional doxorubicin in several randomized trials in metastatic breast cancer, demonstrating decrease cardiac toxicity and a similar efficacy.[63,64] Myocet is currently approved by the European Medicines Agency, but not the FDA, for use in metastatic breast cancer.[65] A phase III trial demonstrated that nonpegylated liposomal doxorubicin had an improved median time to treatment failure, disease progression, and survival time when compared with epirubicin, with similar low rates of cardiotoxicity in the 2 arms.[66] Several small studies have used liposomal doxorubicin in place of conventional doxorubicin in patients with hematologic malignancies at high risk of heart failure owing to advanced age or established CV disease.[67,68] A phase II, single-arm study of nonpegylated liposomal doxorubicin in place of conventional doxorubicin in combination with bleomycin, vinblastine, and dacarbazine in 47 untreated patients with Hodgkin lymphoma older than 69 years of age or 18 to 69 years of age with cardiac disease suggested low cardiotoxicity with this regimen.[67] A phase III trial, which was powered for LVEF changes, randomized 88 individuals with diffuse large B-cell lymphoma to conventional rituximab, cyclophosphamide, doxorubicin, vincristine, and prednisolone (R-CHOP) or the same regimen with liposomal doxorubicin instead of conventional doxorubicin, finding no difference in LVEF, but less of an increase in the natriuretic peptides with liposomal doxorubicin.[68] The GRAALL-SA1 trial compared pegylated liposomal doxorubicin (Doxil) to continuous infusion doxorubicin in combination with vincristine and cyclophosphamide in older individuals with acute lymphoblastic leukemia and a normal LVEF at baseline, finding less toxicity including a trend toward fewer cardiac events, but with no difference in overall survival and a trend toward higher rates of relapse with liposomal doxorubicin compared with continuous infusion doxorubicin.[69] Although further research is needed to guide treatment decisions for individuals at high risk for anthracycline cardiotoxicity, liposomal doxorubicin could be considered in patients at very high risk for heart failure with conventional doxorubicin because of advanced age, cardiac comorbidity, or prior anthracycline treatment.[70,71] Of note, these studies excluded individuals with a low LVEF at baseline or a history of cardiomyopathy or heart failure and these patients would be expected to have the greatest risk from anthracycline therapy and thus potentially the most benefit from cardioprotective strategies if anthrayclines are used.

Continuous Anthracycline Infusion Instead of Bolus Dosing

A continuous anthracycline infusion seeks to decrease the peak plasma levels without decreasing the overall dose administered. In older studies of adults with advanced breast cancer or sarcoma receiving high cumulative anthracycline doses, continuous doxorubicin infusion over 6 to 72 hours compared with bolus dosing over 15 to 20 minutes was associated with attenuated LVEF decreases.[72,73] Whether a continuous infusion is cardioprotective in adults with established heart disease or multiple heart failure risk factors receiving lower cumulative doses of anthracyclines is not known, but is one strategy that can be considered for adults at high risk for heart failure with anthracyclines.[71] As mentioned elsewhere in this article, the GRAALL-SA1 study compared liposomal doxorubicin with continuous infusion doxorubicin with trends toward less toxicity with liposomal doxorubicin but less treatment efficacy compared with continuous infusion doxorubicin in the treatment of older adults with acute lymphocytic leukemia (cardiac and oncologic differences were not statistically significant). Although there is some evidence for continuous infusion doxorubicin to decrease cardiotoxicity in adults, randomized trials of continuous doxorubicin infusion in the pediatric population have not demonstrated cardioprotection compared with bolus dosing.[74,75] A randomized trial of 102 children being treated for acute lymphocytic leukemia showed that continuous infusion led to no changes in long-term cardioprotection or acute lymphocytic leukemia event-free survival.[75]

Neurohormonal Antagonist Therapy and Other Heart Failure Guideline-Directed Medical Therapies

Angiotensin-converting enzyme inhibitors, angiotensin-receptor blockers (ARBs), and beta-blockers are highly effective treatments for cardiomyopathy with reduced LVEF with or without the syndrome of heart failure.[76] Additionally, angiotensin receptor neprilysin inhibitors in place of angiotensin-converting enzyme inhibitors/ARBs, aldosterone antagonists, and sodium-glucose cotransporter-2 inhibitors have demonstrated decreases in mortality in patients with established heart failure with a reduced LVEF and are the now standard of care for established heart failure with a reduced LVEF.[77] Several small studies have evaluated the effect of neurohormonal antagonist therapy started before anthracycline therapy on LVEF. The Prevention of Cardiac Dysfunction during Adjuvant Breast Cancer Therapy (PRADA) single-center study included 130 patients with early breast cancer with planned treatment with adjuvant epirubicin and showed a modest, but statistically significant, attenuation of LVEF decrease compared with placebo at the end of chemotherapy, although there was no difference in LVEF between the groups at 2 years after completion of therapy (with neurohormonal antagonist therapy stopped after completion of chemotherapy).[78,79] Carvedilol initiated before high doses of anthracycline therapy for breast cancer or lymphoma prevented decreases in the LVEF in a single-center study of 50 patients (LVEF of 69% vs LVEF of 52%; $P < .001$).[80] In the OVER-COME trial, a single-center open-label study of 90 patients with hematologic malignancies planned to receive high cumulative anthracycline exposure (80% receiving hematopoietic stem cell transplantation [HSCT]), lisinopril and carvedilol started before anthracycline chemotherapy was associated with a modestly higher LVEF at 6 months compared with control (mean between group difference in LVEF of 3.1%; 95% confidence interval [CI], 0.11–6.1) and a lower incidence of the composite of death or heart failure (6.7% vs 22%; $P = .036$).[81] The single-center CECCY trial randomized 200 patients with HER2–negative breast cancer with planned anthracycline treatment (240 mg/m^2 doxorubicin) 1:1 to carvedilol or placebo with no difference in LVEF at 6 months (primary end point), but with attenuated cardiac Tn elevations and less diastolic dysfunction (secondary end points).[82] A large primary prevention trial in trastuzumab treated participants suggested benefit to carvedilol or lisinopril in the subgroup who received prior anthracyclines (average mean decrease in the LVEF: carvedilol −4.5% ± 0.8; lisinopril −4.0% ± 0.8; placebo −7.7% ± 0.8), with no signal for benefit in the non–anthracycline-treated patients.[83] A recent interim analysis of the SAFE trial found that the ramipril, bisoprolol, and the combination of ramipril and bisoprolol was associated with a higher LVEF and an improved GLS compared with placebo in 174 patients with early breast cancer treated with anthracyclines, but the overall effect sizes were modest and the full report of all 262 randomized individuals is not yet available.[84] A meta-analysis of randomized trials of angiotensin-converting enzyme inhibitors/ARBs or beta-blockers suggested a higher LVEF with cardioprotection with either agent among patients with breast cancer receiving anthracyclines or trastuzumab, although significant heterogeneity among studies was present and the absolute effect sizes were small.[85]

In summary, primary prevention studies using neurohormonal antagonist therapy have shown only modest benefits, especially in populations without multiple cardiac risk factors treated with lower cumulative anthracycline doses. Given the very modest benefits and conflicting results, the routine use of neurohormonal antagonist therapy in all patients is not considered standard of care and is not recommended routinely. A strategy of targeting these medications to those at highest risk, defined either by cumulative anthracycline dose, sequential anthracycline with trastuzumab, comorbid CV disease or multiple risk factors, imaging/biomarkers, or a combination of these, will likely provide greater absolute benefits than routine use in all patients. For example, OVERCOME enrolled individuals treated with high cumulative doses of anthracyclines[81] and Cardinale and colleagues[86] enrolled individuals with an elevated Tn after high-dose chemotherapy. These studies showed a significant benefit of neurohormonal antagonist therapy not only in preventing LVEF decreases after treatment, but also in clinical events. In addition, patients with established CV disease should be treated according to standard guidelines, including neurohormonal antagonist therapy in those with established stage B to D heart failure with a reduced LVEF.[76,77] Ongoing studies are exploring the role of sacubitril-valsartan in the PRADA 2 trial (NCT03760588) and carvedilol in the pediatric population treated with anthracyclines (NCT02717507). As highlighted in a study by Sutton and colleagues,[87] it will be important to understand racial and gender disparities in cardioprotective medication use and cardiac outcomes and investigate strategies to reduce disparities in outcomes.

Statins

Statins decrease oxidative stress in addition to lowering cholesterol. Preclinical studies[88] and observational data[89] suggest that statin therapy may decrease the risk of cardiotoxicity with anthracycline chemotherapy, although the clinical studies published to date have been small.[90,91] To date, there is insufficient evidence to recommend the routine use of statins for the primary prevention of anthracycline cardiotoxicity; however, 2 randomized trials of atorvastatin versus placebo started before anthracycline treatment are ongoing.[92,93] The Preventing Anthracycline Cardiovascular Toxicity with Statins (PREVENT) trial has completed enrollment with 279 patients with breast cancer or lymphoma randomized to atorvastatin or placebo (NCT01988571). Another study, Statins to Prevent Cardiotoxicity from Anthracyclines (STOP-CA) is randomizing 270 participants with lymphoma to atorvastatin or placebo (NCT02943590).

Physical Activity and Other Lifestyle Factors

In the general population, there is a dose-dependent relationship between greater self-reported regular physical activity and a decreased risk of CV events and incident cancer.[94,95] In breast cancer cohort studies, higher self-reported physical activity before, during, or after cancer treatment has been associated with a decreased risk of breast cancer mortality,[96,97] total mortality,[96,97] and fewer CV events.[98,99] Randomized trials of exercise interventions during or after cancer therapy have shown improvements in cardiorespiratory fitness, as assessed by cardiopulmonary exercise testing.[100] Preclinical studies support the role of exercise in decreasing the risk of cardiomyopathy with doxorubicin and have elucidated several potential mechanisms, although clinical trials have been limited by small sample sizes and, thus, the role of exercise on preventing cardiomyopathy or clinical heart failure events remains uncertain.[101] Several ongoing studies are assessing whether exercise interventions at the time of doxorubicin treatment can mitigate the risk of cardiomyopathy and clinical heart failure events.[101] While we await additional studies, physical activity should be strongly encouraged in all survivors of cancer for the myriad of health benefits, including CV health, with at least 150 minutes per week of moderate or strenuous physical activity recommended by multiple organizations including the American Cancer Society,[102] American College of Cardiology/American Heart Association,[103] and the US Department of Health and Human Services.[104] Counseling and interventions to enable smoking cessation, physical activity, healthy diet, and maintenance of a healthy weight in addition to optimal control of hypertension, diabetes, and hyperlipidemia if present (as summarized by the

American Heart Association's Life's Simple 7) may improve CV health as well as decrease the risk of cancer recurrence or new cancers.[105]

CARDIOPROTECTIVE STRATEGIES WITH ANTI–HUMAN-EPIDERMAL GROWTH FACTOR RECEPTOR-2 THERAPY

HER2 comprises 1 of 4 epidermal growth factor receptors: HER1–4. These receptor tyrosine kinases are endogenous protooncogenes and promote cell proliferation and survival. HER2 is overexpressed in approximately 20% to 25% of breast cancers. Before the development of anti- HER2 therapy, HER2 expressions was associated with a worse prognosis. Trastuzumab is a humanized monoclonal antibody that functions to trigger HER2 internalization and promote HER2 degradation. Since the approval of trastuzumab in 1998, the prognosis of HER2+ breast cancer has significantly improved. Several large-scale clinical trials reported nearly a 33% decrease in overall mortality and a 50% decrease in the disease recurrence in those who received trastuzumab in addition to adjuvant chemotherapy regimen for treatment of early stage HER2+ breast cancer.[106]

Despite the unequivocal efficacy of trastuzumab in decreasing the morbidity and mortality associated with HER2+ breast cancers, clinical application is most limited by left ventricular (LV) dysfunction and heart failure. The HER2/ErbB2 signaling pathway is important for cardiomyocyte repair in response to anthracyclines and thus it is not surprising,in retrospect, that concomitant anthracycline and trastuzumab therapy was associated with New York Heart Association functional class III or IV (severe) heart failure in 16% of patients with metastatic breast cancer treated with the combination.[107] Fortunately, with strict criteria for withholding trastuzumab in participants with prior cardiac disease or with LVEF reductions after adjuvant chemotherapy and protocols for holding or discontinuing trastuzumab according to LVEF monitoring, heart failure occurs in only 1% to 4% and asymptomatic reductions in LVEF in 10% to 15% of participants in clinical trial populations.[24,108,109] Sequential treatment with anthracyclines followed by anti-HER2 therapy is associated with the higher risk of LVEF decreased compared with anthracyclines only or anti-HER2 therapy without prior anthracycline therapy.[13,14] Consistent with the hypothesis that HER2 signaling is important for cardiomyocyte response anthracyclines, a shorter the time interval between completion of anthracycline therapy and initiation of trastuzumab seems to be associated with higher incidence of LVEF decreases.[110]

The current management of trastuzumab-induced cardiotoxicity favors pausing trastuzumab therapy until there is a recovery of cardiac function versus discontinuing the drug altogether in those with a persistently low LVEF. However, such interruptions are associated with an increased risk of disease recurrence and worse outcomes.[111] Given the efficacy of trastuzumab in the management of HER2+ breast cancer, it is important to identify cardioprotective strategies that decrease the risk of cardiac dysfunction and define clinically meaningful improvements for management of cardiotoxicity.

Neurohormonal Antagonist Therapy

Several trials have evaluated the role of neurohormonal blockade with angiotensin-converting enzyme inhibitors, ARBs, or beta-blockers for the prevention of LVEF decreases in those receiving trastuzumab for treatment of HER2+ breast cancer. The Multidisciplinary Approach to Novel Therapies in Cardio-Oncology Research (MANTICORE 101-Breast) trial randomized 94 women with HER2+ breast cancer with planned adjuvant trastuzumab therapy (77% had received nonanthracycline chemotherapy regimen) to perindopril, bisoprolol, or placebo for the duration of their trastuzumab therapy. The primary outcome was change in LV end-diastolic volume index on cardiac magnetic resonance imaging, from baseline to completion of adjuvant anti-HER2 therapy. Although there was no difference in the primary end point among the 3 groups at the completion of trastuzumab treatment, there was a statistically significant difference in the secondary end point (a decrease in LVEF on cardiac magnetic resonance imaging) among the study groups (1% in bisoprolol group vs 3% in perindopril group vs 5% in placebo group; $P = .001$). Importantly, there were significantly fewer interruptions in trastuzumab therapy owing to the incidence of cardiac dysfunction among those who received treatment with perindopril (9% of angiotensin-converting enzyme inhibitor–treated patients) or bisoprolol (9% of patients) compared with those in the placebo group (30% of those in placebo group).

This clinically important finding of fewer interruptions in trastuzumab treatment was also seen in a randomized, double-blind, placebo-controlled trial of 468 patients with early stage HER2+ breast cancer randomized to lisinopril, carvedilol, or placebo.[83] There was no significant difference in the primary end point of decline in the LVEF of 10% or more in those with normal LV function or a decrease in the LVEF of 5% or more in those with reduced systolic function (LVEF of <50%) in the entire study cohort. However, in a prespecified subgroup analysis of those with prior anthracycline treatment, both carvedilol and lisinopril were associateed with a lower incidence of cardiotoxicity and fewer interruptions in trastuzumab therapy. .

In a randomized trial of candesartan or placebo during trastuzumab therapy in 206 women with early stage HER2+ breast cancer, all of whom had completed anthracycline-based chemotherapy regimens, there was no difference in the primary end point defined as a decrease in the LVEF by more than 15% points from baseline or an LVEF less than 45%.[112]

In summary, given 1 neutral study of candesartan and signals for benefit coming only for secondary end points or subgroup analyses, the routine use of neurohormonal antagonist therapy for the primary prevention of trastuzumab cardiotoxicity cannot be recommended for all patients. There may be a role for lisinopril or carvedilol in individuals treated with sequential anthracyclines followed by trastuzumab, especially if additional cardiac risk factors are present, although additional studies would be useful.

Safety of Anti–Human-Epidermal Growth Factor Receptor-2 Therapy in Those with Mildly Reduced Left Ventricular Ejection Fraction and No Heart Failure Symptoms

Given the efficacy of trastuzumab in treatment of HER2+ breast cancer, 2 recent studies have investigated the safety and feasibility of continuing anti-HER2 targeted therapies while using optimized neurohormonal blockade (carvedilol ± ramipril or candesartan) as a part of standard guideline-directed medical therapy in patients with HER2+ breast cancer and preexisting LV dysfunction with stage B heart failure and an LVEF of 40% to 50%.[113,114]

In the SAFE-HEaRT trial, 30 patients with stage I to IV HER2+ breast cancer with a baseline of LVEF 40% to 49%, without symptoms of heart failure who were either already receiving or were planned to receive anti-HER2+ therapy were treated with carvedilol and ramipril or candesartan.[113] Of the 30 patients, 27 (90%) met the primary end point of completing their planned HER2-targeted therapies without developing a clinically significant cardiac event, defined as successful completion of planned HER2 treatment without incidence of a cardiac event (new heart failure symptoms, cardiac arrhythmia, myocardial infarction, sudden cardiac death, or death owing to CV causes) or developing asymptomatic decline in LV function (a decrease in the LVEF by >10% points from

baseline and/or an LVEF of <35%). This observation was was also seen in the SCHOLAR pilot study, in which 20 patients with early stage breast cancer and mild to moderate trastuzumab-induced cardiotoxicity were treated with maximally tolerated doses of angiotensin-converting enzyme inhibitors (ramipril) with or without beta-blockers (carvedilol), allowing 18 of 20 (90%) of the study patients to receive all planned trastuzumab doses without developing overt heart failure symptoms or an LVEF of less than 40%.[114] Further research with large-scale, randomized studies and long-term follow-up are needed to further evaluate whether the benefit associated with the completion of planned anti-HER2 treatment justifies this risk.

SHORTER DURATION OF HUMAN-EPIDERMAL GROWTH FACTOR RECEPTOR-2 TARGETED THERAPIES

Although the benefits of treatment with trastuzumab in patients with HER2+ breast cancer have been well-established, the optimal duration of HER2–targeted therapy continues to be a topic of debate. Determining the optimal duration of HER2–targeted therapy is of particular importance, because longer durations of trastuzumab therapy have been associated with a higher incidence of cardiotoxic side effects in some studies.[115] The landmark oncology trials investigating the efficacy and safety of trastuzumab therapy for the treatment of HER2+ breast cancer used a 12-month treatment duration, which has since become the standard of care.[106] Two large randomized, noninferiority trials compared 6 months with 12 months of trastuzumab therapy.[116,117] Despite having similar numerical results in disease-free survival (hazard ratio, 1.08; 95% CI, 0.93–1.25) in the PHARE trial and a hazard ratio of 1.07 (90% CI, 0.93–1.24) in the PERSEPHONE trial. These studies used different prespecified noninferiority cutoffs and, thus, came to different conclusions regarding noninferiority. At this point, 12 months of anti-HER2 therapy remains the standard of care; however, the benefit of 12 months versus 6 months seems to be modest based on the existing literature and thus patient centered shared decision making may be appropriate when cardiotoxicity is present.

CARDIOPROTECTIVE STRATEGIES WITH RADIATION

RT has been linked to various CV outcomes such as coronary disease, heart failure, valvular disease, pericarditis, and conduction abnormalities.

These effects are mediated in part by microvascular endothelial damage and fibrosis.[118] A population-based case control study from Sweden and Denmark demonstrated a linear relationship between the mean heart dose and major coronary events in patients receiving RT for breast cancer, with the risk increasing within the first 5 years and persisting until the third decade after treatment.[16] Other studies have shown a similar relationship between the mean dose to the heart and heart failure in patients undergoing RT for breast cancer and Hodgkin's lymphoma.[17,18]

Contemporary advances in RT protocols have allowed the implementation of cardiac-sparing techniques to minimize the radiation dose to the heart and surrounding vascular structures, including deep inspiration breath hold, partial breast (rather than whole breast) irradiation, and other methods to improve localization of treatment while simultaneously minimizing the risk of cardiotoxicity.[119,120] However, radiation to the heart is not eliminated, and thus a certain degree of risk is still present. Proton therapy decreases cardiopulmonary risk in the treatment of esophageal cancers.[121,122] The ongoing RADCOMP Consortium Trial is currently examining the comparative efficacy of proton versus photon therapy in breast cancer with cardiac toxicity as a secondary end point.[123]

Although observational studies have shown that traditional risk factors for atherosclerotic disease are associated with an increased risk of CV events after RT, there are no randomized trials to date examining interventions which may decrease the number of cardiac events in those undergoing RT.[29] Thus, further research is needed to identify effective interventions and the ideal threshold for intervention in this population at greater risk, particularly younger individuals or those without a high predicted 10-year atherosclerotic CV events risk that would not currently be recommended to receive aggressive primary prevention interventions, such as statin therapy, if it were not for their cancer treatment.

CARDIOPROTECTIVE STRATEGIES WITH HEMATOPOIETIC CELL TRANSPLANTATION

HSCT is associated with an increased risk of CV events, such as heart failure, atherosclerotic CV events, and arrhythmias, and the predictors of CV complications with HSCT is impacted by age at the time of transplantation, the presence of preexisting CV risk factors (ie, hypertension, diabetes, hyperlipidemia), treatment with a cardiotoxic chemotherapy regimen before HSCT, the type of stem cell transplant (autologous vs allogenic), and the intensity of conditioning regimen.[31,124] Furthermore, complications of HSCT such as hepatic veno-oclusive disease, thrombotic microangiopathy, and graft-versus-host disease can all cause cardiac injury and have been associated individually with adverse CV outcomes.[125]

Late CV complications are among the most common causes of nonrelapse mortality. In a single-center retrospective cohort study, Chow and colleagues[126] reported a significantly increased risk of CV death (adjusted incidence rate difference, 3.6 per 1000 person-years; 95% CI, 1.7–5.5), with an increased incidence of ischemic heart disease, cardiomyopathy, stroke, and arrhythmias in HSCT recipients compared with matched controls in the general population. Armenian and colleagues[31] reported a 4.5-fold increased risk of congestive heart failure (standardized incidence ratio, 4.5) in autologous HSCT recipients compared with the general population, with the incidence rate for heart failure in this population increasing to 9.1% at 15 years.

There are very few randomized controlled trials evaluating the impact of cardioprotective strategies in attenuating HSCT-associated cardiotoxicity . In the OVERCOME trial of 90 participants with hematologic malignancies (80% underwent HSCT), randomization to enalapril and carvedilol versus usual care was associated with a lesser incidence of the combined event of death or heart failure (6.7% vs 22%; $P = .036$) and of death, heart failure, or a final LVEF of less than 45% (6.7% vs 24.4%; $P = .02$).[81] Although further large-scale studies with long-term follow-up are needed, the results of this study suggest a promising cardioprotective role of neurohormonal blockade in this population. Studies of CV monitoring and prevention strategies in long-term survivors treated with HSCT are also needed.

CARDIOPROTECTIVE STRATEGIES: VASCULAR ENDOTHELIAL GROWTH FACTOR INHIBITORS

Since it was first proposed by Dr Judah Folkman, the concept of "antiangiogenesis" has transformed the treatment of a wide range of malignancies by targeting signaling pathways such as VEGF thereby halting tumor growth and progression. This family of agents encompasses monoclonal antibodies against VEGF and its receptors, decoy VEGF receptors and small molecule tyrosine kinase inhibitors (TKIs). Treatment with VEGF inhibitors has improved outcomes significantly, with higher rates of progression-free and overall survival in a wide array of malignancies including metastatic colorectal cancer, ovarian cancer, renal cell carcinoma and non–small cell lung cancer.[127]

However, the improved oncologic outcomes seen with VEGF-targeted therapies come at the cost of adverse CV effects as these agents are known to be associated with higher incident rates of hypertension, cardiomyopathy, cardiac ischemia, thromboembolism, QT prolongation, and arrhythmias. Prior studies have estimated that up to 55% of patients develop hypertension and up to 10% of patients develop cardiomyopathy with VEGF-targeted therapies.[128,129]

Prior studies have reported conflicting results when it comes to the optimal antihypertensive agent for the management of VEGF inhibitor–mediated hypertension. In one of the largest retrospective studies to date, McKay and associates[130] conducted a retrospective study of 4736 patients with metastatic renal cell carcinoma enrolled in phase II and III clinical trials finding improved overall survival for those who received angiotensin-converting enzyme inhibitors or ARBs compared with those treated with other antihypertensive agents such as beta-blockers, calcium channel blockers (CCB), or diuretics (adjusted hazard ratio, 0.838; 95% CI, 0.731–0.960; $P = .0105$) and those without any antihypertensive treatment (adjusted hazard ratio, 0.810; 95% CI, 0.707–0.929; $P = .0026$). In subgroup analyses, there was a significant improvement in overall survival for those who received ACEIs or ARBs versus compared with nonusers (adjusted hazard ratio, 0.737; 95% CI, 0.640–0.848; $P < .0001$) in patients who received VEGF-targeted therapies (n = 3511). In a subsequent single-center, retrospective study, Bottinor and colleagues[131] demonstrated a statistically significant attenuation of increase in the mean systolic blood pressure for patients who had received treatment with ACEIs or ARBs before the initiation of VEGF inhibitor therapy compared with other antihypertensive therapies in a cohort of 795 patients. In contrast, Waliany and colleagues[132] found that CCB and potassium-sparing diuretics were noted to be more effective in treatment of TKI-associated hypertension compared with other antihypertensive agents (beta-blockers, angiotensin-converting enzyme inhibitors, thiazide, and loop diuretics) in a different single-center retrospective review. The role of prophylactic calcium channel antagonism in VEGF-TKI–mediated hypertension was investigated by Langenberg and colleagues[133] in one of the few prospective studies to date on this topic. This double-blind, randomized study sought to investigate whether prophylaxis with CCB affected dose reductions or therapy withdrawal in 126 patients with advanced solid organ malignancies who were planned to receive cediranib, a potent VEGF-TKI. Study participants who received antihypertensive prophylaxis received low dose CCB 3 to 7 days before initiating therapy with cediranib for those who had a screening blood pressure of 110/70 mm Hg or higher; those with a screening blood pressure less than 110/70 mm Hg received their prophylactic CCB dose on the same days as their first dose of cediranib. Although there was no significant difference in dose reductions or interruptions in cediranib therapy with CCB prophylaxis, the overall incidence of severe hypertension was lower in those who received antihypertensive prophylaxis. This study also used a standardized hypertension treatment protocol for all patients. Further studies are needed to assess which antihypertensive agents and dosing strategies are associated with improved CV and oncologic outcomes.

CARDIOPROTECTIVE STRATEGIES WITH FLUOROPYRIMIDINES

Fluoropyrimidines, such as 5-fluorouracil and capecitabine, belong to the antimetabolite class of chemotherapeutic agents that are widely used worldwide for treatment of a broad range of solid organ malignancies including head and neck, esophageal, gastric, colorectal, and breast cancers. These agents can cause coronary artery vasospasm, endothelial injury, and direct myocardial toxicity, contributing to the observed incidence of acute coronary syndromes, myocardial infraction, arrhythmias, heart failure, cardiogenic shock, and even rare cases of cardiac arrest/sudden cardiac death.[134] Predominantly reported via retrospective studies, the incidence of cardiotoxicity owing to 5-fluorouracil or capecitabine use is highly variable and ranges anywhere from 0.5% to 19.0%, depending on the definitions of cardiotoxicity, specific study design, and cancer regimen.[134–136] A recent single-center retrospective review suggested that vasospasm occurred in 2% of the population and there was no difference in mortality between those with and without vasospasm.[137] Current understanding of risk factors or risk predictors of 5-fluorouracil cardiotoxicity is limited and primary prevention is not recommended for all patients. In the presence of symptoms concerning for cardiotoxicity, current practice recommends the immediate discontinuation of fluoropyrimidine therapy and the initiation of antianginal treatment. However, in a case series of 11 patients with suspected fluoropyrimidine-mediated coronary vasospasm, all patients were able to continue with fluoropyrimidine-based chemotherapy regimen using a multipronged approach of transitioning to a bolus 5-fluorouracil infusion from continuous infusion, concurrent treatment with long-acting nitrates and CCB for the duration of the chemotherapy course and close monitoring in an inpatient telemetry-capable unit for 24 hours after treatment.[138]

CARDIOPROTECTIVE STRATEGIES WITH BCR-ABL TYROSINE KINASE INHIBITORS

Chronic myeloid leukemia is a myeloproliferative disorder resulting from a chromosomal transloca-tion of the ABL gene from chromosome 9 and the BCR gene on chromosome 22, leading to the formation of a fusion gene, BCR-ABL protein causing aberrant TK activity. Imatinib, the first BCR-ABL TKI, revolutionized the management of chronic myeloid leukemia, with an excellent safety profile and very low risk of cardiac events. Howev-er, many patients managed with imatinib lose their hematological response, necessitating manage-ment with more potent and less selective TKIs such as nilotinib, dasatinib, ponatinib, and bosuti-nib, with variable inhibition of non–BCR-Abl TKs and varied CV toxicity.

The randomized ENESTnd trial showed improved molecular remission, but more CV events in patients treated with nilotinib versus ima-tinib as first-line therapy.[139] Mechanistically, niloti-nib has been associated with increases in blood pressure, cholesterol levels, glucose, thrombosis mediators such as P-selectin, and platelet adhe-sive function and endogenous thrombin levels, as well as QT prolongation, in vivo.[139–141] Arterial vascular events such as myocardial infarction, stroke, and lower extremity ischemia occurred in approximately 8% of patients in clinical trials of ponatinib, leading to a Black Box warning on the US FDA label for ponatinib and restriction of use to those with progressive disease on another BCR-Abl TKI.[20,142]

Nilotinib-related CV events are higher in those with CV risk factors and prevalent CV disease, and established risk stratification tools may be helpful to guide decisions about TKI selection, car-diology referral, and cardioprotective medications. Using the SCORE chart (includes sex, age, smok-ing status, systolic pressure, and cholesterol), the cumulative incidence of atherosclerotic events at 48 months after initiation of nilotinib was zero in the low-risk patients compared with 10% in the moderate-risk category and 29% in the high-risk group.[143] The Framingham Risk Score has also been shown to be predictive of nilotinib-associated CV events.[139] Taken together, these data suggest that atherosclerotic CV events pre-diction tools used for primary prevention in general population are useful in risk stratification for TKI-mediated ischemic events as well.

CARDIOPROTECTIVE STRATEGIES WITH IMMUNE CHECKPOINT INHIBITORS

The ability of certain types of cancers to avoid host immunosurveillance relies on the activation of various immune checkpoint pathways, which serve to dampen or suppress the host immune response to immunogenic stimuli. Cytotoxic T lymphocyte-associated protein-4 and programmed cell death protein-1 are types of inhibitory receptors that are expressed on T lymphocytes. The binding of these receptors to their corresponding ligands on either host antigen presenting cells or tumor cells pre-vents T-cell activation thereby downregulating the host immune response. By upregulating expression of these negative modulators of host immune response such as programmed cell death 1 ligand-1, tumor cells can escape detection and resultant T-cell–mediated destruction, leading to uninhibited tumor growth and overall progres-sion.[144] The advent of ICIs nearly a decade ago has transformed the field of oncology and altered the clinical course and treatment outcomes for pa-tients with various types of advanced malignancies. Since the initial landmark trials, several ICIs have been approved by the FDA and are currently widely used in management of advanced melanoma, non–small cell lung cancers, renal cell carcinoma, uro-thelial cancer, and refractory Hodgkin's lymphoma, among others.

Despite the significant benefits for some pa-tients, a wide range of immune-related adverse events can affect multiple organ systems, including the skin, gastrointestinal, pulmonary, endocrine, and CV systems, with manifestations ranging from fatigue or mild rash to severe colitis. Occurring in as many as 70% to 90% of patients undergoing treatment with these agents, most of these immune-mediated toxicities can either be reversed or at least well-controlled with glucocor-ticoid therapy.[145] ICI myocarditis is rare (incidence rate ranging from 0.27% to 2.00%), although serious, because it is associated with CV death, cardiogenic shock, or life-threatening arrhythmias in up to 50% of cases.[21,146] Most of the ICI myocarditis cases have been noted to occur early after the initiation of ICI therapy. Combination ICI therapy has been observed to be the predominant and most well-established risk factor for ICI-mediated myocarditis thus far, with a nearly 4-fold increased risk of toxicity with combination therapy as opposed to monotherapy. Although several other theoretic risk factors such as comor-bid CV disease, concurrent use of other non-ICI cardiotoxic chemotherapy agents, underlying autoimmune disease, and genetic factors have been postulated to increase the risk of ICI-mediated myocarditis, further research is needed to identify risk factors for ICI myocarditis. Once suspected, immediate evaluation using a combination of cardiac biomarkers, telemetry monitoring, cardiac magnetic resonance imaging, and/or endomyocardial biopsy should be initiated to help establish the diagnosis of myocarditis and exclude other etiologies. Owing to a dearth of prospective studies on this topic, the management principles of ICI-mediated cardiotoxicity are guided by retrospective analyses and expert opinions. The current standard of care for the treatment of ICI-associated cardiotoxicity includes the immediate discontinuation of ICI therapy, supportive therapy for management of cardiac complications (ie, arrhythmias, volume overload, shock), and the initiation of high-dose intravenous steroids with higher starting dose of steroids associated with lower rates of major adverse cardiac events in observational studies.[21,147] For patients with an inadequate response to corticosteroid therapy, immunosuppressive agents such as mycophenolate mofetil, intravenous immunoglobulin, antithymocyte globulin, and abatacept have been used to mitigate the T-cell response and treat ICI-mediated myocarditis.[148,149]

Although ICI-mediated cardiotoxicity occurs less frequently than other types of infusion-related adverse events (gastrointestinal vs endocrine adverse events) and considered to be a rare clinical entity, it has been associated with major adverse cardiac events and higher case fatality rates, when present. Further research in the form of prospective studies is needed to quantify the true incidence of ICI-mediated cardiotoxicity, identify patients who are at higher risk of developing cardiotoxic side effects and define optimal treatment strategies.

CLINICS CARE POINTS

- Assess cardiac risk by considering treatment regimen, prevalent cardiovascular disease and cardiac risk factors.

- Prevalent cardiovascular disease should be managed according to standard cardiovascular guidelines.

- Consider cardio-oncology referral for optimization and risk stratification if multiple cardiovascular risk factors or a treatment regimen with high risk of cardiac events.

REFERENCES

1. Siegel RL, Miller KD, Fuchs HE, et al. Cancer Statistics, 2021. CA Cancer J Clin 2021;71:7–33.
2. Bradshaw PT, Stevens J, Khankari N, et al. Cardiovascular disease mortality among breast cancer survivors. Epidemiology 2016;27:6–13.
3. Hanrahan EO, Gonzalez-Angulo AM, Giordano SH, et al. Overall survival and cause-specific mortality of patients with stage T1a,bN0M0 breast carcinoma. J Clin Oncol 2007;25:4952–60.
4. Virani SS, Alonso A, Benjamin EJ, et al. American Heart Association Council on E, Prevention Statistics C and Stroke Statistics S. Heart Disease and Stroke Statistics-2020 update: a report from the American Heart Association. Circulation 2020; 141:e139–596.
5. Armenian SH, Xu L, Ky B, et al. Cardiovascular disease among survivors of adult-onset cancer: a community-based retrospective cohort study. J Clin Oncol 2016;34:1122–30.
6. Strongman H, Gadd S, Matthews A, et al. Medium and long-term risks of specific cardiovascular diseases in survivors of 20 adult cancers: a population-based cohort study using multiple linked UK electronic health records databases. Lancet 2019;394:1041–54.
7. Swain SM, Whaley FS, Ewer MS. Congestive heart failure in patients treated with doxorubicin: a retrospective analysis of three trials. Cancer 2003;97: 2869–79.
8. Von Hoff DD, Layard MW, Basa P, et al. Risk factors for doxorubicin-induced congestive heart failure. Ann Intern Med 1979;91:710–7.
9. Narayan HK, French B, Khan AM, et al. Noninvasive measures of ventricular-arterial coupling and circumferential strain predict cancer therapeutics-related cardiac dysfunction. JACC Cardiovasc Imaging 2016;9:1131–41.
10. Cardinale D, Colombo A, Bacchiani G, et al. Early detection of anthracycline cardiotoxicity and improvement with heart failure therapy. Circulation 2015;131:1981–8.
11. van Nimwegen FA, Schaapveld M, Janus CP, et al. Cardiovascular disease after Hodgkin lymphoma treatment: 40-year disease risk. JAMA Intern Med 2015;175:1007–17.
12. Chow EJ, Chen Y, Kremer LC, et al. Individual prediction of heart failure among childhood cancer survivors. J Clin Oncol 2015;33:394–402.
13. Thavendiranathan P, Abdel-Qadir H, Fischer HD, et al. Risk-imaging mismatch in cardiac imaging practices for women receiving systemic therapy for early-stage breast cancer: a population-based cohort study. J Clin Oncol 2018;36:2980–7.
14. Narayan HK, Finkelman B, French B, et al. Detailed echocardiographic phenotyping in breast cancer

patients: associations with ejection fraction decline, recovery, and heart failure symptoms over 3 years of follow-up. Circulation 2017;135:1397–412.

15. Miller KD, O'Neill A, Gradishar W, et al. Double-Blind Phase III Trial of adjuvant chemotherapy with and without bevacizumab in patients with lymph node-positive and high-risk lymph node-negative breast cancer (E5103). J Clin Oncol 2018;36:2621–9.

16. Darby SC, Ewertz M, Hall P. Ischemic heart disease after breast cancer radiotherapy. N Engl J Med 2013;368:2527.

17. Saiki H, Petersen IA, Scott CG, et al. Risk of heart failure with preserved ejection fraction in older women after contemporary radiotherapy for breast cancer. Circulation 2017;135:1388–96.

18. van Nimwegen FA, Ntentas G, Darby SC, et al. Risk of heart failure in survivors of Hodgkin lymphoma: effects of cardiac exposure to radiation and anthracyclines. Blood 2017;129:2257–65.

19. Atkins KM, Rawal B, Chaunzwa TL, et al. Cardiac radiation dose, cardiac disease, and mortality in patients with lung cancer. J Am Coll Cardiol 2019; 73:2976–87.

20. Dorer DJ, Knickerbocker RK, Baccarani M, et al. Impact of dose intensity of ponatinib on selected adverse events: multivariate analyses from a pooled population of clinical trial patients. Leuk Res 2016;48:84–91.

21. Mahmood SS, Fradley MG, Cohen JV, et al. Myocarditis in patients treated with immune checkpoint inhibitors. J Am Coll Cardiol 2018;71:1755–64.

22. Romond EH, Jeong JH, Rastogi P, et al. Seven-year follow-up assessment of cardiac function in NSABP B-31, a randomized trial comparing doxorubicin and cyclophosphamide followed by paclitaxel (ACP) with ACP plus trastuzumab as adjuvant therapy for patients with node-positive, human epidermal growth factor receptor 2-positive breast cancer. J Clin Oncol 2012; 30:3792–9.

23. Ezaz G, Long JB, Gross CP, et al. Risk prediction model for heart failure and cardiomyopathy after adjuvant trastuzumab therapy for breast cancer. J Am Heart Assoc 2014;3:e000472.

24. Perez EA, Suman VJ, Davidson NE, et al. Cardiac safety analysis of doxorubicin and cyclophosphamide followed by paclitaxel with or without trastuzumab in the North Central Cancer Treatment Group N9831 adjuvant breast cancer trial. J Clin Oncol 2008;26:1231–8.

25. Pinder MC, Duan Z, Goodwin JS, et al. Congestive heart failure in older women treated with adjuvant anthracycline chemotherapy for breast cancer. J Clin Oncol 2007;25:3808–15.

26. Advani PP, Ballman KV, Dockter TJ, et al. Long-term cardiac safety analysis of NCCTG N9831

(Alliance) adjuvant trastuzumab trial. J Clin Oncol 2016;34:581–7.

27. Chavez-MacGregor M, Zhang N, Buchholz TA, et al. Trastuzumab-related cardiotoxicity among older patients with breast cancer. J Clin Oncol 2013;31:4222–8.

28. Hooning MJ, Botma A, Aleman BM, et al. Long-term risk of cardiovascular disease in 10-year survivors of breast cancer. J Natl Cancer Inst 2007; 99:365–75.

29. Armstrong GT, Oeffinger KC, Chen Y, et al. Modifiable risk factors and major cardiac events among adult survivors of childhood cancer. J Clin Oncol 2013;31:3673–80.

30. Leger KJ, Cushing-Haugen K, Hansen JA, et al. Clinical and Genetic Determinants of Cardiomyopathy Risk among Hematopoietic Cell Transplantation Survivors. Biol Blood Marrow Transplant 2016;22:1094–101.

31. Armenian SH, Sun CL, Shannon T, et al. Incidence and predictors of congestive heart failure after autologous hematopoietic cell transplantation. Blood 2011;118:6023–9.

32. Tichelli A, Bucher C, Rovo A, et al. Premature cardiovascular disease after allogeneic hematopoietic stem-cell transplantation. Blood 2007;110: 3463–71.

33. Kenzik KM, Balentine C, Richman J, et al. New-Onset Cardiovascular Morbidity in Older Adults With Stage I to III Colorectal Cancer. J Clin Oncol 2018;36:609–16.

34. Cardinale D, Sandri MT, Colombo A, et al. Prognostic value of troponin I in cardiac risk stratification of cancer patients undergoing high-dose chemotherapy. Circulation 2004;109:2749–54.

35. Sawaya H, Sebag IA, Plana JC, et al. Assessment of echocardiography and biomarkers for the extended prediction of cardiotoxicity in patients treated with anthracyclines, taxanes, and trastuzumab. Circ Cardiovasc Imaging 2012;5:596–603.

36. Ky B, Putt M, Sawaya H, et al. Early increases in multiple biomarkers predict subsequent cardiotoxicity in patients with breast cancer treated with doxorubicin, taxanes, and trastuzumab. J Am Coll Cardiol 2014;63:809–16.

37. Garrone O, Crosetto N, Lo Nigro C, et al. Prediction of anthracycline cardiotoxicity after chemotherapy by biomarkers kinetic analysis. Cardiovasc Toxicol 2012;12:135–42.

38. Katsurada K, Ichida M, Sakuragi M, et al. High-sensitivity troponin T as a marker to predict cardiotoxicity in breast cancer patients with adjuvant trastuzumab therapy. SpringerPlus 2014;3:620.

39. Auner HW, Tinchon C, Linkesch W, et al. Prolonged monitoring of troponin T for the detection of anthracycline cardiotoxicity in adults with hematological malignancies. Ann Hematol 2003;82:218–22.

40. Lipshultz SE, Rifai N, Sallan SE, et al. Predictive value of cardiac troponin T in pediatric patients at risk for myocardial injury. Circulation 1997;96: 2641–8.

41. Lipshultz SE, Rifai N, Dalton VM, et al. The effect of dexrazoxane on myocardial injury in doxorubicin-treated children with acute lymphoblastic leukemia. N Engl J Med 2004;351:145–53.

42. Lipshultz SE, Miller TL, Scully RE, et al. Changes in cardiac biomarkers during doxorubicin treatment of pediatric patients with high-risk acute lymphoblastic leukemia: associations with long-term echocardiographic outcomes. J Clin Oncol 2012;30: 1042–9.

43. Lenihan DJ, Stevens PL, Massey M, et al. The utility of point-of-care biomarkers to detect cardiotoxicity during anthracycline chemotherapy: a feasibility study. J Card Fail 2016;22:433–8.

44. Thavendiranathan P, Poulin F, Lim KD, et al. Use of myocardial strain imaging by echocardiography for the early detection of cardiotoxicity in patients during and after cancer chemotherapy: a systematic review. J Am Coll Cardiol 2014;63:2751–68.

45. Thavendiranathan P, Negishi T, Somerset E, et al. Strain-Guided Management of Potentially Cardiotoxic Cancer Therapy. J Am Coll Cardiol 2021;77: 392–401.

46. Chow EJ, Chen Y, Hudson MM, et al. Prediction of ischemic heart disease and stroke in survivors of childhood cancer. J Clin Oncol 2018;36: 44–52.

47. Upshaw JN, Ruthazer R, Miller KD, et al. Personalized decision making in early stage breast cancer: applying clinical prediction models for anthracycline cardiotoxicity and breast cancer mortality demonstrates substantial heterogeneity of benefit-harm trade-off. Clin Breast Cancer 2019;19: 259–67.

48. Abdel-Qadir H, Thavendiranathan P, Austin PC, et al. Development and validation of a multivariable prediction model for major adverse cardiovascular events after early stage breast cancer: a population-based cohort study. Eur Heart J 2019; 40:3913–20.

49. Zhang S, Liu X, Bawa-Khalfe T, et al. Identification of the molecular basis of doxorubicin-induced cardiotoxicity. Nat Med 2012;18:1639–42.

50. Finkelman BS, Putt M, Wang T, et al. Arginine-nitric oxide metabolites and cardiac dysfunction in patients with breast cancer. J Am Coll Cardiol 2017; 70:152–62.

51. ZINECARD (dexrazoxane) [package insert] U.S. Food and Drug Administration website. Available at: https://www.accessdata.fda.gov. Accessed November 2019.

52. Speyer JL, Green MD, Zeleniuch-Jacquotte A, et al. ICRF-187 permits longer treatment with doxorubicin in women with breast cancer. J Clin Oncol 1992;10:117–27.

53. Swain SM, Whaley FS, Gerber MC, et al. Cardioprotection with dexrazoxane for doxorubicin-containing therapy in advanced breast cancer. J Clin Oncol 1997;15:1318–32.

54. Tebbi CK, London WB, Friedman D, et al. Dexrazoxane-associated risk for acute myeloid leukemia/myelodysplastic syndrome and other secondary malignancies in pediatric Hodgkin's disease. J Clin Oncol 2007;25:493–500.

55. Asselin BL, Devidas M, Chen L, et al. Cardioprotection and safety of dexrazoxane in patients treated for newly diagnosed T-Cell acute lymphoblastic leukemia or advanced-stage lymphoblastic non-Hodgkin lymphoma: a report of the children's oncology group randomized trial pediatric oncology group 9404. J Clin Oncol 2016;34:854–62.

56. Chow EJ, Asselin BL, Schwartz CL, et al. Late mortality after dexrazoxane treatment: a report from the children's oncology group. J Clin Oncol 2015;33: 2639–45.

57. Shaikh F, Dupuis LL, Alexander S, et al. Cardioprotection and second malignant neoplasms associated with dexrazoxane in children receiving anthracycline chemotherapy: a systematic review and meta-analysis. J Natl Cancer Inst 2016;108.

58. Seif AE, Walker DM, Li Y, et al. Dexrazoxane exposure and risk of secondary acute myeloid leukemia in pediatric oncology patients. Pediatr Blood Cancer 2015;62:704–9.

59. Macedo AVS, Hajjar LA, Lyon AR, et al. Efficacy of dexrazoxane in preventing anthracycline cardiotoxicity in breast cancer. JACC: CardioOncol 2019;1:68–79.

60. Jones RL, Wagner AJ, Kawai A, et al. Prospective evaluation of doxorubicin cardiotoxicity in patients with advanced soft-tissue sarcoma treated in the ANNOUNCE Phase III randomized trial. Clin Cancer Res 2021;27:3861–6.

61. Cardioxane (dexrazoxane). European Medicines Agency website. 2017. Available at: https://www.ema.europa.eu/en/medicines/human/referrals/cardioxane. Accessed February 2022.

62. DOXIL (doxorubicin HCl liposome injection) [package insert] U.S. Food and Drug Administration website. 2007. Available at: https://www.accessdata.fda.gov. Accessed November 2019.

63. Batist G, Ramakrishnan G, Rao CS, et al. Reduced cardiotoxicity and preserved antitumor efficacy of liposome-encapsulated doxorubicin and cyclophosphamide compared with conventional doxorubicin and cyclophosphamide in a randomized, multicenter trial of metastatic breast cancer. J Clin Oncol 2001;19:1444–54.

64. Harris L, Batist G, Belt R, et al. Liposome-encapsulated doxorubicin compared with conventional

doxorubicin in a randomized multicenter trial as first-line therapy of metastatic breast carcinoma. Cancer 2002;94:25–36.

65. Myocet (doxorubicin). European Medicines Agency website. Available at: https://www.ema. europa.eu/en/medicines/human/EPAR/myocet. Accessed November 2019.

66. Chan S, Davidson N, Juozaityte E, et al. Phase III trial of liposomal doxorubicin and cyclophosphamide compared with epirubicin and cyclophosphamide as first-line therapy for metastatic breast cancer. Ann Oncol 2004;15:1527–34.

67. Salvi F, Luminari S, Tucci A, et al. Bleomycin, vinblastine and dacarbazine combined with non-pegylated liposomal doxorubicin (MBVD) in elderly (>/=70 years) or cardiopathic patients with Hodgkin lymphoma: a phase-II study from Fondazione Italiana Linfomi (FIL). Leuk Lymphoma 2019;1–9.

68. Fridrik MA, Jaeger U, Petzer A, et al. Cardiotoxicity with rituximab, cyclophosphamide, non-pegylated liposomal doxorubicin, vincristine and prednisolone compared to rituximab, cyclophosphamide, doxorubicin, vincristine, and prednisolone in frontline treatment of patients with diffuse large B-cell lymphoma: a randomised phase-III study from the Austrian Cancer Drug Therapy Working Group [Arbeitsgemeinschaft Medikamentose Tumortherapie AGMT](NHL-14). Eur J Cancer 2016;58:112–21.

69. Hunault-Berger M, Leguay T, Thomas X, et al. A randomized study of pegylated liposomal doxorubicin versus continuous-infusion doxorubicin in elderly patients with acute lymphoblastic leukemia: the GRAALL-SA1 study. Haematologica 2011;96: 245–52.

70. Network NCC. NCCN Guidelines version 5.2021. Diffuse Large B-Cell Lymphoma. Available at: nccn.org. Accessed February 2022.

71. Armenian SH, Lacchetti C, Barac A, et al. Prevention and monitoring of cardiac dysfunction in survivors of adult cancers: American Society of Clinical Oncology clinical practice guideline. J Clin Oncol 2017;35:893–911.

72. Shapira J, Gotfried M, Lishner M, et al. Reduced cardiotoxicity of doxorubicin by a 6-hour infusion regimen. A prospective randomized evaluation. Cancer 1990;65:870–3.

73. Casper ES, Gaynor JJ, Hajdu SI, et al. A prospective randomized trial of adjuvant chemotherapy with bolus versus continuous infusion of doxorubicin in patients with high-grade extremity soft tissue sarcoma and an analysis of prognostic factors. Cancer 1991;68:1221–9.

74. Lipshultz SE, Giantris AL, Lipsitz SR, et al. Doxorubicin administration by continuous infusion is not cardioprotective: the Dana-Farber 91-01 Acute

Lymphoblastic Leukemia protocol. J Clin Oncol 2002;20:1677–82.

75. Lipshultz SE, Miller TL, Lipsitz SR, et al. Continuous versus bolus infusion of doxorubicin in children with ALL: long-term cardiac outcomes. Pediatrics 2012;130:1003–11.

76. Yancy CW, Jessup M, Bozkurt B, et al. 2017 ACC/AHA/HFSA focused update of the 2013 ACCF/AHA guideline for the management of heart failure: a report of the American College of Cardiology/American Heart Association Task Force on Clinical Practice Guidelines and the Heart Failure Society of America. J Card Fail 2017;22(9):659–69.

77. McDonagh TA, Metra M, Adamo M, et al. 2021 ESC Guidelines for the diagnosis and treatment of acute and chronic heart failure. Eur Heart J 2021;42(36): 3599–726.

78. Gulati G, Heck SL, Ree AH, et al. Prevention of cardiac dysfunction during adjuvant breast cancer therapy (PRADA): a 2 x 2 factorial, randomized, placebo-controlled, double-blind clinical trial of candesartan and metoprolol. Eur Heart J 2016;37: 1671–80.

79. Heck SL, Mecinaj A, Ree AH, et al. Prevention of Cardiac Dysfunction During Adjuvant Breast Cancer Therapy (PRADA): extended follow-up of a 2x2 factorial, randomized, placebo-controlled, double-blind clinical trial of candesartan and metoprolol. Circulation 2021;143:2431–40.

80. Kalay N, Basar E, Ozdogru I, et al. Protective effects of carvedilol against anthracycline-induced cardiomyopathy. J Am Coll Cardiol 2006;48: 2258–62.

81. Bosch X, Rovira M, Sitges M, et al. Enalapril and carvedilol for preventing chemotherapy-induced left ventricular systolic dysfunction in patients with malignant hemopathies: the OVERCOME trial (preventiOn of left Ventricular dysfunction with Enalapril and caRvedilol in patients submitted to intensive ChemOtherapy for the treatment of Malignant hEmopathies). J Am Coll Cardiol 2013;61:2355–62.

82. Avila MS, Ayub-Ferreira SM, de Barros Wanderley MR, et al. Carvedilol for prevention of chemotherapy-related cardiotoxicity: the CECCY Trial. J Am Coll Cardiol 2018;71:2281–90.

83. Guglin M, Krischer J, Tamura R, et al. Randomized trial of lisinopril versus carvedilol to prevent trastuzumab cardiotoxicity in patients with breast cancer. J Am Coll Cardiol 2019;73:2859–68.

84. Livi L, Barletta G, Martella F, et al. Cardioprotective strategy for patients with nonmetastatic breast cancer who are receiving an anthracycline-based chemotherapy: a randomized clinical trial. JAMA Oncol 2021;7(10):1544–9.

85. Lewinter C, Nielsen TH, Edfors LR, et al. A systematic review and meta-analysis of beta-blockers and renin-angiotensin system inhibitors for preventing

left ventricular dysfunction due to anthracyclines or trastuzumab in patients with breast cancer. Eur Heart J 2021. https://doi.org/10.1093/eurheartj/ehab843.

86. Cardinale D, Colombo A, Sandri MT, et al. Prevention of high-dose chemotherapy-induced cardiotoxicity in high-risk patients by angiotensin-converting enzyme inhibition. Circulation 2006;114:2474–81.

87. Sutton AL, Felix AS, Bandyopadhyay D, et al. Cardioprotective medication use in Black and white breast cancer survivors. Breast Cancer Res Treat 2021;188:769–78.

88. Riad A, Bien S, Westermann D, et al. Pretreatment with statin attenuates the cardiotoxicity of Doxorubicin in mice. Cancer Res 2009;69:695–9.

89. Seicean S, Seicean A, Plana JC, et al. Effect of statin therapy on the risk for incident heart failure in patients with breast cancer receiving anthracycline chemotherapy: an observational clinical cohort study. J Am Coll Cardiol 2012;60:2384–90.

90. Acar Z, Kale A, Turgut M, et al. Efficiency of atorvastatin in the protection of anthracycline-induced cardiomyopathy. J Am Coll Cardiol 2011;58:988–9.

91. Nabati M, Janbabai G, Esmailian J, et al. Effect of Rosuvastatin in preventing chemotherapy-induced cardiotoxicity in women with breast cancer: a randomized, single-blind, placebo-controlled trial. J Cardiovasc Pharmacol Ther 2019;24:233–41.

92. U.S. National Institutes of Health, National Library of Medicine. Clinicaltrials.gov. Preventing Anthracycline Cardiovascular Toxicity With Statins (PREVENT). Available at: https://clinicaltrials.gov/ct2/show/NCT01988571. Accessed November 4, 2019.

93. U.S. National Institutes of Health, National Library of Medicine. Clinicaltrials.gov. STOP-CA (Statins TO Prevent the Cardiotoxicity From Anthracyclines). Available at: https://clinicaltrials.gov/ct2/show/NCT02943590. Accessed November 4, 2019.

94. Eijsvogels TM, Molossi S, Lee DC, et al. Exercise at the extremes: the amount of exercise to reduce cardiovascular events. J Am Coll Cardiol 2016;67:316–29.

95. Wen CP, Wai JP, Tsai MK, et al. Minimum amount of physical activity for reduced mortality and extended life expectancy: a prospective cohort study. Lancet 2011;378:1244–53.

96. Holmes MD, Chen WY, Feskanich D, et al. Physical activity and survival after breast cancer diagnosis. JAMA 2005;293:2479–86.

97. Irwin ML, Smith AW, McTiernan A, et al. Influence of pre- and postdiagnosis physical activity on mortality in breast cancer survivors: the health, eating, activity, and lifestyle study. J Clin Oncol 2008;26:3958–64.

98. Jones LW, Habel LA, Weltzien E, et al. Exercise and risk of cardiovascular events in women with non-metastatic breast cancer. J Clin Oncol 2016;34:2743–9.

99. Okwuosa TM, Ray RM, Palomo A, et al. Pre-diagnosis exercise and cardiovascular events in primary breast cancer. JACC CardioOncology 2019;1:41–50.

100. Scott JM, Zabor EC, Schwitzer E, et al. Efficacy of exercise therapy on cardiorespiratory fitness in patients with cancer: a systematic review and meta-analysis. J Clin Oncol 2018;36:2297–305.

101. Naaktgeboren WR, Binyam D, Stuiver MM, et al. Efficacy of physical exercise to offset anthracycline-induced cardiotoxicity: a systematic review and meta-analysis of clinical and preclinical studies. J Am Heart Assoc 2021;10:e021580.

102. Rock CL, Doyle C, Demark-Wahnefried W, et al. Nutrition and physical activity guidelines for cancer survivors. CA: a Cancer J clinicians 2012;62:243–74.

103. Arnett DK, Blumenthal RS, Albert MA, et al. 2019 ACC/AHA guideline on the primary prevention of cardiovascular disease: executive summary: a report of the American College of Cardiology/American Heart Association Task Force on Clinical Practice Guidelines. J Am Coll Cardiol 2019;74:1376–414.

104. Powell KE, King AC, Buchner DM, et al. The Scientific Foundation for the Physical Activity Guidelines for Americans, 2nd Edition. J Phys Act Health 2018;1–11.

105. Han L, You D, Ma W, et al. National Trends in American Heart Association Revised Life's Simple 7 Metrics Associated With Risk of Mortality Among US Adults. JAMA Netw Open 2019;2:e1913131.

106. Romond EH, Perez EA, Bryant J, et al. Trastuzumab plus adjuvant chemotherapy for operable HER2-positive breast cancer. N Engl J Med 2005;353:1673–84.

107. Slamon DJ, Leyland-Jones B, Shak S, et al. Use of chemotherapy plus a monoclonal antibody against HER2 for metastatic breast cancer that overexpresses HER2. N Engl J Med 2001;344:783–92.

108. Procter M, Suter TM, de Azambuja E, et al. Longer-term assessment of trastuzumab-related cardiac adverse events in the Herceptin Adjuvant (HERA) trial. J Clin Oncol 2010;28:3422–8.

109. Tan-Chiu E, Yothers G, Romond E, et al. Assessment of cardiac dysfunction in a randomized trial comparing doxorubicin and cyclophosphamide followed by paclitaxel, with or without trastuzumab as adjuvant therapy in node-positive, human epidermal growth factor receptor 2-overexpressing breast cancer: NSABP B-31. J Clin Oncol 2005;23:7811–9.

110. Rayson D, Richel D, Chia S, et al. Anthracycline-trastuzumab regimens for HER2/neu-overexpressing

breast cancer: current experience and future strategies. Ann Oncol 2008;19:1530–9.

111. Rushton M, Lima I, Tuna M, et al. Impact of stopping trastuzumab in early breast cancer: a population-based study in Ontario, Canada. J Natl Cancer Inst 2020;112:1222–30.

112. Boekhout AH, Gietema JA, Milojkovic Kerklaan B, et al. Angiotensin II-receptor inhibition with candesartan to prevent trastuzumab-related cardiotoxic effects in patients with early breast cancer: a randomized clinical trial. JAMA Oncol 2016;2:1030–7.

113. Lynce F, Barac A, Geng X, et al. Prospective evaluation of the cardiac safety of HER2-targeted therapies in patients with HER2-positive breast cancer and compromised heart function: the SAFE-HEaRt study. Breast Cancer Res Treat 2019;175:595–603.

114. Leong DP, Cosman T, Alhussein MM, et al. Safety of continuing trastuzumab despite mild cardiotoxicity: a phase I trial. JACC CardioOncol 2019;1:1–10.

115. Gyawali B, Niraula S. Duration of adjuvant trastuzumab in HER2 positive breast cancer: overall and disease free survival results from meta-analyses of randomized controlled trials. Cancer Treat Rev 2017;60:18–23.

116. Earl HM, Hiller L, Vallier AL, et al. 6 versus 12 months of adjuvant trastuzumab for HER2-positive early breast cancer (PERSEPHONE): 4-year disease-free survival results of a randomised phase 3 non-inferiority trial. Lancet 2019;393:2599–612.

117. Pivot X, Romieu G, Debled M, et al. 6 months versus 12 months of adjuvant trastuzumab in early breast cancer (PHARE): final analysis of a multicentre, open-label, phase 3 randomised trial. Lancet 2019;393:2591–8.

118. Stewart FA, Seemann I, Hoving S, et al. Understanding radiation-induced cardiovascular damage and strategies for intervention. Clin Oncol 2013;25:617–24.

119. Lai J, Hu S, Luo Y, et al. Meta-analysis of deep inspiration breath hold (DIBH) versus free breathing (FB) in postoperative radiotherapy for left-side breast cancer. Breast Cancer 2020;27:299–307.

120. Everett AS, Hoppe BS, Louis D, et al. Comparison of techniques for involved-site radiation therapy in patients with lower mediastinal lymphoma. Pract Radiat Oncol 2019;9:426–34.

121. Wang X, Palaskas NL, Yusuf SW, et al. Incidence and onset of severe cardiac events after radiotherapy for esophageal cancer. J Thorac Oncol 2020;15:1682–90.

122. Lin SH, Hobbs BP, Verma V, et al. Randomized Phase IIB trial of proton beam therapy versus intensity-modulated radiation therapy for locally advanced esophageal cancer. J Clin Oncol 2020;38:1569–79.

123. Bekelman JE, Lu H, Pugh S, et al. Pragmatic randomised clinical trial of proton versus photon therapy for patients with non-metastatic breast cancer: the Radiotherapy Comparative Effectiveness (RadComp) Consortium trial protocol. BMJ Open 2019;9:e025556.

124. Baker JK, Shank-Coviello J, Zhou B, et al. Cardiotoxicity in hematopoietic stem cell transplant: keeping the beat. Clin Lymphoma Myeloma Leuk 2020;20:244–251 e4.

125. Rackley C, Schultz KR, Goldman FD, et al. Cardiac manifestations of graft-versus-host disease. Biol Blood Marrow Transplant 2005;11:773–80.

126. Chow EJ, Mueller BA, Baker KS, et al. Cardiovascular hospitalizations and mortality among recipients of hematopoietic stem cell transplantation. Ann Intern Med 2011;155:21–32.

127. Ferrara N, Adamis AP. Ten years of anti-vascular endothelial growth factor therapy. Nat Rev Drug Discov 2016;15:385–403.

128. Hall PS, Harshman LC, Srinivas S, et al. The frequency and severity of cardiovascular toxicity from targeted therapy in advanced renal cell carcinoma patients. JACC Heart Fail 2013;1:72–8.

129. Narayan V, Keefe S, Haas N, et al. Prospective Evaluation of sunitinib-induced cardiotoxicity in patients with metastatic renal cell carcinoma. Clin Cancer Res 2017;23:3601–9.

130. McKay RR, Rodriguez GE, Lin X, et al. Angiotensin system inhibitors and survival outcomes in patients with metastatic renal cell carcinoma. Clin Cancer Res 2015;21:2471–9.

131. Bottinor WJ, Shuey MM, Manouchehri A, et al. Renin-angiotensin-aldosterone system modulates blood pressure response during vascular endothelial growth factor receptor inhibition. JACC CardioOncol 2019;1:14–23.

132. Waliany S, Sainani KL, Park LS, et al. Increase in blood pressure associated with tyrosine kinase inhibitors targeting vascular endothelial growth factor. JACC CardioOncol 2019;1:24–36.

133. Langenberg MH, van Herpen CM, De Bono J, et al. Effective strategies for management of hypertension after vascular endothelial growth factor signaling inhibition therapy: results from a phase II randomized, factorial, double-blind study of Cediranib in patients with advanced solid tumors. J Clin Oncol 2009;27:6152–9.

134. Polk A, Vistisen K, Vaage-Nilsen M, et al. A systematic review of the pathophysiology of 5-fluorouracil-induced cardiotoxicity. BMC Pharmacol Toxicol 2014;15:47.

135. Upshaw JN, O'Neill A, Carver JR, et al. Fluoropyrimidine cardiotoxicity: time for a contemporaneous appraisal. Clin colorectal Cancer 2019;18:44–51.

136. Wacker A, Lersch C, Scherpinski U, et al. High incidence of angina pectoris in patients treated with

5-fluorouracil. A planned surveillance study with 102 patients. Oncology 2003;65:108–12.

137. Zafar A, Drobni ZD, Mosarla R, et al. The incidence, risk factors, and outcomes with 5-fluorouracil-associated coronary vasospasm. JACC CardioOncol 2021;3:101–9.

138. Clasen SC, Ky B, O'Quinn R, et al. Fluoropyrimidine-induced cardiac toxicity: challenging the current paradigm. J Gastrointest Oncol 2017;8:970–9.

139. Hochhaus A, Saglio G, Hughes TP, et al. Long-term benefits and risks of frontline nilotinib vs imatinib for chronic myeloid leukemia in chronic phase: 5-year update of the randomized ENESTnd trial. Leukemia 2016;30:1044–54.

140. Alhawiti N, Burbury KL, Kwa FA, et al. The tyrosine kinase inhibitor, nilotinib potentiates a prothrombotic state. Thromb Res 2016;145:54–64.

141. Bocchia M, Galimberti S, Aprile L, et al. Genetic predisposition and induced pro-inflammatory/pro-oxidative status may play a role in increased atherothrombotic events in nilotinib treated chronic myeloid leukemia patients. Oncotarget 2016;7: 72311–21.

142. Cortes JE, Kim DW, Pinilla-Ibarz J, et al. A phase 2 trial of ponatinib in Philadelphia chromosome-positive leukemias. N Engl J Med 2013;369: 1783–96.

143. Breccia M, Molica M, Zacheo I, et al. Application of systematic coronary risk evaluation chart to identify chronic myeloid leukemia patients at risk of cardiovascular diseases during nilotinib treatment. Ann Hematol 2015;94:393–7.

144. Granier C, De Guillebon E, Blanc C, et al. Mechanisms of action and rationale for the use of checkpoint inhibitors in cancer. ESMO Open 2017;2: e000213.

145. Postow MA, Sidlow R, Hellmann MD. Immune-related adverse events associated with immune checkpoint blockade. N Engl J Med 2018;378: 158–68.

146. Salem JE, Manouchehri A, Moey M, et al. Cardiovascular toxicities associated with immune checkpoint inhibitors: an observational, retrospective, pharmacovigilance study. Lancet Oncol 2018;19: 1579–89.

147. Haanen J, Carbonnel F, Robert C, et al. Management of toxicities from immunotherapy: ESMO Clinical Practice Guidelines for diagnosis, treatment and follow-up. Ann Oncol 2017;28:iv119–42.

148. Esfahani K, Buhlaiga N, Thebault P, et al. Alemtuzumab for immune-related myocarditis due to PD-1 therapy. N Engl J Med 2019;380:2375–6.

149. Salem JE, Allenbach Y, Vozy A, et al. Abatacept for severe immune checkpoint inhibitor-associated myocarditis. N Engl J Med 2019;380:2377–9.

Radiation-Induced Cardiac Dysfunction
Optimizing Radiation Delivery and Postradiation Care

Lauren N. Pedersen, PhD[a], Menka Khoobchandani, PhD[a],
Randall Brenneman, MD, PhD[a,c], Joshua D. Mitchell, MD, MSCI[b,c,d],
Carmen Bergom, MD, PhD[a,b,c],*

KEYWORDS

- Radiation • Cancer • Electronic medical record • Breast cancer • Lung cancer
- Deep inspiration breath hold • Implementation science • Radiation-induced cardiac dysfunction

KEY POINTS

- A significant proportion of patients with cancers in the thoracic region who receive radiation exposure to the heart as part of their cancer radiation therapy (RT) will develop radiation-induced cardiac dysfunction (RICD).
- RICD may be mitigated by using heart-sparing RT techniques (such as deep inspiratory breath hold, prone patient positioning if appropriate, and so on) to keep the incidental dose to the heart and cardiac substructures as low as reasonably possible.
- In the pre-RT period, efficient identification of patients with preexisting cardiovascular disease or cardiometabolic risk factors, who are therefore at elevated risk of RICD, can be achieved through focused history taking and potentially via automated identification using electronic medical record (EMR)-based strategies.
- Coronary artery calcification (CAC) is an indicator of atherosclerotic burden in the general population and is correlated with cardiac events after RT. Assessment for CAC on RT planning CTs and posttreatment surveillance CTs may be leveraged for risk assessment as well as post-RT cardio-oncological follow-up.
- Post-RT EMR notifications to treating physicians may help to address the issue of patients with thoracic cancer lost to follow-up to assist with postradiation screening and surveillance.

INTRODUCTION

Relative survival rates for patients with cancer have dramatically increased over the last 5 decades, owing in large part to concerted efforts in both early detection and improved treatment modalities.[1] Radiation therapy (RT) is a hallmark of modern cancer treatment, with more than half of all patients with cancer receiving RT at some point during their care. RT is a critical component of treatment of many cancers of the thoracic region (ie, breast, lung, and esophageal cancers, lymphomas). Thoracic RT frequently results in incidental radiation to the heart, and studies have

Funding: This work was supported by NIH R01HL147884 (C. Bergom).
[a] Department of Radiation Oncology, Washington University School of Medicine, 4921 Parkview Place, St. Louis, MO 63110, USA; [b] Cardio-Oncology Center of Excellence, Washington University in St. Louis, St Louis, MO, USA; [c] Alvin J. Siteman Center, Washington University in St. Louis, St Louis, MO, USA; [d] Division of Cardiology, Department of Medicine, Washington University in St. Louis, St Louis, MO, USA
* Corresponding author. Department of Radiation Oncology, Washington University School of Medicine, 4921 Parkview Place, St. Louis, MO 63110.
E-mail address: cbergom@wustl.edu

demonstrated that radiation doses to the heart or certain heart structures correlate with cardiac outcomes and/or survival.[2,3] Indeed, more than one-third of patients receiving cardiac radiation exposure as part of their RT may experience radiation-induced cardiac dysfunction (RICD) and/or premature mortality.[4] RICD encompasses several cardiac abnormalities that can occur acutely or as late side effects of RT.[2,4–6] Often, RICD is recognized years after RT exposure, manifesting in a variety of disparate phenotypes, including but not limited to, coronary artery and/or valvular heart disease, abnormal cardiac conduction, microvascular dysfunction, pericardial disease, myocardial fibrosis, and/or heart failure (**Table 1**).[7–11] Recent data in patients with lung and esophageal cancer, who tend to receive higher doses of cardiac radiation, indicate that cardiac toxicity greater than or equal to grade 3 can occur in more than 10% of patients in the first 2 years following completion of therapy.[4,12,13]

Concurrent improvements in adjuvant therapy following definitive treatment of thoracic cancers, such as adjuvant immunotherapy for non–small cell lung cancer, have altered the natural history of the disease such that more patients are living to experience late cardiac RT-induced sequelae.

Although all factors increasing the risk of RICD are not yet identified, research has demonstrated that the presence of cardiac risk factors, including the presence of coronary artery calcifications, radiation dose received to the heart and/or cardiac substructures, and a handful of other factors can increase the risk of RICD.[4,14–24] In addition, there are several radiation techniques and technologies that can decrease cardiac exposure during RT treatment. Thus, the process of minimizing radiation dose and identifying those at highest risk is a multistep process, requiring integration of RT planning and delivery details contributing to heart dose, other potentially cardiotoxic systemic therapies delivered to the patient, and the patient's

Table 1
Clinical manifestations of radiation-induced cardiac dysfunction

CVD Pathology	Comments	Screening/Evaluation
Pericardial disease	Acute pericarditis is uncommon in the modern treatment era. Pericardial effusion can occur in as many as 36% of patients undergoing high-dose RT. Constrictive pericarditis can be seen years later in 7%–20% of patients receiving high-dose RT	Echocardiography is generally the initial screening test CT/MRI are helpful for further evaluation
Cardiomyopathy	Patients are at increased risk for systolic and diastolic heart failure, although diastolic heart failure is significantly more likely	Echocardiography approximately every 5 y Natriuretic peptides may also be useful
Coronary artery disease/ischemia	Review of available CT scans for CAC can aid with early detection of CAD to help target preventive therapy. In patients without known CAD, further ischemic evaluation should be considered at regular intervals based on the radiation received and other cardiac risk factors	ECG, CAC, CTA, stress echocardiography
Conduction abnormalities	Many types of conduction abnormalities have been reported after cardiac radiation exposure, including prolonged QTc, supraventricular arrhythmias, differing degrees of AV block, and ventricular tachycardia	ECG
Valvular heart disease	Aortic valve is most commonly involved; patients are at risk for stenosis and regurgitation	Echocardiogram approximately every 5 y

Abbreviations: AV, atrioventricular; CAC, coronary artery calcification; CAD, coronary artery disease; CT, computed tomography; CTA, computed tomographic angiography; ECG, electrocardiography; QTc, duration of the QT interval adjusted for heart rate.
Data from Refs.[25,42,59,70]

cardiometabolic health.[2,25–27] Herein, the authors review current evidence regarding elements of RT delivery and a patient's cardiometabolic health that may modulate RICD. The authors then discuss how automated surveillance of RICD risk factors within the electronic medical record (EMR) environment may be an implementation strategy to better detect and treat RICD.

ELEMENTS OF RADIATION THERAPY DELIVERY IMPACTING RADIATION-INDUCED CARDIAC DYSFUNCTION RISK

Improvements in RT treatment delivery, such as daily image guidance and highly conformal RT delivery techniques, have resulted in significant reductions in heart RT doses for patients with cancers located in the thoracic region (**Fig. 1**). Despite these improvements, some degree of cardiac dose, typically assessed as radiation to the entire heart contour, is often unavoidable for many patients with tumors/targets near the heart. Much of the data regarding RICD have been obtained from patients with left-sided breast cancer and lymphoma because these cancers were historically treated with radiation fields resulting in some degree of heart dose. Late follow-up of these patients quantified the risk per gray of mean heart dose as increasing the relative risk

of major cardiac events/heart disease by 4% to 16%.[15,19,28] Other studies have found the risk of RICD in patients with thoracic cancer to be 1.5 to 3 times higher compared with patients with cancer who did not receive thoracic RT.[29] The cellular mechanisms underlying RICD, whose investigation has been aided by the use of preclinical models and image-guided RT, are well-reviewed elsewhere, but briefly summarized in **Fig. 2**.[2,5,7,25,30–32] In developing treatment plans that result in heart doses as low as reasonably achievable to reduce a patient's risk for RICD, radiation oncologists should consider (1) patient and radiation target anatomy, (2) the specific cardiac substructures receiving dosage, (3) the potential use of patient respiratory control techniques and patient positioning to displace the heart relative to the radiation field, (4) the dose constraints and risks for radiation exposure to nearby organs-at-risk, and (5) the RT treatment modality (eg, photons and/or protons).

Whole heart and cardiac substructure dose. Guidelines from the Quantitative Analysis of Normal Tissue Effects in the Clinic (QUANTEC) report suggest that a whole heart volume receiving 25 Gy of less than 10% reduces RICD in the form of long-term cardiac death.[33] Because there is no threshold radiation dose identified below which there is no risk of RICD, and mean heart dose

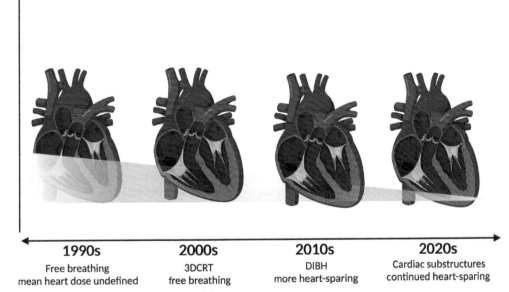

Fig. 1. Advances in RT delivery in recent decades. In the last 3 decades, the introduction of 3D conformal RT (3DCRT) and additional heart-sparing techniques have reduced the mean heart doses delivered to patients with many thoracic cancers. At present, some radiation oncologists are also starting to track the dose delivered to specific cardiac substructures, in addition to the whole heart, which, when coupled with clinical outcomes, will assist in knowledge of ideal dose constraints to these substructures. Abbreviations: DIBH, deep inspiratory breath holds; 3DCRT, 3-dimensional conformal radiation therapy. (Created with BioRender.com.)

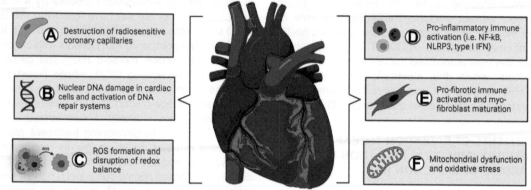

Fig. 2. Cellular mechanisms of RICD. Cardiotoxic effects of radiation are imparted through both direct and indirect means. (*A*) Coronary endothelial cells, and in particular capillary endothelial cells, are relatively radiosensitive, and destruction of coronary capillaries is thought to be a pivotal consequence of radiation, because it reduces blood supply to the myocardium and may promote thrombosis. (*B*) In all cell types, RT directly imparts damage to nuclear DNA and also enhances production of (*C*) reactive oxygen species (ROS), which preferentially degrade the protective endcaps of DNA called telomeres. (*D*) Following genomic damage, apoptotic and proinflammatory (P2X, P2Y, nuclear factor [NF]-κB, NLRP3) pathways are often activated. (*E*) Proinflammatory responses provoked by radiation are often followed by a subsequent anti-inflammatory phase, the aim of which is tissue repair and stabilization through fibrogenesis. (*F*) Radiation is destructive to mitochondrial DNA and disrupts mitochondrial oxidative metabolism, redox balance, and apoptotic signaling. Abbreviations: IFN, interferon. (Created with BioRender.com.)

can correlate with cardiac outcomes, many radiation oncologists use mean heart dose constraints to analyze potential RT treatment plans. For example, recent cooperative group breast cancer trials such as Alliance A221505 and NSABP-B51 have goals for mean heart doses less than 3 to 5 Gy. However, recent evidence also indicates that radiation delivered to certain cardiac substructures may be a better indicator of future RICD compared with mean heart dose.[3] As mean heart dose in some studies only weakly correlates with mean dose delivered to cardiac substructures, it can also be helpful for radiation oncologists to identify which cardiac substructures are receiving incidental radiation dosage.[33] In one study using an unbiased approach to assess dose-sensitive cardiac regions that correlated with survival in greater than 1100 patients with lung cancer, the dose to an area in the base of the heart including the aorta, the origin of the coronary arteries, and the sinoatrial node was most influential on patient mortality.[34] The left anterior descending artery (LAD) has also been identified as a critical substructure whose radiation may associate with subsequent cardiac events and survival,[2,33] as have other cardiac regions.[3]

Given these findings, computed tomographic (CT) scan-based manual contouring of the heart for cardiac substructures can be helpful in RT planning.[35] Manually contouring cardiac substructures is a challenging and time-consuming procedure that is all the more challenging with

non-contrast CT simulation scans.[35] Automatic segmentation based on validated cardiac atlases and facilitated by deep learning models represents an alternative to manual contouring that shows promise in optimizing pre-RT planning.[36,37] A recent comparison of atlas versus deep learning automatic segmentation applied to cardiac substructures as well as organs-at-risk in patients with breast cancer suggests that deep learning models may be the most reliable and robust of advanced contouring techniques.[36,38] Studies suggest that cardiac substructure-sparing plans can lead to reduced doses to structures such as the LAD and left ventricle in some patients.[39] As these methods and/or additional techniques to track dose to cardiac substructures become more widespread and adopted, additional evidence on doses to substructures and cardiac outcomes will help to inform ideal dose constraints for cardiac substructures.

Patient respiratory control. The heart is a dynamic structure, changing position with each cardiac cycle, as well as being displaced by changes associated with the respiratory cycle. The latter change can be exploited to increase the distance between the chest wall and anterior portion of the heart by timing radiation with an inspiratory cycle. We recently reviewed the advantages of using deep inspiratory breath holds (DIBH) in patients with breast cancer receiving RT.[40] Compared with free-breathing plans, planning performed with DIBH demonstrated reductions in mean heart dose and also mean LAD dose, given the LAD's close proximity to the chest wall.[40] The most common methods of DIBH are voluntary DIBH and moderate DIBH, in which a spirometer or other active breathing control device is used to guide a patient's breathing.[40] Use of DIBH depends on both a patient's ability to comply with the breathing instructions (ie, voluntary DIBH) as well as having sufficient pulmonary reserve to breath-hold for a time period suitable for RT delivery. Voluntary DIBH seems to be more well tolerated by patients and may decrease the time needed for both simulation and daily setup.[41,42]

Implementation of either DIBH method necessitates acquisition of at least 2 planning CT scans, one acquired during free breathing and one during DIBH. Often the decision regarding the use of DIBH is made at the time of the RT planning simulation CT scan. The decision is patient and context dependent; it cannot be reliably predicted solely from pulmonary function tests and/or diagnostic imaging. In addition, not all centers have DIBH technology available.[43]

Patient positioning. In patients with breast cancer, RT treatment in the prone position may reduce heart RT dose by physically increasing the distance between the anterior portion of the heart and the chest wall deep to the treated breast.[40] Paradoxically, in some patients prone positioning may exacerbate heart RT dose through displacement of the heart anteriorly due to gravity, which may adversely affect the heart-sparing potential of this technique.[44] Important considerations for prone versus supine patient positioning are the patient's breast volume and which breast is affected.[45] In addition to these considerations, radiation oncologists may choose to combine positional changes and DIBH to maximally spare the heart during RT. Mulliez and colleagues[46] reported that prone positioning with DIBH reduced mean heart dose by 40% compared with prone shallow breathing and that prone DIBH was at least as favorable as supine DIBH in regard to heart dose. Like DIBH, use of prone positioning is typically empirical and determined at the time of simulation with comparison to supine scans and measurement of the left ventricular wall to chest wall distance on axial CT slices. Prone positioning depends on the patient's ability to tolerate lying prone for at least 15 to 20 minutes both for simulation and daily treatments.[8]

RT modality. Most commonly, RT is delivered with high-energy photons (X-rays). Photon irradiation can be administered using 3D conformal RT (3DCRT) techniques, where CT scans are used to determine the shape and arrangement of beams to minimize doses to adjacent organs-at-risk while adequately covering the target volumes. Photon RT can also be administered using intensity-modulated radiation therapy (IMRT) or volumetric-modulated arc therapy (VMAT), where inverse planning with computers determines multiple beams/arcs with varying intensities that be administered to better spare organs at risk from high doses of radiation while adequately dosing the radiation targets. Although IMRT/VMAT can decrease high-dose volumes to many organs-at-risk, it often can result in more areas receiving lower radiation doses. The clinical implications of cardiac dose heterogeneity, that is, higher point doses restricted to smaller volumes versus lower point doses with higher cardiac integral dose, have not been well established.

Irradiation using protons is also an option at some centers. Protons are charged particles that, due to their Bragg peak properties, can result in near elimination of exit doses, which can decrease radiation exposure to organs near the targeted volumes.[47] Proton treatments are not widely used due to increased cost, limited availability of centers, and a lack of data for many tumor sites demonstrating superior outcomes or reduction in severe toxicities versus photon-based treatment. Proton therapy in breast cancer treatment has been found to significantly spare cardiac substructures compared with photon IMRT or VMAT.[48,49] Furthermore, mathematical modeling of cardiac-related morbidity in a cohort of 41 patients with breast cancer receiving RT suggests that proton therapy can reduce RICD risk compared with modern photon therapy.[50] Similar cardiac-sparing advantages using proton therapy have been demonstrated in patients with stage 3 non–small cell lung cancer.[51]

OTHER FACTORS IMPACTING RADIATION-INDUCED CARDIAC DYSFUNCTION RISK

Several additional factors beyond cardiac radiation itself impact a patient's ultimate risk for RICD. Many patients with thoracic cancers receive concurrent or sequential systemic chemo- and/or immunotherapy that can increase risk for future cardiotoxicity. Concurrent and/or sequential treatment strategies have specific benefits; for example, RT may beneficially prime the immune system toward an enhanced antitumor response during immunotherapy, and chemotherapy can act as a radiosensitizer in many settings.[52] Despite these advantages, evidence suggests that concurrent and/or sequential cancer treatments should be carefully planned to minimize RICD and other side effects. A patient's existing cardiometabolic health, which includes both existing cardiac diagnoses and cardiometabolic risk factors, including factors such as smoking, dyslipidemia, hypertension, body mass index greater than 30 kg/m^2, and/or diabetes mellitus, can increase the absolute risk of future cardiac dysfunction in patients with cancer after cardiac radiation exposure.[14,15,19,53–55] It is currently routine for cardiometabolic data to be acquired in patients with cancer during initial history and physical examination, as well as in survivorship clinics during long-term follow-up; however, these data are not always routinely used to guide patient referrals to cardiology/cardio-oncology post-RT.

Concurrent and/or sequential cancer therapies. Just as is the case for RT, immunotherapy, chemotherapy, and other targeted systemic therapies are each independently linked to cardiac dysfunction.[56–58] Indeed, recommendations from the National Comprehensive Cancer Network acknowledge both trastuzumab and anthracycline treatment as cardiac risk factors. When assessed at a median of 10 years posttreatment, breast cancer survivors receiving chemotherapy with or without RT were found to have elevated risk for left ventricular dysfunction.[59] Furthermore, the observed association between chemotherapy and future cardiac dysfunction persisted after adjustment for cardiometabolic risk factors.[59] Dolladille and colleagues[60] recently described increased rates of late left ventricular systolic dysfunction and heart failure in patients with cancer treated with immune checkpoint inhibitors. In particular, nivolumab has been reported to elicit increased cardiac adverse events compared with other immune checkpoint inhibitors.[61]

Of great interest is the potential for RT and other concurrent/sequential cancer treatments to be additive or synergistic in their impact on cardiac dysfunction. Preclinical models suggest that concurrent RT and immune checkpoint blockade (eg, anti-PD-1 therapy) exacerbates cardiac dysfunction, potentially through shared immune axes.[62,63] Studies in patients with cancer also report a greater incidence of RICD in patients with thoracic cancer treated with anthracycline chemotherapy compared with those treated with RT alone.[64] Findings from Hardy and colleagues[65] suggest that chemoradiation and chemotherapy treatments may have differential impacts on the heart, with the former increasing a patient's risk for heart failure and ischemic heart disease and the latter increasing risk for heart failure and conduction disorders. Guidelines from the American Society of Clinical Oncology state that patients receiving both low-dose anthracycline and low-dose RT (<30 Gy) are at high risk for cardiac dysfunction.[8] Other guidelines also note that anthracycline treatment increases the risk of RICD after cardiac radiation exposure.[8–10,27]

Patient cardiometabolic health. Patients with thoracic cancer often enter primary cancer treatment with one or more clinically diagnosed cardiovascular diseases (CVD) or cardiometabolic risk factors; in fact, between 27% and 43% of patients with lung cancer have one or more forms of CVD or cardiometabolic risk factors by the time of RT.[66] As discussed earlier, current evidence suggests that existing CVD and cardiometabolic risk factors increase a patient's risk for RICD. Predictive mathematical modeling constructed by Kim and colleagues[14] suggests that existing cardiometabolic dysfunction (hypertension, age, body mass index, dyslipidemia, diabetes mellitus, myocardial infarction, peripheral arterial disease, heart failure, stroke) is associated with the risk of cardiovascular outcomes after cancer treatment in a patient with breast cancer. In agreement with this modeling, a longitudinal study of greater than 10,000 patients with thoracic cancer performed by Armstrong and colleagues[64] demonstrated that patients with two or more CVD risk factors had greater risk of future cardiovascular events. In particular, smoking has been found to elevate the risk of cardiac mortality and/or myocardial infarction after RT by more than 3-fold.[15,53]

In addition to traditional cardiometabolic risk factors, coronary artery calcification (CAC) score may be of specific importance to the determination of RICD risk. In the general population, CAC is a validated marker of overall atherosclerotic burden and is a strong predictor of future cardiovascular events.[67] In patients with cancer receiving RT, CAC measured by planning CT is correlated with future occurrence of adverse cardiac event.[68,69] Furthermore, CAC observed during the post-RT period may be more predictive of RICD than traditional risk scores, such as the Framingham risk score.[70]

AUTOMATED ELECTRONIC MEDICAL RECORD TRACKING AND PHYSICIAN NOTIFICATION AS A POTENTIAL STRATEGY TO BETTER DETECT AND TREAT RADIATION-INDUCED CARDIAC DYSFUNCTION

Multiple organizations have set forth imaging screening guidelines and consensus recommendations for patients with thoracic cancer receiving RT,[3,8–10,27] which are meant to guide health care providers in their detection and treatment of RICD. Despite these guidelines, survey data gathered by Amin and colleagues[66] between 2017 and 2019 indicated that 69% of radiation oncologists perceived a lack of evidence for the type and timing of cardiac monitoring in patients with thoracic cancer. Greater than 40% of respondents indicated that they did not have an established referral plan if CAC was observed on a patient's planning CT,[66] which may result in preventative therapies such as statins being overlooked. These responses highlight the importance of developing strategies that aid radiation oncologists and treating physicians in detecting RICD risk and in planning subsequent care appropriately.

EMR tracking and surveillance of RICD risk factors may serve as a potential strategy to mitigate the challenges identified by Amin and colleagues[66] and others. Indeed, EMRs present a unique opportunity to integrate seemingly unrelated data points, such as cardiometabolic risk factors, and present these points to cardiology and/or oncology physicians via automatically triggered reminders. This concept was recently demonstrated in a non-cancer population; EMR alerts to cardiologists increased the optimal dosing of statin prescription to patients with underlying atherosclerotic CVD.[71]

The ability to use EMRs to create alerts and notifications from new guidelines depends on several factors, such as the ability to personalize and create new reminders within the available EMR framework and the readiness for the organization to implement such changes. **Fig. 3** provides a visual framework for the use of EMRs to track and notify health care providers of cancer treatment attributes and patient cardiometabolic health factors that may impact risk for RICD. In the pre-RT period, EMRs could "flag" existing CVD and/or cardiometabolic risk factors that have been identified at previous wellness visits. In the case that some pertinent health information is not available, radiation oncologists may deem it necessary to have patients with thoracic cancer screened according to best practices.[27] In addition, efforts to readily identify patients with baseline CAC on their radiation planning or cancer staging CT scans can identify those with underlying CAD who may benefit from cardiovascular preventive therapy. In this area, artificial intelligence shows great promise in its ability to automatically screen non-gated CT scans for the presence of coronary artery calcium to improve CAC reporting and subsequent targeting of preventive therapies.[72] Radiation oncologists can further supplement the EMR by specific inclusion of heart and cardiac substructure dosimetry in completion of therapy records to assist in further risk stratification and coordination between treatment teams. In the post-RT period, EMRs can alert treating physicians to a patient's prior RT as well as elements of their RT delivery that may impact RICD risk, as detailed earlier. As previously stated, many patients with thoracic cancer will not develop clinically overt

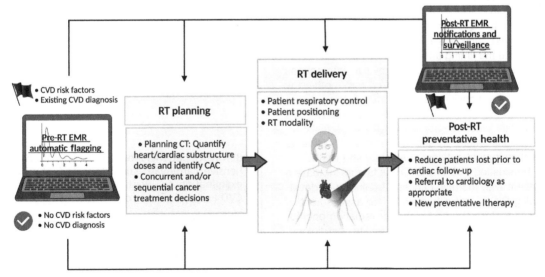

Fig. 3. Health implementation strategies to improve the detection and treatment of RICD. In the pre-RT period, EMRs indicating the presence of cardiovascular disease (CVD) and/or cardiometabolic risk factors can identify the need for cardiovascular health optimization. Likewise, identification of coronary artery calcification (CAC) on RT planning CTs can inform cardiac care. Cardiac doses can be minimized by tracking doses and using cardiac-sparing techniques based on individual patient factors. In the post-RT period, automated EMR notifications to treating physicians concerning elements of a patient's RT and cardiometabolic health can reduce patients lost to follow-up, aid in the appropriate referral of patients to cardiologists, and inform the use of cardiac therapies to minimize clinical effects of cardiac radiation exposure. (Created with BioRender.com.)

RICD for many years after treatment; therefore, automated EMR notifications directed to treating physicians in the post-RT period may help to address the issue of patients lost to follow-up before the occurrence of a cardiac event.

DISCUSSION AND SUMMARY

A significant proportion of patients with thoracic cancer receiving RT will develop some form of RICD. There is currently no standardized method by which to risk stratify patients with thoracic cancer for RICD; however, current data suggest that risk is impacted by several factors that are both radiation dependent and independent. Screening and surveillance for these factors in both the pre-RT and post-RT periods may be a useful tool for radiation oncologists, cardiologists, and cardio-oncologists seeking to refine the prevention, detection, and/or treatment of RICD.

Current evidence suggests that the dose of radiation delivered to cardiac substructures may better predict risk for RICD compared with mean heart dose. However, more work is needed to determine which specific substructures are most critical to this relationship and what dose constraints should be ideal for planning purposes. As this body of knowledge grows, simultaneous advances in atlas- and deep-learning-based cardiac segmentation can aid radiation oncologists in planning RT that minimizes substructure doses. It may be the case for some patients that important substructures cannot be completely avoided during RT, and this information can be used to optimize the timing and frequency of post-RT cardio-oncological follow-up. Likewise, interactions between RT and chemo- and/or immunotherapy should be considered when determining future risk for RICD. Additional investigation is needed to further elucidate additive and/or synergistic interactions among RT and other primary treatments as they impact anticancer efficacy and RICD.

Preexisting CVD and CVD risk factors increase a patient with thoracic cancer's likelihood of developing RICD, and a framework for assessment of these factors can be helpful for radiation oncologists to risk stratify and refer to cardiology/cardio-oncology to optimize cardiac health as appropriate. Identification of CAC is predictive of future cardiovascular risk in the general population and should be considered a similar tool in patients with thoracic cancer receiving RT. Automatic flagging of patient medical records for CVD, cardiometabolic risk factors, and CAC may be an effective strategy for identifying the need for cardio-oncological referral in these patients. Future longitudinal investigations are needed to elucidate the efficacy of such strategies within different thoracic cancer patient populations receiving RT and in different health care settings.

There are several challenges and opportunities for researchers as we seek to better understand, prevent, and treat RICD. Contrary to the tactics used to minimize RT exposure in patients with cancer, localized high-dose RT is now being used at several centers worldwide to treat refractory ventricular tachycardia.[73] Although the original rationale for using RT for this indication stemmed from the hypothesis that RT would create transmural fibrotic scarring in the treated area, additional preclinical studies now indicate that other mechanisms[74,75] may play a role in the dramatic reduction in ventricular tachycardia events seen after targeted treatment with high doses of cardiac RT.[76] Analysis of long-term data from patients treated with these focal high-dose RT treatments may lead to new insights into RICD mechanisms, as well as the radiation-induced remodeling that occurs in hearts with compromised function at the time of treatment. Such studies, coupled with ongoing research using preclinical models and patient samples, may also lead to the identification of biomarkers for earlier RICD detection and subsequent intervention. Finally, more research is needed to identify strategies that promote cardiac microvascular and cellular resilience following radiation injury, thereby revealing therapeutics to prevent and/or treat RICD. These future studies, coupled with the implementation interventions noted earlier, have the potential to improve the therapeutic ratio of RT by minimizing the incidence and severity of RICD.

CLINICS CARE POINTS

- Before RT, patients should undergo a comprehensive cardiovascular history and physical examination to identify and treat existing CVD and optimize cardiovascular risk factors.

- The heart should be contoured for RT planning, with consideration of contouring and tracking doses to cardiac substructures. In addition, the planning CT should be used to identify CAC as a marker of existing coronary artery disease.

- Heart-sparing techniques (eg, respiratory gating, deep inspiration breath hold, prone positioning, or proton RT) should be considered for RT delivery.

- In the post-RT period, patients should undergo regular cardiovascular history and physical examination as well as screening for CVD per existing recommendations. EMR notifications addressing patient's history of RT and cardiometabolic health is a potential strategy to reduce patients lost to follow-up and to aid in appropriate patient referral to cardiologists.

REFERENCES

1. American Cancer Society. Cancer Treatment & Survivorship Facts & Figures 2019-2021. Atlanta: American Cancer Society; 2019. Available at: https://www.cancer.org/research/cancer-facts-statistics/survivor-facts-figures.html.
2. Zorn SR, Rayan D, Brown SA, et al. Radiation-induced cardiotoxicity: from bench to bedside and beyond. Adv Oncol 2021;1:1–13.
3. Bergom C, Bradley JA, Ng AK, et al. Past, present, and future of radiation-induced cardiotoxicity: refinements in targeting, surveillance, and risk stratification. JACC CardioOncol 2021;3(3):343–59.
4. Wang H, Wei H, Zheng Q, et al. Radiation-induced heart disease: a review of classification, mechanism and prevention. Int J Biol Sci 2019;15(10):2128–38.
5. Schlaak RA, SenthilKumar G, Boerma M, et al. Advances in preclinical research models of radiation-induced cardiac toxicity. Cancers (Basel) 2020;12(2):415.
6. Suchorska WM. Radiobiological models in prediction of radiation cardiotoxicity. Rep Pract Oncol Radiother 2020;25(1):46–9.
7. Jaworski C, Mariani JA, Wheeler G, et al. Cardiac complications of thoracic irradiation. J Am Coll Cardiol 2013;61(23):2319–28.
8. Armenian SH, Lacchetti C, Lenihan D. Prevention and Monitoring of Cardiac Dysfunction in Survivors of Adult Cancers: American Society of Clinical Oncology Clinical Practice Guideline Summary. J Oncol Pract 2017;35(8):893–911.
9. Curigliano G, Lenihan D, Fradley M, et al. Management of cardiac disease in cancer patients throughout oncological treatment: ESMO consensus recommendations. Ann Oncol 2020;31(2):171–90.
10. Lancellotti P, Nkomo VT, Badano LP, et al. Expert consensus for multi-modality imaging evaluation of cardiovascular complications of radiotherapy in adults: a report from the European Association of Cardiovascular Imaging and the American Society of Echocardiography. Eur Heart J Card Img 2013;14(8):721–40.
11. Desai MY, Windecker S, Lancellotti P, et al. Prevention, diagnosis, and management of radiation-associated cardiac disease: JACC scientific expert panel. J Am Coll Cardiol 2019;74:905–27.
12. Beukema JC, van Luijk P, Widder J, et al. Is cardiac toxicity a relevant issue in the radiation treatment of esophageal cancer? Radiother Oncol 2015;114(1):85–90.
13. Dess RT, Sun YL, Matuszak MM, et al. Cardiac events after radiation therapy: combined analysis of prospective multicenter trials for locally advanced non-small-cell lung cancer. J Clin Oncol 2017;35(13):1395–402.
14. Kim D, Park MS, Youn JC, et al. Development and validation of a risk score model for predicting the cardiovascular outcomes after breast Cancer therapy: the CHEMO-RADIAT score. J Am Heart Assoc 2021;10(16):e021931.
15. Taylor C, Correa C, Duane FK, et al. Estimating the risks of breast cancer radiotherapy: evidence from modern radiation doses to the lungs and heart and from previous randomized trials. J Clin Oncol 2017;35(15):1641–9.
16. Virani SS, Alonso A, Aparicio HJ, et al. Heart disease and stroke statistics-2021 update a report from the american heart association. Circulation 2021;143(8):e254–743.
17. Andrews J, Psaltis PJ, Bartolo BAD, et al. Coronary arterial calcification: a review of mechanisms, promoters and imaging. Trends Cardiovasc Med 2018;28(8):491–501.
18. Cutter DJ, Schaapveld M, Darby SC, et al. Risk of valvular heart disease after treatment for Hodgkin lymphoma. J Natl Cancer Inst 2015;107(4):djv008.
19. Darby SC, Ewertz M, McGale P, et al. Risk of ischemic heart disease in women after radiotherapy for breast cancer. N Engl J Med 2013;368(11):987–98.
20. Liu LK, Ouyang W, Zhao X, et al. Pathogenesis and prevention of radiation-induced myocardial fibrosis. Asian Pac J Cancer Prev 2017;18(3):583–7.
21. Madan R, Benson R, Sharma DN, et al. Radiation induced heart disease: Pathogenesis, management and review literature. J Egypt Natl Canc Inst 2015;27(4):187–93.
22. Veinot JP, Edwards WD. Pathology of radiation-induced heart disease: a surgical and autopsy study of 27 cases. Hum Pathol 1996;27(8):766–73.
23. Wethal T, Lund MB, Edvardsen T, et al. Valvular dysfunction and left ventricular changes in Hodgkin's lymphoma survivors. A longitudinal study. Br J Cancer 2009;101(4):575–81.
24. Yusuf SW, Sami S, Daher IN. Radiation-induced heart disease: a clinical update. Cardiol Res Pract 2011;2011:317659.
25. Ell P, Martin JM, Cehic DA, et al. Cardiotoxicity of radiation therapy: mechanisms, management, and mitigation. Curr Treat Options Oncol 2021;22(8):70.
26. Salomaa S, Jung T. Roadmap for research on individual radiosensitivity and radiosusceptibility - the MELODI view on research needs. Int J Radiat Biol 2020;96(3):277–9.

27. Mitchell JD, Cehic DA. Cardiovascular manifestation from therapeutic radiation. JACC-CardioOncol 2021; 3(3):360–80.

28. van den Bogaard VA, Ta BD, van der Schaaf A, et al. Validation and modification of a prediction model for acute cardiac events in patients with breast cancer treated with radiotherapy based on three-dimensional dose distributions to cardiac substructures. J Clin Oncol 2017;35(11):1171–8.

29. Raghunathan D, Khilji MI, Hassan SA, et al. Radiation-induced cardiovascular disease. Curr Atheroscler Rep 2017;19(5):22.

30. Livingston K, Schlaak RA, Puckett LL, et al. The role of mitochondrial dysfunction in radiation-induced heart disease: from bench to bedside. Front Cardiovasc Med 2020;7:20.

31. Gujral DM, Lloyd G, Bhattacharyya S. Radiation-induced valvular heart disease. Heart 2016;102(4): 269–76.

32. Ganatra S, Chatur S, Nohria A. How to diagnose and manage radiation cardiotoxicity. JACC CardioOncol 2020;2(4):655–60.

33. Beaton L, Bergman A, Nichol A, et al. Cardiac death after breast radiotherapy and the QUANTEC cardiac guidelines. Clin Transl Radiat Oncol 2019; 19:39–45.

34. McWilliam A, Kennedy J, Hodgson C, et al. Radiation dose to heart base linked with poorer survival in lung cancer patients. Eur J Cancer 2017;85:106–13.

35. Zhou J, Liu Y, Huang L, et al. Validation and comparison of four models to calculate pretest probability of obstructive coronary artery disease in a Chinese population: A coronary computed tomographic angiography study. J Cardiovasc Comput Tomogr 2017;11(4):317–23.

36. Choi MS, Choi BS, Chung SY, et al. Clinical evaluation of atlas- and deep learning-based automatic segmentation of multiple organs and clinical target volumes for breast cancer. Radiother Oncol 2020; 153:139–45.

37. Zhou R, Liao Z, Pan T, et al. Cardiac atlas development and validation for automatic segmentation of cardiac substructures. Radiother Oncol 2017; 122(1):66–71.

38. Henke LE, Olsen JR, Contreras JA, et al. Stereotactic MR-guided online adaptive radiation therapy (SMART) for Ultracentral thorax malignancies: results of a phase 1 trial. Adv Radiat Oncol 2019; 4(1):201–9.

39. Morris ED, Aldridge K, Ghanem AI, et al. Incorporating sensitive cardiac structure sparing into radiation therapy planning. J Appl Clin Med Phys 2020; 21(11):195–204.

40. Bergom C, Currey A, Desai N, et al. Deep inspiration breath hold: techniques and advantages for cardiac sparing during breast cancer irradiation. Front Oncol 2018;8:87.

41. Bartlett FR, Colgan RM, Donovan EM, et al. Voluntary breath-hold technique for reducing heart dose in left breast radiotherapy. J Vis Exp 2014;89:51578.

42. Bartlett FR, Yarnold JR, Kirby AM. Breast radiotherapy and heart disease - where are we now? Clin Oncol-Uk 2013;25(12):687–9.

43. Desai N, Currey AD, Kelly TR, et al. Nationwide trends in heart-sparing techniques utilized in radiation therapy for breast cancer. Int J Radiat Oncol 2018;102(3):E599.

44. Chino JP, Marks LB. Prone positioning causes the heart to be displaced anteriorly within the thorax: Implications for breast cancer treatment. Int J Radiat Oncol 2008;70(3):916–20.

45. Kirby AM, Evans PM, Donovan EM, et al. Prone versus supine positioning for whole and partial-breast radiotherapy: a comparison of non-target tissue dosimetry. Radiother Oncol 2010;96(2):178–84.

46. Mulliez T, Veldeman L, Speleers B, et al. Heart dose reduction by prone deep inspiration breath hold in left-sided breast irradiation. Radiother Oncol 2015; 114(1):79–84.

47. Levin WP, Kooy H, Loeffler JS, et al. Proton beam therapy. Br J Cancer 2005;93(8):849–54.

48. Fagundes MA, Robison B, Price SG, et al. High-dose rectal sparing with transperineal injection of hydrogel spacer in intensity modulated proton therapy for localized prostate cancer. Int J Radiat Oncol 2015;93(3):E230.

49. Loap P, Tkatchenko N, Goudjil F, et al. Cardiac substructure exposure in breast radiotherapy: a comparison between intensity modulated proton therapy and volumetric modulated arc therapy. Acta Oncol 2021;60(8):1038–44.

50. Stick LB, Yu J, Maraldo MV, et al. Joint estimation of cardiac toxicity and recurrence risks after comprehensive nodal photon versus proton therapy for breast cancer. Int J Radiat Oncol 2017;97(4): 754–61.

51. Ferris MJ, Martin KS, Switchenko JM, et al. Sparing cardiac substructures with optimized volumetric modulated arc therapy and intensity modulated proton therapy in thoracic radiation for locally advanced non-small cell lung cancer. Pract Radiat Oncol 2019; 9(5):E473–81.

52. Jagodinsky JC, Harari PM, Morris ZS. The promise of combining radiation therapy with immunotherapy. Int J Radiat Oncol 2020;108(1):6–16.

53. Hooning MJ, Botma A, Aleman BMP, et al. Long-term risk of cardiovascular disease in 10-year survivors of breast cancer. J Natl Cancer Inst 2007;99: 365–75.

54. Wethal T, Nedregaard B, Andersen R, et al. Atherosclerotic lesions in lymphoma survivors treated with radiotherapy. Radiother Oncol 2014;110:448–54.

55. Atkins KM, Chaunzwa TL, Lamba N, et al. Association of left anterior descending coronary artery

radiation dose with major adverse cardiac events and mortality in patients with non–small cell lung cancer. JAMA Oncol 2021;7:206–19.

56. Heinzerling L, Ott PA, Hodi FS, et al. Cardiotoxicity associated with CTLA4 and PD1 blocking immunotherapy. J Immunother Cancer 2016;4:50.

57. McGowan JV, Chung R, Maulik A, et al. Anthracycline chemotherapy and cardiotoxicity. Cardiovasc Drugs Ther 2017;31(1):63–75.

58. Cho H, Lee S, Sim SH, et al. Cumulative incidence of chemotherapy-induced cardiotoxicity during a 2-year follow-up period in breast cancer patients. Breast Cancer Res Treat 2020;182(2):333–43.

59. Boerman LM, Maass SWMC, van der Meer P, et al. Long-term outcome of cardiac function in a population-based cohort of breast cancer survivors: a cross-sectional study. Eur J Cancer 2017;81: 56–65.

60. Dolladille C, Ederhy S, Sassier M, et al. Immune checkpoint inhibitor rechallenge after immune-related adverse events in patients with cancer. JAMA Oncol 2020;6(6):865–71.

61. Mascolo A, Scavone C, Ferrajolo C, et al. Immune checkpoint inhibitors and cardiotoxicity: an analysis of spontaneous reports in eudravigilance. Drug Saf 2021;44(9):957–71.

62. Myers CJ, Lu B. Decreased survival after combining thoracic irradiation and an Anti-PD-1 Antibody correlated with increased T-cell infiltration into cardiac and lung tissues. Int J Radiat Oncol 2017;99(5): 1129–36.

63. Du SS, Zhou L, Alexander GS, et al. PD-1 modulates radiation-induced cardiac toxicity through cytotoxic T lymphocytes. J Thorac Oncol 2018;13(4):510–20.

64. Armstrong GT, Oeffinger KC, Chen Y, et al. Modifiable risk factors and major cardiac events among adult survivors of childhood cancer. J Clin Oncol 2013;31(29):3673–80.

65. Hardy D, Liu CC, Cormier JN, et al. Cardiac toxicity in association with chemotherapy and radiation therapy in a large cohort of older patients with non-small-cell lung cancer. Ann Oncol 2010;21(9): 1825–33.

66. Amin NP, Desai N, Kim SM, et al. Cardiac monitoring for thoracic radiation therapy: survey of practice patterns in the United States. Am J Clin Oncol 2020;43(4):249–56.

67. Yeboah J, McClelland RL, Polonsky TS, et al. Comparison of novel risk markers for improvement in cardiovascular risk assessment in intermediate-risk individuals. JAMA 2012;308(8):788–95.

68. Roos CTG, van den Bogaard VAB, Greuter MJW, et al. Is the coronary artery calcium score associated with acute coronary events in breast cancer patients treated with radiotherapy? Radiother Oncol 2018;126(1):170–6.

69. Tjessem KH, Bosse G, Fossa K, et al. Coronary calcium score in 12-year breast cancer survivors after adjuvant radiotherapy with low to moderate heart exposure - Relationship to cardiac radiation dose and cardiovascular risk factors. Radiother Oncol 2015;114(3):328–34.

70. Tomizawa N. Could coronary calcification identified at non-gated chest CT be a predictor for cardiovascular events in breast cancer patients? Int J Cardiol 2019;282:108–9.

71. Adusumalli S, Westover JE, Jacoby DS, et al. Effect of passive choice and active choice interventions in the electronic health record to cardiologists on statin prescribing a cluster randomized clinical trial. JAMA Cardiol 2021;6(1):40–8.

72. Eng D, Chute C, Khandwala N, et al. Automated coronary calcium scoring using deep learning with multicenter external validation. NPJ Digital Med 2021;4:88.

73. van der Ree MH, Blanck O, Limpens J, et al. Cardiac radioablation—a systematic review. Heart Rhythm 2020;17:1381–92.

74. Zhang DM, Szymanski J, Bergom C, et al. Leveraging radiobiology for arrhythmia management: a new treatment paradigm? Clin Oncol (R Coll Radiol) 2021;33(11):723–34.

75. Zhang DM, Navara R, Yin T, et al. Cardiac radiotherapy induces electrical conduction reprogramming in the absence of transmural fibrosis. Nat Commun 2021;12(1):5558.

76. Robinson CG, Samson PP, Moore KMS, et al. Phase I/II trial of electrophysiology-guided noninvasive cardiac radioablation for ventricular tachycardia. Circulation 2019;139(3):313–21.

Understanding Myocardial Metabolism in the Context of Cardio-Oncology

Jing Liu, MD, PhD[a], Zsu-Zsu Chen, MD[b], Jagvi Patel, BS[a], Aarti Asnani, MD[a],*

KEYWORDS

- Myocardial metabolism • Cardio-oncology • Chemotherapy • Metabolic disorders • Heart failure

KEY POINTS

- Metabolic pathways implicated in the pathogenesis of anthracycline-associated cardiotoxicity include DNA damage, glucose metabolism disorders, and mitochondrial and iron metabolism dysfunction.
- Chemotherapeutics targeting tumor metabolism have the potential to adversely affect the heart.
- New biomarkers and cardioprotective strategies are needed for the early diagnosis of cancer therapy-induced cardiovascular events.

INTRODUCTION

Cardiovascular diseases (CVD) that develop during or after cancer therapy have become a major cause of morbidity and mortality in cancer survivors. To optimize the outcomes of patients with cancer with pre-existing CVD or those that develop CVD as a consequence of therapy, a new cardiology subspecialty named "cardio-oncology" has boomed over the past decade. Cardio-oncology is focused on the prevention, diagnosis, treatment, and follow-up of CVD that arises in the setting of cancer therapy.[1,2] Cancer treatments include traditional and targeted therapies, radiotherapy, immunotherapy, surgery, and stem cell transplant. Among these, chemotherapy is a mainstay of treatment of various cancers such as malignant lymphoma and small cell lung cancer.[3,4] However, chemotherapy-induced cardiotoxicity is a serious complication that can be life threatening and limits the clinical use of various chemotherapeutic agents, particularly those of the anthracycline class.[3]

Molecular mechanisms of chemotherapy-induced cardiotoxicity are complex, including the generation of reactive oxygen species (ROS) and increased oxidative stress, DNA damage, iron metabolism dysfunction, and mitochondrial disorders.[5–8] Recent studies in cancer cell metabolism provide unprecedented opportunities for a new understanding of myocardial metabolism and may offer new approaches for the treatment of CVD. A deeper understanding of the molecular mechanisms underlying both tumor and myocardial metabolism during cancer treatment may lead to the development of personalized treatment regimens with the goal of limiting cardiotoxicity.[9]

In this review, we will discuss the role of metabolism in anthracycline cardiomyopathy, the potential metabolic effects of newer cancer treatments, and proposed areas of overlap between myocardial and tumor metabolic pathways.

ANTHRACYCLINES AND MYOCARDIAL METABOLISM

Traditional chemotherapies target cells at different phases of the cell cycle. Anthracyclines are antitumor antibiotics that interfere with enzymes involved in DNA replication and are capable of

[a] Division of Cardiovascular Medicine, Department of Medicine, Beth Israel Deaconess Medical Center, Harvard Medical School, 330 Brookline Ave, Boston, MA 02215, USA; [b] Division of Endocrinology, Diabetes, and Metabolism, Department of Medicine, Beth Israel Deaconess Medical Center, Harvard Medical School, 330 Brookline Ave, Boston, MA 02215, USA
* Corresponding author. Center for Life Science, 3 Blackfan Circle, Room 911, Boston, MA 02115.
E-mail address: aasnani@bidmc.harvard.edu

Heart Failure Clin 18 (2022) 415–424
https://doi.org/10.1016/j.hfc.2022.02.004
1551-7136/22/© 2022 Elsevier Inc. All rights reserved.

cytotoxicity regardless of the cell cycle phase.[10,11] Anthracyclines are thought to inhibit the proliferation of rapidly dividing cells through multiple mechanisms, including their ability to intercalate between and cross-link DNA strands, to alkylate DNA, and to interfere with topoisomerase II.[12–14] As a result, DNA unwinding and strand separation are prevented, thereby blocking DNA replication and transcription. In addition, anthracyclines generate highly reactive free radicals which can result in abundant damage to DNA and to the plasma membrane through lipid oxidation.[15–18] Despite their cytostatic and cytotoxic effects against a wide variety of solid tumors and hematologic malignancies, their clinical use is hindered by tumor resistance and toxicity to healthy tissues. The major toxic side effect of anthracyclines in patients with cancer relates to their cardiotoxic properties.[19] Doxorubicin (DOX) is a highly effective chemotherapeutic drug belonging to the nonselective class I anthracycline family,[20] which is widely used for the treatment of solid tumors as well as leukemia and lymphoma.[21,22] However, its clinical use is limited by its cumulative cardiotoxicity, which can lead to myocardial dysfunction and ultimately heart failure in many patients.[23–25]

Compared with other tissues, the heart is particularly susceptible to metabolic toxicities due to its high bioenergetic needs and dependence on ATP to sustain contractile function, basal metabolic processes, and ionic homeostasis. In the normal adult heart, fatty acids are the main substrate used to provide energy (~50%-70%), with the remainder being derived from glycolysis and GTP formation in the tricarboxylic acid (TCA) cycle.[26] Under normal conditions, glucose metabolism and fatty acid metabolism work together to provide ATP; however, during pathologic conditions such as anthracycline cardiomyopathy, fatty acid and glucose metabolism can switch. While this switch is compensatory early on, persistent glycolysis is maladaptive and leads to energetic failure.[27] Animal studies have shown that cardiac insulin resistance is a putative early marker of heart stress.[28] Consistent with these preclinical findings, inhibition of glucose uptake consequent to insulin signaling desensitization is a clinical risk factor for heart failure, and disruption of cardiac metabolic adaptation has been associated with worse prognosis.[29,30] In line with these observations, Taegtmeyer and colleagues have proposed insulin resistance as a physiologic adaptation to nonischemic cardiac injury, protecting cardiomyocytes from substrate overload in dysregulated metabolic states. Impairment of insulin signaling has been reported to reduce glucose uptake and activate fatty acid oxidation in an AMPK-dependent manner. AMPK triggers long-term catabolic pathways that generate ATP, including fatty acid oxidation and glycolysis, while downregulating processes that are dispensable for short-term cell survival, such as the biosynthetic metabolism that rapidly consumes the ATP pool.[30–33] DOX-mediated disruption of AMPK drives metabolic disarrangements and cellular substrate overload. Experimental evidence shows that DOX-induced AMPK inhibition increases glucose uptake after 2 weeks of treatment, probably due to concomitant expression of GLUT1, an insulin-independent glucose transporter normally absent in the adult heart.[34,35]

Mitochondrial dysfunction and oxidative stress have also been demonstrated to play a central role in DOX-induced cardiotoxicity.[36,37] As a consequence of its accumulation within mitochondria, DOX uncouples mitochondrial respiratory chain complexes, eventually impairing ATP production.[38] Thus, DOX cardiotoxicity directly contributes to ATP deficiency, altering mitochondrial energy metabolism and bioenergetics.[39] DOX also forms adducts with mitochondrial DNA and binds to other biomolecules like the mitochondrial abundant phospholipid cardiolipin. Mitochondrial DNA oxidation has been postulated to be cardioselective and cumulative,[40] thereby contributing to the development of heart failure.[41] Once DOX accumulates in mitochondria, it can initiate the production of intramitochondrial ROS and reactive nitrogen species (RNS) by various, mainly nonenzymatic mechanisms, leading to the activation of cell death pathways.[42] For instance, the activation of various molecular signals downstream of AMPK can influence the Bcl-2/Bax apoptosis pathway. By altering the Bcl-2/Bax ratio, downstream activation of caspases leads to apoptosis.[11] In parallel, increased ROS production induces the activation of pro-inflammatory transcription factor NF-κB and inducible nitric oxide synthase.[43] The diffusion-limited reaction of superoxide and nitric oxide forms peroxynitrite, a potent oxidant that further potentiates the initiation of cell death.[44] Impaired mitochondrial biogenesis contributes to DOX cardiotoxicity in preclinical models,[45–47] and defects in anaplerosis have been described in other types of heart failure.[48] Our group and others have demonstrated that the measurement of plasma metabolites in oncology patients has the potential to provide insights into cellular metabolism, specifically mitochondrial metabolism.[49,50] In our study, we assessed the role of intermediary metabolism in 38 women with breast cancer treated with anthracyclines and trastuzumab. Using targeted mass spectrometry to measure 71 metabolites in the plasma, we identified changes in citric acid and aconitic acid that differentiated patients who developed cardiotoxicity from those who did not. In patients with cardiotoxicity, the magnitude of change in citric acid at 3 months correlated with the change in left ventricular ejection fraction (LVEF) and absolute LVEF at 9 months. Patients with cardiotoxicity also demonstrated more pronounced changes in purine and pyrimidine metabolism. Although further mechanistic work is needed to validate these findings, early metabolic changes may provide insight into the mechanisms associated with the development of chemotherapy-associated cardiotoxicity.[51]

Impairment of cellular iron metabolism is another major contributor to DOX-induced cardiotoxicity.[52,53] Iron accumulation into mitochondria has been linked to ferroptosis, a recently described form of iron-dependent cell death, which is morphologically, biochemically, and genetically distinct from apoptosis, necrosis, and autophagy. Ferroptosis is characterized by mitochondrial iron accumulation and lipid peroxidation.[54] In a study by Fang and colleagues, mice defective for canonical activators of necroptosis or apoptosis or both (Ripk3$^{-/-}$, Mlkl$^{-/-}$, or Fadd$^{-/-}$ Mlkl$^{-/-}$, respectively), showed typical hallmarks of ferroptosis in cardiomyocytes after DOX administration. This study demonstrated that ferroptosis is triggered by heme oxygenase-1-mediated heme degradation through an Nrf2-dependent mechanism that drastically induces iron overload in mitochondria, thereby activating ferroptosis.[55] In addition, DOX can interact with iron directly to form a complex that results in iron cycling between the ferrous [Fe(II)] and ferric [Fe(III)] forms, leading to additional ROS production.[56] DOX-induced oxidative stress is further aggravated by the interaction with iron and/or inhibition of antioxidant mechanisms by DOX. Taken together, several metabolic mechanisms contribute to the pathogenesis of anthracycline cardiotoxicity, as summarized in **Fig. 1** and **Table 1**.

EPIGENETIC REGULATION IN CANCER AND MYOCARDIAL METABOLISM

Epigenetics refers to heritable modifications to the genome that occur independently of variations in the DNA sequence, including DNA methylation, histone modifications, and various RNA-mediated processes.[57,58] Epigenetic mechanisms are required to maintain normal growth, development, and homeostatic gene expression in different organs. Abnormal epigenetic regulation may lead to tumorigenesis and the development of cancer. For instance, DNA hypomethylation, histone modification, and miRNAs have been reported to be involved in the development of breast, prostate, lung, and colon cancer.[59,60] The recognition of epigenetic abnormalities driving tumor growth has led to the development of specific treatments targeting epigenetics in cancer.[61] Histone acetylation, a well-studied posttranslational histone modification, is controlled by the opposing activities of histone acetyltransferases (HATs) and histone deacetylases (HDACs).[62] In many patients with cancer, a high level of HDACs is associated with advanced disease and poor outcomes in patients. Inhibition of HDACs can induce tumor cell apoptosis, growth arrest, senescence, differentiation, and immunogenicity, and inhibit angiogenesis.[63] The most successful clinical application of HDAC inhibitors (HDACis) has been the use of vorinostat and romidepsin against refractory cutaneous and peripheral T cell lymphoma.[63] In addition to these two FDA-approved agents, HDAC1, -2, and -3 are frequently overexpressed in human tumors, and knockdown of HDAC1 or -2 is sufficient to reduce tumor growth in vivo in the preclinic model. These studies provide a strong rationale for the development of class– or isoform-specific inhibitors for the treatment of cancer. However, acetylation has been reported to be involved in DOX-associated cardiotoxicity through the activity of HDACs and HATs.[64] Activation or overexpression of HDACs, including SIRT1, SIRT3, and HDAC6, can prevent DOX cardiotoxicity via many molecular pathways.[64] As an emerging therapeutic strategy, extensive research has focused on the combined application of HDAC inhibitors and chemotherapy drugs. Of note, several HDAC inhibitors are reported to mitigate cardiotoxicity. A more sophisticated understanding of the role of acetylation in DOX-associated cardiotoxicity may provide insight into new strategies to improve treatment outcomes in patients with cancer and CVD.

CURRENT NEWER AGENTS IN CANCER THERAPY AFFECT METABOLISM, SPECIFICALLY MYOCARDIAL METABOLISM

As opposed to traditional cytotoxic chemotherapies, which are highly effective but can cause nonspecific damage to both cancer and healthy cells, newer hormonal therapies and targeted therapies are tailored to specific molecular pathways overexpressed by cancer cells. There is increasing recognition that those newer therapies also cause metabolic toxicities, as described in **Table 1**.

It is known that breast cancer and prostate cancer are driven partly by sex hormones, and treatment of those diseases is often based on hormone-modifying therapy.[65] Studies showed

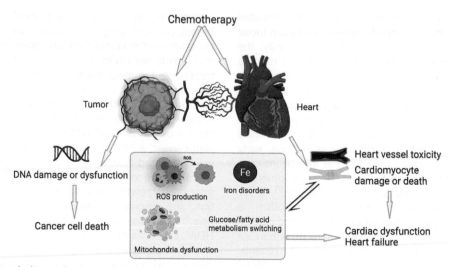

Fig. 1. Metabolic mechanisms of chemotherapy-induced cardiac side effects.

that androgen suppression therapy is currently used in 50% of patients with prostate cancer and has robust efficacy, but accumulating evidence suggests that this therapy may lead to abnormal cardiometabolic parameters including increased LDL cholesterol, visceral fat, and insulin resistance, as well as decreased lean body mass and glucose tolerance.[66] Several population-based observational studies suggest an increased risk of cardiovascular events, including myocardial infarction, stroke, hypertension, arrhythmia, and sudden cardiac death.[67,68] This increased risk has been observed primarily in patients treated with gonadotropin-releasing hormone (GnRH) agonists rather than antagonists,[69–71] which differ primarily in their effects on follicle-stimulating hormone (FSH) and downstream testosterone signaling. GnRH agonists, such as leuprolide, bind to GnRH receptors in the pituitary gland, thereby causing an initial increase in GnRH. This leads to the release of FSH and luteinizing hormone (LH), an LH-mediated increase in testosterone production in the testes, and a subsequent negative feedback loop to the pituitary gland. The end result is the downregulation of GnRH receptors in the pituitary gland, decreased LH levels, and castrate levels of testosterone. On the other hand, GnRH antagonists cause rapid inhibition of FSH and LH leading to an immediate decrease in testosterone levels. The different kinetics of testosterone release and suppression has been proposed as one possible explanation for the more prominent association between androgen suppression therapy and cardiovascular events in patients treated with FSH agonists compared with those treated with FSH antagonists. However, the association between FSH

signaling and cardiovascular risk in patients treated with androgen suppression therapy has not been definitively established from a mechanistic point of view, representing an unmet need that should be addressed in future studies.

The development of successful molecular targeted therapies relies on the understanding of signal transduction pathways. The phosphatidylinositol 3-kinase (PI3K)/mammalian target of rapamycin (mTOR) signaling pathway plays an important role in essential cellular functions, including cell growth, proliferation, differentiation, metabolism, survival, and angiogenesis.[72] Some inhibitors of this pathway have been approved by the Food and Drug Administration after their efficiency and safety have been shown for the treatment of various types of cancer, particularly breast cancer.[72,73] However, metabolic side effects reported in clinical trials of PI3K/Akt/mTOR inhibitors include hyperglycemia and hyperlipidemia, with elevations in both low-density lipoprotein (LDL) cholesterol and triglycerides.[74] In a review summarizing data from 341 patients treated in 12 phase I trials of PI3K/AKT/mTOR inhibitors, 298 patients (87.4%) developed hyperglycemia. Hyperglycemia was grade 1 in 217 (72.8%) and grade 2 in 61 (20.5%) patients, respectively. Grade ≥3 hyperglycemia was seen in 6.7% of patients (n = 20).[74] Interestingly, mice lacking functional PI3Kγ showed preserved cardiac function after chronic low-dose DOX treatment and were protected against DOX-induced cardiotoxicity. Blockade of PI3Kγ may, therefore, provide a dual therapeutic advantage in cancer therapy by simultaneously preventing anthracyclines cardiotoxicity and reducing tumor growth, although hyperglycemia remains a clinical concern in patients receiving PI3K inhibitors.[75]

Table 1
Current cancer agents inducing cardiac related side effects

Categories	Representative Drugs	Cancer Treatment	Mechanisms	Cardiac Side Effects
Antibiotics: Anthracyclines	Doxorubicin Epirubicin Daunorubicin	Lymphoma/Leukemia/ Breast cancer	Interfere with enzymes involved in copying DNA during the cell cycle.	Cardiomyopathy/Heart failure
Antimetabolites	5-fluorouracil (5-FU)	Breast/colon/rectal pancreatic/stomach cancer	Inhibition of thymidylate synthase (TS) and incorporation of its metabolites into RNA and DNA	Ischemia, dilated cardiomyopathy, ventricular arrhythmia, and sudden cardiac death
Alkylating agents	Cyclophosphamide	Multiple myeloma/ sarcoma/breast cancer	Damage DNA of cancer cells	Fatal hemorrhagic myocarditis/ Cardiomyopathy
PI3K/Akt/mTOR inhibitors	Alpelisib/idelalisib/ copanlisib	Breast cancer	Inhibition of cell proliferation, growth, cell size, metabolism, and motility	Hyperglycemia and hyperlipidemia
Hormone inhibitors	Anastrozole/exemestane/ letrozole, and Leuprolide/Goserelin	Breast/prostate/ endometrial (uterine) cancers	Preventing the body from making the hormone or making the cancer cells unable to use the hormone that they need to grow	Increased LDL cholesterol, insulin resistance, myocardial infarction, stroke, arrhythmia, and sudden cardiac death
BCR-ABL inhibitors	Imatinib	Leukemia	Causing the arrest of growth or apoptosis in hematopoietic cells that express BCR-ABL	Cardiac dysfunction with some agents
Anti-VEGF/anti-angiogenesis	Bevacizumab	Gastrointestinal cancer	Blocking the activity of proangiogenic factors which help cancer cell growth	Hypertension
Anti-HER2	Trastuzumab	Breast cancer	Blocking the HER2 receptors from receiving the growth signals in HER2-positive breast cancer.	Cardiac dysfunction

In addition to hormonal therapies, targeted therapies including tyrosine kinase inhibitors (TKIs) have become first-line therapy for most patients with chronic myelogenous leukemia (CML), as well as other solid organ cancers including non-small cell lung cancer, liver, and thyroid.[76] Oral small molecules targeting BCR-ABL for the treatment of CML include imatinib, dasatinib, nilotinib, bosutinib, and ponatinib. These TKIs may cause cardiovascular and/or metabolic complications, either through on-target or off-target toxicities. The variability in cardiovascular phenotypes observed clinically in patients receiving the same TKI agents suggests that cardiovascular toxicity may result from interactions between each patient's cardiovascular risk factors, genetic predisposition, and specific targets affected by each TKI.[77]

Tumor hypoxia is a central driver of pathologic tumor growth, metastasis, and chemoresistance. Therefore, targeting hypoxia signaling pathways has emerged as a new therapeutic approach for cancer treatment. Though efficacious, these therapies are associated with significant cardiovascular toxicities, ranging from hypertension to cardiomyopathy.[78] For instance, vascular endothelial growth factor (VEGF), which is induced under conditions of hypoxia in mammalian cells, is a potent angiogenic factor and an endothelial-cell specific mitogen.[79] Under normal conditions, VEGF signaling results in vasodilation, vascular permeability, and endothelial cell homeostasis, which are important processes during embryogenesis, wound healing, and hypoxia adaptation. However, abnormal VEGF signaling leads to pathologic tumor growth and invasion and is an important driver of malignancy in both primary tumors and metastatic cancers by facilitating tumor cell intravasation and dissemination. Therefore, anti-VEGF therapies are now part of the growing armamentarium for cancer and represent the first-line standard of care for many types of malignancies. Furthermore, it is expected that an increasing number of patients will be eligible for these therapies in the coming years. Though efficacious, especially in patients with limited treatment options, VEGF inhibitors are associated with cardiovascular complications, which can lead to dose reduction or early cessation.

Recent studies have found that targeting Bcl2-associated athanogene-3 (BAG3) is a highly effective treatment of cancer.[80] BAG3 is an ideal cancer target because (a) it can promote survival through multiple cell pathways; (b) its expression is induced by stress and growth factors found in cancer cells; (c) high levels of expression correlate directly with chemoresistance; and (d) high levels of BAG3 predict a poor outcome in a variety of cancers, including thyroid, breast, liver, leukemias, and metastatic melanoma.[81–84] However, BAG3 is an evolutionarily conserved protein that is expressed at high levels in the heart. In the heart, BAG3 inhibits apoptosis, promotes autophagy, couples the β-adrenergic receptor with the L-type Ca2+ channel, and maintains the structure of the sarcomere. Therefore, the development of BAG3 inhibitors to treat cancer may be changeling given its complex role in the heart and in cancer. Modalities that enable tissue-specific delivery of BAG3 inhibitors, for instance, may be a direction for future study.

INTERACTION BETWEEN TUMOR AND MYOCARDIAL METABOLISM

Cancer cells activate their metabolism to promote growth, proliferation, and long-term maintenance. The characteristic metabolic hallmark of cancer metabolism is enhanced uptake and utilization of glucose and increased lactate secretion, even in the presence of oxygen and completely functioning mitochondria (aerobic glycolysis). This phenomenon is known as the Warburg effect and was first described in 1926.[85] Under normal conditions, fatty acids are the main source of energy in the heart, while under certain conditions, the main source of energy shifts to glucose whereby pyruvate converts into lactate, to meet the energy demand. The Warburg effect is the energy shift from oxidative phosphorylation to glycolysis in the presence of oxygen. This effect is observed in tumors as well as in various kinds of myocardial injuries including chemotherapy cardiomyopathy. If glycolysis is more dominant than glucose oxidation, the 2 pathways uncouple, contributing to the severity of heart failure.[86]

Cancer therapies cause CVD and metabolic disorders which in turn have been shown to be a risk factor for subsequent CVD and cancer.[87] Recent studies have demonstrated that exercise can improve cardiovascular outcomes in patients with cancer and also indicated that dietary modification has beneficial cardiovascular outcomes in animal models with cancer.[88,89] A recent large prospective observational cohort study showed that higher levels of physical activity before cancer diagnosis were associated with lower risks of CV events in women with breast cancer.[75] Exercise in patients with cancer is not only thought to be safe, but it has been also shown to improve quality of life and aerobic fitness while reducing the risk of cancer recurrence and all-cause mortality.[90] Taken together, preclinical and clinical studies suggest that exercise and dietary modification are unlikely to be harmful and may mitigate the cardio-vascular risks associated with cancer and cancer therapy.

Increasing evidence suggests that metabolic reprogramming plays an important role in cardiac adaptation during cancer.[91] First, chemotherapeutics targeting tumor metabolism often adversely affect the heart. Metabolic phenotypes in cancers evolve as the disease progresses, resulting in variable efficacy of therapies and severity of cardiovascular side effects. Secondly, cardiac cells share many of the same stress response pathways and metabolic strategies with cancer cells, such as glucose and fatty acid uptake, suggesting that metabolic alterations during tumor progression affect nonmalignant tissue such as heart. Therefore, understanding the complex interactions between cancer cells metabolism and cardiac cells metabolism can enable the development of new therapeutic strategies and yield improvements in mortality from both CVD and cancer.[92]

FUTURE DIRECTIONS

Currently, the potential effects of blocking metabolic pathways in tumor cells on the development of cardiovascular toxicity are not well understood, particularly for newer cancer treatments such as targeted and hormonal therapies. Additionally, cardioprotective therapies that modulate cardiac metabolism have not been extensively studied in the setting of cancer treatment. Recent clinical trials have shown that sodium–glucose co-transport 2 (SGLT2) inhibitors have dramatic beneficial cardiovascular outcomes. These include a reduced incidence of cardiovascular death and heart failure hospitalization in patients with and without diabetes as well as those with and without prevalent heart failure. Accordingly, SGLT2 inhibitors might be a promising cardioprotective therapy for patients undergoing treatment of cancer. Importantly, there is a need to elucidate the mechanisms involved in cross-talk between cardiac and cancer cells. The identification of biomarkers, whether in the blood or by novel imaging techniques, and characterization of cardiac metabolic changes during cancer therapy will be important for the early diagnosis of cardiotoxicity and subsequent intervention. Thus, interdisciplinary collaborations among cardiologists, oncologists, and basic science researchers will be necessary to advance the field and identify metabolic vulnerabilities for the development of novel therapeutics.

FUNDING SUPPORT

This work is supported by a grant from the National Institutes of Health (K08HL145019 to Dr A. Asnani). Dr Z.-Z. Chen is funded by the National Institute of Diabetes and Digestive and Kidney Diseases (K23DK127073). Dr J. Liu is supported by an American Heart Association Postdoctoral Fellowship (#20POST35210968).

CONFLICT OF INTEREST

No conflict of interest was declared.

REFERENCES

1. Chang HM, Moudgil R, Scarabelli T, et al. Cardiovascular complications of cancer therapy: best practices in diagnosis, prevention, and management: part 1. J Am Coll Cardiol 2017;70(20):2536–51.
2. Chang HM, Moudgil R, Scarabelli T, et al. Cardiovascular complications of cancer therapy: best practices in diagnosis, prevention, and management: part 2. J Am Coll Cardiol 2017;70(20):2552–65.
3. Bovelli D, Plataniotis G, Roila F, et al. Cardiotoxicity of chemotherapeutic agents and radiotherapy-related heart disease: ESMO Clinical Practice Guidelines. Ann Oncol 2010;21(Suppl 5):v277–82.
4. Lyon AR, Yousaf N, Battisti NML, et al. Immune checkpoint inhibitors and cardiovascular toxicity. Lancet Oncol 2018;19(9):e447–58.
5. Carrasco R, Castillo RL, Gormaz JG, et al. Role of oxidative stress in the mechanisms of anthracycline-induced cardiotoxicity: effects of preventive strategies. Oxid Med Cell Longev 2021; 2021:8863789.
6. Kværner AS, Minaguchi J, Yamani NE, et al. DNA damage in blood cells in relation to chemotherapy and nutritional status in colorectal cancer patients-A pilot study. DNA Repair (Amst) 2018;63:16–24.
7. Ahmad J. Iron deficiency anemia is common in patients receiving chemotherapy. Blood 2015; 126(23):4559.
8. Guigni BA, Callahan DM, Tourville TW, et al. Skeletal muscle atrophy and dysfunction in breast cancer patients: role for chemotherapy-derived oxidant stress. Am J Physiol Cell Physiol 2018;315(5): C744–56.
9. Kalyanaraman B. Teaching the basics of cancer metabolism: developing antitumor strategies by exploiting the differences between normal and cancer cell metabolism. Redox Biol 2017;12:833–42.
10. Edwardson DW, Narendrula R, Chewchuk S, et al. Role of drug metabolism in the cytotoxicity and clinical efficacy of anthracyclines. Curr Drug Metab 2015;16(6):412–26.
11. Tacar O, Sriamornsak P, Dass CR. Doxorubicin: an update on anticancer molecular action, toxicity and

novel drug delivery systems. J Pharm Pharmacol 2013;65(2):157–70.

12. Gewirtz DA. A critical evaluation of the mechanisms of action proposed for the antitumor effects of the anthracycline antibiotics adriamycin and daunorubicin. Biochem Pharmacol 1999;57(7):727–41.

13. Sinha BK, Politi PM. Anthracyclines. Cancer Chemother Biol Response Modif 1990;11:45–57.

14. Hande KR. Topoisomerase I.I. Inhibitors. Update Cancer Ther 2008;3:13–26.

15. Muindi J, Sinha BK, Gianni L, et al. Thiol-dependent DNA damage produced by anthracycline-iron complexes. The structure-activity relationships and molecular mechanisms. Mol Pharmacol 1985;27(3): 356–65.

16. Mizutani H. Mechanism of DNA damage and apoptosis induced by anticancer drugs through generation of reactive oxygen species. Yakugaku Zasshi 2007;127(11):1837–42.

17. Sawyer DB, Peng X, Chen B, et al. Mechanisms of anthracycline cardiac injury: can we identify strategies for cardioprotection? Prog Cardiovasc Dis 2010;53(2):105–13.

18. Westman EL, Canova MJ, Radhi IJ, et al. Bacterial inactivation of the anticancer drug doxorubicin. Chem Biol 2012;19(10):1255–64.

19. Volkova M, Russell R. Anthracycline cardiotoxicity: prevalence, pathogenesis and treatment. Curr Cardiol Rev 2011;7(4):214–20.

20. Carvalho C, Santos RX, Cardoso S, et al. Doxorubicin: the good, the bad and the ugly effect. Curr Med Chem 2009;16(25):3267–85.

21. Weiss RB. The anthracyclines: will we ever find a better doxorubicin? Semin Oncol 1992;19(6): 670–86.

22. Cortes-Funes H, Coronado C. Role of anthracyclines in the era of targeted therapy. Cardiovasc Toxicol 2007;7(2):56–60.

23. Singal PK, Li T, Kumar D, et al. Adriamycin-induced heart failure: mechanism and modulation. Mol Cell Biochem 2000;207(1–2):77–86.

24. Cardinale D, Colombo A, Bacchiani G, et al. Early detection of anthracycline cardiotoxicity and improvement with heart failure therapy. Circulation 2015;131(22):1981–8.

25. Colombo A, Cipolla C, Beggiato M, et al. Cardiac toxicity of anticancer agents. Curr Cardiol Rep 2013;15(5):362.

26. Lopaschuk GD, Belke DD, Gamble J, et al. Regulation of fatty acid oxidation in the mammalican heart in health and disease. Biochim Biophys Acta 1994; 1213:263–76.

27. Stanley WC, Recchia FA, Lopaschuk GD. Myocardial substrate metabolism in the normal and failing heart. Physiol Rev 2005;85(3):1093–129.

28. Zhang L, Jaswal JS, Ussher JR, et al. Cardiac insulin-resistance and decreased mitochondrial energy production precede the development of systolic heart failure after pressure-overload hypertrophy. Circ Heart Fail 2013;6(5):1039–48.

29. Witteles RM, Fowler MB. Insulin-resistant cardiomyopathy clinical evidence, mechanisms, and treatment options. J Am Coll Cardiol 2008;51(2): 93–102.

30. Russo M, Della Sala A, Tocchetti CG, et al. Metabolic aspects of anthracycline cardiotoxicity. Curr Treat Options Oncol 2021;22(2):18.

31. Taegtmeyer H, Beauloye C, Harmancey R, et al. Insulin resistance protects the heart from fuel overload in dysregulated metabolic states. Am J Physiol Heart Circ Physiol 2013;305(12):H1693–7.

32. Long YC, Cheng Z, Copps KD, et al. Insulin receptor substrates Irs1 and Irs2 coordinate skeletal muscle growth and metabolism via the Akt and AMPK pathways. Mol Cell Biol 2011;31(3):430–41.

33. Hardie DG. AMP-activated protein kinase: a master switch in glucose and lipid metabolism. Rev Endocr Metab Disord 2004;5(2):119–25.

34. Gratia S, Kay L, Potenza L, et al. Inhibition of AMPK signalling by doxorubicin: at the crossroads of the cardiac responses to energetic, oxidative, and genotoxic stress. Cardiovasc Res 2012;95(3):290–9.

35. Bulten BF, Sollini M, Boni R, et al. Cardiac molecular pathways influenced by doxorubicin treatment in mice. Sci Rep 2019;9(1):2514.

36. Osataphan N, Phrommintikul A, Chattipakorn SC, et al. Effects of doxorubicin-induced cardiotoxicity on cardiac mitochondrial dynamics and mitochondrial function: Insights for future interventions. J Cell Mol Med 2020;24(12):6534–57.

37. Varga ZV, Ferdinandy P, Liaudet L, et al. Drug-induced mitochondrial dysfunction and cardiotoxicity. Am J Physiol Heart Circ Physiol 2015;309(9): H1453–67.

38. Goormaghtigh E, Chatelain P, Caspers J, et al. Evidence of a complex between adriamycin derivatives and cardiolipin: possible role in cardiotoxicity. Biochem Pharmacol 1980;29(21):3003–10.

39. Trites MJ, Clugston RD. The role of adipose triglyceride lipase in lipid and glucose homeostasis: lessons from transgenic mice. Lipids Health Dis 2019;18(1): 204.

40. Serrano J, Palmeira CM, Kuehl DW, et al. Cardioselective and cumulative oxidation of mitochondrial DNA following subchronic doxorubicin administration. Biochim Biophys Acta 1999;1411(1):201–5.

41. Lauritzen KH, Kleppa L, Aronsen JM, et al. Impaired dynamics and function of mitochondria caused by mtDNA toxicity leads to heart failure. Am J Physiol Heart Circ Physiol 2015;309(3):H434–49.

42. Mukhopadhyay P, Rajesh M, Yoshihiro K, et al. Simple quantitative detection of mitochondrial superoxide producton in live cells. Biochem Biophys Res Commun 2007;358(1):203–8.

Mukhopadhyay P, Rajesh M, Batkai S, et al. Role of superoxide, nitric oxide, and peroxynitrite in doxorubicin-induced cell death in vivo and in vitro. Am J Physiol Heart Circ Physiol 2009;296(5): H1466–83.

Pacher P, Liaudet L, Bai P, et al. Potent metalloporphyrin peroxynitrite decomposition catalyst protects against the development of doxorubicin-induced cardiac dysfunction. Circulation 2003;107(6): 896–904.

Danz ED, Skramsted J, Henry N, et al. Resveratrol prevents doxorubicin cardiotoxicity through mitochondrial stabilization and the Sirt1 pathway. Free Radic Biol Med 2009;46(12):1589–97.

Jirkovsky E, Popelova O, Krivakova-Stankova P, et al. Chronic anthracycline cardiotoxicity: molecular and functional analysis with focus on nuclear factor erythroid 2-related factor 2 and mitochondrial biogenesis pathways. J Pharmacol Exp Ther 2012; 343(2):468–78.

Guo J, Guo Q, Fang H, et al. Cardioprotection against doxorubicin by metallothionein is associated with preservation of mitochondrial biogenesis involving PGC1alpha pathway. Eur J Pharmacol 2014;737:117–24.

Abel ED. Cardiac metabolism in heart failure: implications beyond ATP production. In: Doenst T, Nguyen TD, editors. Circ Res 2013;113(6):709–24.

Thompson Legault J, Strittmatter L, Tardif J, et al. A metabolic signature of mitochondrial dysfunction revealed through a monogenic form of Leigh syndrome. Cell Rep 2015;13(5):981–9.

Roberts LD, Boström P, O'Sullivan JF, et al. β-Aminoisobutyric acid induces browning of white fat and hepatic β-oxidation and is inversely correlated with cardiometabolic risk factors. Cell Metab 2014; 19(1):96–108.

Asnani A, Shi X, Farrell L, et al. Changes in citric acid cycle and nucleoside metabolism are associated with anthracycline cardiotoxicity in patients with breast cancer. J Cardiovasc Transl Res 2020; 13(3):349–56.

Berthiaume JM, Wallace KB. Adriamycin-induced oxidative mitochondrial cardiotoxicity. Cell Biol Toxicol 2007;23(1):15–25.

Myers C. The role of iron in doxorubicin-induced cardiomyopathy. Semin Oncol 1998;25(4 Suppl 10): 10–4.

Stockwell BR, Friedmann Angeli JP, Bayir H, et al. Ferroptosis: a regulated cell death nexus linking metabolism, redox biology, and disease. Cell 2017; 171(2):273–85.

Fang X, Wang H, Han D, et al. Ferroptosis as a target for protection against cardiomyopathy. Proc Natl Acad Sci U S A 2019;116(7):2672–80.

Ichikawa Y, Ghanefar M, Bayeva M, et al. Cardiotoxicity of doxorubicin is mediated through mitochondrial iron accumulation. J Clin Invest 2014;124(2):617–30.

57. Gibney ER, Nolan CM. Epigenetics and gene expression. Heredity (Edinb) 2010;105(1):4–13.

58. Cavalli G, Heard E. Advances in epigenetics link genetics to the environment and disease. Nature 2019; 571(7766):489–99.

59. Bates SEN. Epigenetic therapies for cancer. Engl J Med 2020;383(7):650–63.

60. Chen QW, Zhu XY, Li YY, et al. Epigenetic regulation and cancer (review). Oncol Rep 2014;31(2):523–32.

61. Yoo CB, Jones PA. Epigenetic therapy of cancer: past, present and future. Nat Rev Drug Discov 2006;5(1):37–50.

62. Li Y, Seto E. HDACs and HDAC Inhibitors in Cancer Development and Therapy. Cold Spring Harb Perspect Med 2016;6(10):a026831.

63. West AC, Johnstone RW. New and emerging HDAC inhibitors for cancer treatment. J Clin Invest 2014; 124(1):30–9.

64. Li D, Yang Y, Wang S, et al. Role of acetylation in doxorubicin-induced cardiotoxicity. Redox Biol 2021;46:102089.

65. Redig AJ, Munshi HG. Care of the cancer survivor: metabolic syndrome after hormone-modifying therapy. Am J Med 2010;123(1):87.e1-6.

66. Bhatia N, Santos M, Jones LW, et al. Cardiovascular effects of androgen deprivation therapy for the treatment of prostate cancer: ABCDE steps to reduce cardiovascular disease in patients with prostate cancer. Circulation 2016;133:537–41.

67. Hu JR, Duncan MS, Morgans AK, et al. Cardiovascular effects of androgen deprivation therapy in prostate cancer: contemporary meta-analyses. Arterioscler Thromb Vasc Biol 2020;40(3):e55–64.

68. Keating NL, O'Malley AJ, Smith MR. Diabetes and cardiovascular disease during androgen deprivation therapy for prostate cancer. J Clin Oncol 2006; 24(27):4448–56.

69. Zhao J, Zhu S, Sun L, et al. Androgen deprivation therapy for prostate cancer is associated with cardiovascular morbidity and mortality: a meta-analysis of population-based observational studies. PLoS One 2014;9:e107516.

70. Nguyen PL, Je Y, Schutz FA, et al. Association of androgen deprivation therapy with cardiovascular death in patients with prostate cancer: a meta-analysis of randomized trials. JAMA 2011;306: 2359–66.

71. Bosco C, Bosnyak Z, Malmberg A, et al. Quantifying observational evidence for risk of fatal and nonfatal cardiovascular disease following androgen deprivation therapy for prostate cancer: a meta-analysis. Eur Urol 2015;68:386–96.

72. Alzahrani AS. PI3K/Akt/mTOR inhibitors in cancer: at the bench and bedside. Semin Cancer Biol 2019;59: 125–32.

73. Hillmann P, Fabbro D. PI3K/mTOR Pathway Inhibition: Opportunities in Oncology and Rare Genetic Diseases. Int J Mol Sci 2019;20(22):5792.

74. Khan KH, Wong M, Rihawi K, et al. Hyperglycemia and phosphatidylinositol 3-kinase/protein kinase B/mammalian target of rapamycin (PI3K/AKT/mTOR) inhibitors in phase I trials: incidence, predictive factors, and management. Oncologist 2016;21(7):855–60.

75. Li M, Sala V, De Santis MC, et al. Phosphoinositide 3-kinase gamma inhibition protects from anthracycline cardiotoxicity and reduces tumor growth. Circulation 2018;138(7):696–711.

76. Druker BJ, Talpaz M, Resta DJ, et al. Efficacy and safety of a specific inhibitor of the BCR-ABL tyrosine kinase in chronic myeloid leukemia. N Engl J Med 2001;344(14):1031–7.

77. Brown S-A, Nhola L, Herrmann J. Cardiovascular toxicities of small molecule tyrosine kinase inhibitors: an opportunity for systems-based approaches. Clin Pharmacol Ther 2017;101(1):65–80.

78. Baik AH. Hypoxia signaling and oxygen metabolism in cardio-oncology. J Mol Cell Cardiol 2022;165:64–75.

79. Shibuya M. Vascular endothelial growth factor (VEGF) and its receptor (VEGFR) signaling in angiogenesis: a crucial target for anti- and pro-angiogenic therapies. Genes Cancer 2011;2(12):1097–105.

80. Kirk JA, Cheung JY, Feldman AM. Therapeutic targeting of BAG3: considering its complexity in cancer and heart disease. J Clin Invest 2021;131(16):e149415.

81. Meng X, Kong DH, Li N, et al. Knockdown of BAG3 induces epithelial-mesenchymal transition in thyroid cancer cells through ZEB1 activation. Cell Death Dis 2014;5(2):e1092.

82. Shields S, Conroy E, O'Grady T, et al. BAG3 promotes tumour cell proliferation by regulating EGFR signal transduction pathways in triple negative breast cancer. Oncotarget 2018;9(21):15673–90.

83. Xiao H, Tong R, Cheng S, et al. BAG3 and HIF coexpression detected by immunohistochem correlated with prognosis in hepatocellular ca noma after liver transplantation. Biomed Res 2014;2014:516518.

84. Guerriero L, Chong K, Franco R, et al. BAG3 pr expression in melanoma metastatic lymph no correlates with patients' survival. Cell Death 2014;5(4):e1173.

85. Jang M, Kim SS, Lee J. Cancer cell metabolism plications for therapeutic targets. Exp Mol 2013;45(10):e45.

86. Liberti MV, Locasale JW. The warburg effect: does it benefit cancer cells? Trends Biochem 2016;41(3):211–8.

87. Esposito K, Chiodini P, Colao A, et al. Metabolic drome and risk of cancer: a systematic review meta-analysis. Diabetes Care 2012;35(11):2402–

88. Okwuosa TM, Ray RM, Palomo A, et al. Pre-d nosis exercise and cardiovascular events in prin breast cancer: women's health initiative. JACC dioOncol 2019;1(1):41–50.

89. Das M, Ellies LG, Kumar D, et al. Time-restric feeding normalizes hyperinsulinemia to inl breast cancer in obese postmenopausal mo models. Nat Commun 2021;12(1):565.

90. Zimmerman A, Planek MIC, Chu C, et al. Exerc cancer and cardiovascular disease: what should nicians advise? Cardiovasc Endocrinol Metab 2(10(2):62–71.

91. Koelwyn GJ, Newman AAC, Afonso MS, et Myocardial infarction accelerates breast cancer innate immune reprogramming. Nat Med 2020 1452–8.

92. Karlstaedt A, Barrett M, Hu R, et al. Car oncology: understanding the intersections betw cardiac metabolism and cancer biology. JA Basic Transl Sci 2021;6(8):705–18.

Intracellular Signaling Pathways Mediating Tyrosine Kinase Inhibitor Cardiotoxicity

Shane S. Scott, MS[a], Ashley N. Greenlee, BS[a], Anna Matzko[a],
Matthew Stein[a], Michael T. Naughton[a], Taborah Z. Zaramo, BS[a],
Ethan J. Schwendeman, BS[a], Somayya J. Mohammad, MS[a],
Mamadou Diallo[a], Rohith Revan[a], Gabriel Shimmin, BS[a],
Shwetabh Tarun, BA[a], Joel Ferrall, BS[a], Thai H. Ho, MD, PhD[b],
Sakima A. Smith, MD, MPH[a,c,*]

KEYWORDS

- Tyrosine kinase inhibitors (TKIs) • Cardiotoxicity • Arrhythmias • Cardio-oncology
- Intracellular signaling • Phosphoinositide 3-kinase (PI3K) signaling
- Vascular endothelial growth factor receptor (VEGFR)
- Hypertension 5' AMP-activated protein kinase (AMPK)

KEY POINTS

- Tyrosine kinase inhibitor (TKI) therapy has markedly improved survivorship of patients with cancer; however, these novel therapies also target specific signaling pathways integral to normal cardiovascular physiology, promoting cardiotoxicity.
- The pathophysiology of TKI-induced cardiovascular complications involves a complex interplay of changes in the balance of endothelin-1 (ET-1) and nitric oxide (NO), inhibition of vascular endothelial growth factor receptor (VEGFR) and phosphoinositide 3-kinase (PI3K)/protein kinase B (Akt) signaling, dysregulation of cardiac ion channels, and cardiomyocyte apoptosis, all of which contribute to the development of systolic dysfunction and heart failure (HF).
- TKI-induced cardiotoxicity is potentially treatable with angiotensin-converting enzyme inhibitors (ACEIs), non-dihydropyridine calcium channel blockers, and beta (β)-blockers. Notably, the β-blocker nebivolol increases NO signaling and may be of particular interest. However, clinical trials are required to assess the efficacy of these cardioprotective agents against TKI-mediated hypertension (HTN), arrhythmias, and HF.
- Deeper insight into the signaling pathways underlying TKI-associated cardiotoxic sequelae may lead to recognition of new kinase pathways integral to cardiovascular biology, development of novel therapies, and effective cardioprotective treatments.

[a] Dorothy M. Davis Heart and Lung Research Institute, The Ohio State University College of Medicine, Columbus, OH 43210, USA; [b] Division of Medical Oncology, Department of Internal Medicine, Mayo Clinic Arizona, Phoenix, AZ 85054, USA; [c] Division of Cardiology, Department of Internal Medicine, The Ohio State University Wexner Medical Center, Columbus, OH 43210, USA
* Corresponding author. Dorothy M. Davis Heart and Lung Research Institute Wexner Medical Center, The Ohio State University, 473 West 12th Avenue, Suite 200, Columbus, OH 43210.
E-mail address: Sakima.Smith@osumc.edu
Twitter: @Shane_S_Scott (S.S.S.); @Sakima_Lab (S.A.S.)

Heart Failure Clin 18 (2022) 425–442
https://doi.org/10.1016/j.hfc.2022.02.003
1551-7136/22/© 2022 Elsevier Inc. All rights reserved.

INTRODUCTION

Tyrosine kinase inhibitor (TKI) therapy has improved the survival of several cancers in the United States, including metastatic renal cell carcinoma (mRCC), hepatocellular carcinoma, thyroid cancer, colorectal cancer, and chronic myeloid leukemia (CML).[1–5] Although TKIs have remained effective treatment options, frequent cardiac adverse effects (AEs) have been recognized (**Fig. 1**). Hypertension (HTN), QT prolongation, arrhythmias, left ventricular systolic dysfunction (LVSD), and heart failure (HF) are among the most common cardiac AEs reported.[2,4,6] The incidence of cancer increases with age, and the cardiotoxicity of TKIs is especially relevant among cancer patients with cancer who have preexisting cardiac dysfunction, risk factors, and/or previous treatment with cardiotoxic chemotherapy.[6,7] Clinical trials assessing the efficacy of TKIs often exclude patients with poor cardiac function, as such the reported incidence of cardiac AEs in these trials may not accurately reflect patient comorbidities. Therefore, to decrease cardiac morbidity while increasing quality of life in cancer survivors, cardiologists and oncologists must be familiar with the cardiotoxicity profiles of these emerging cancer therapies and the mechanisms that mediate their effects.

TKI-induced cardiotoxicity is mediated through the inhibition of target receptors such as vascular endothelial growth factor (VEGF), platelet-derived growth factor (PDGF), and stem cell factor (c-KIT) receptors on nontarget cells.[4,8] Inhibition of these highly expressed receptors on cancer cells is effective in reducing cancer growth and progression. However, the inhibition of these receptors on cell types in the cardiovascular system, from cardiomyocytes to fibroblasts, and endothelial cells (ECs) promotes cardiovascular injury.[2] It has been hypothesized that VEGF/VEGF receptor (VEGFR) inhibition along with subsequent changes in the balance of endothelin-1 (ET-1) and nitric oxide (NO) is responsible for HTN, the most common cardiac AE associated with TKI use, and can lead to dose reductions of therapy.[2,4,9] Furthermore, current evidence suggests that the "off"-target effects of TKIs on cardiomyocyte receptors lead to dysregulation of ion channel function and turnover, contributing to increased incidence of arrhythmias in treatment recipients.[4,6,10,11] Concurrent or sequential use of TKIs in patients with previous or concurrent exposure to other cancer drugs (eg, anthracyclines, 5-fluorouracil) may exacerbate cardiac injury, accelerating morbidity and the development of HF (**Table 1**).[4,12]

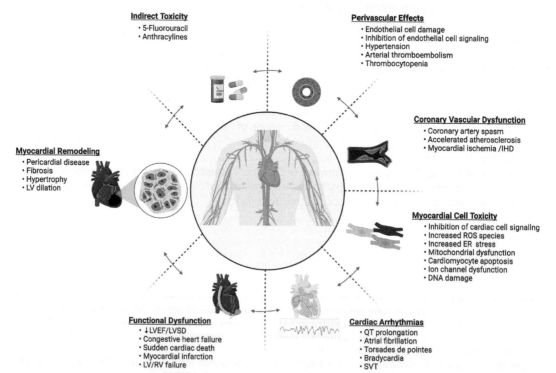

Fig. 1. Consequences and mechanisms of direct and indirect tyrosine kinase inhibitor (TKI)-induced cardiotoxicity. *Abbreviations*: ER, endoplasmic reticulum; IHD, ischemic heart disease; LV/RV, left ventricle/right ventricle; LVSD, left ventricular systolic dysfunction; ROS, reactive oxygen species; SVT, supraventricular tachycardia. (Created with BioRender.com.)

Table 1
Selected tyrosine kinase inhibitors, their receptor targets, cardiotoxicity incidence and proposed cardiotoxic signaling mechanisms

Agents	Receptor Target(s)	Cardiotoxicity	Preclinical Models	Proposed Cardiotoxic Signaling Mechanisms	Reference
Axitinib[a] (Inlyta)	VEGFR-1, -2, -3 PDGFR-α/β c-KIT	HTN AT QT Pericarditis LVSD	NA	NA	25,26,47
Cabozantinib[a] (Cabometyx)	VEGFR-2 CDK RET	HTN AT ↓ LVEF	NA	Inhibition of VEGFR-2 signaling leads to decreased expression of endothelial NO synthase and diminished NO synthesis, which disrupts the balance of NO and ET-1 promoting vasoconstriction, increased peripheral resistance, and increased blood pressure.[a]	26,47
Dasatinib[b] (Sprycel)	c-KIT PDGFR-/β EphA2 ABL BRAF Src kinase	CHF LVSD QT Thrombocytopenia HTN MI	Rat primary cardiomyocytes	Activation of ER stress response signaling leads to cellular apoptosis.	26,72,96
Gefitinib (Iressa)	EGFR1 (ERBB1)	MI	H9c2 ventricular cardiomyocytes	Increased expression of BNP and β-MHC along with decreased levels of α-MHC, promotes cardiac hypertrophy in vivo and in vitro due to activation of cardiac apoptosis and oxidative stress pathways (ie, increased caspase-3, p53 and HO1).	97,99
Imatinib (Gleevec)	c-KIT Bcr-Abl PDGFR-α/β	HTN QT IHD CHF LVSD	Rat primary cardiomyocytes	Activation of ER stress pathways, mitochondrial dysfunction, and increased ROS precipitates cellular apoptosis and necrosis in cultured cells and murine hearts. Increased expression of protein kinase Cδ (PKCδ), a kinase with pro-apoptotic effects in the heart.	26,34,95,96,100

(continued on next page)

Table 1
(continued)

Agents	Receptor Target(s)	Cardiotoxicity	Preclinical Models	Proposed Cardiotoxic Signaling Mechanisms	Reference
Lapatinib (Tykerb)	EGFR1 (ERBB1) ERBB2	HTN QT ↓ LVEF LVSD	NA	Increased ratio of pro-apoptotic BCL-X_S to BCL-X_L proteins, which may lead to ATP depletion, reduced cardiac contractility, and cardiac cell death via mitochondrial induced apoptosis.	26,99,100
Nilotinib (Tasigna)	Bcr-Abl DDR1/2 PDGFR-α/β c-KIT	HTN QT IHD SCD	Rat primary cardiomyocytes	Activation of ER stress response pathways leading to cell death. Direct inhibition of hERG potassium channels reduce I_{Kr} promoting QT prolongation and arrhythmias.	26,72,96
Pazopanib[a,b] (Votrient)	VEGFR-1, -2, -3 PDGFR-α/β c-KIT FGFR1/3 MCSFR-1 B-RAF	HTN AF HF *Torsades de pointes* AT LVSD	Atrial HL-1 cells; C57BL/6 Mice	Inhibition of VEGFR on cardiomyocytes reduces PI3K/Akt signaling leading to activation of proapoptotic pathways. Inhibition of FGFR-1 and -2 results in impaired cardiac response to stress and reduced contractility.	2,26,47
Ponatinib[a] (Iclusig)	Bcr-Abl FLT3 c-KIT VEGFR-2 PDGFR Src kinase FGFR1-3	HTN QT HF MI LVSD	hiPSC-induced cardiomyocytes; Zebrafish; NRVMs	Increased accumulation of ROS and mitochondrial dysfunction. Inhibition of cardiac Akt and Erk pro-survival signaling pathways leads to cardiomyocyte apoptosis.	26

	Targets	Cardiotoxicity	Model systems	Mechanism	References
Sunitinib[a,b] (Sutent)	VEGFR-1, -2, -3 PDGFR-α/β RET c-KIT FLT3 CSF-1R	HTN HF QT ↓ LVEF LVSD	NRVMs; Swiss-webster Mice; Rat H9c2 cardiomyocytes; C57BL/6J mice	Inhibition of AMPK-mTOR signaling, ATP depletion, and impaired energy homeostasis promotes cardiomyocyte autophagy and death and contributes to LVSD. Inhibition of the RSK protein promotes mitochondrial dysfunction, which increases the release of cytochrome C (cyto C), and activation of caspase 9. Increased cyto C and activated caspase 9 initiates the mitochondrial apoptotic pathway *in vitro* and *in vivo*. Induction of cardiomyocyte apoptosis in presence of underlying cardiac pathology (HTN).	26,55,100,89,95,100
Sorafenib[a,b] (Nexavar)	VEGFR-1, -2, -3 PDGFR-β B-RAF/C-RAF c-KIT FLT3	HTN HF MI QTc CHF LVEF AT	Zebrafish; NRVMs	Inhibition of Ras/Raf/Mek/Erk signaling pathway promotes mitochondrial dysfunction and apoptosis, which reduces cardiac cell survival. Increased activated CaMKII (ie, phosphorylated, and oxidized CaMKII), and ROS expression leads to pre-ventricular contractions and dysregulation in Ca²⁺ homeostasis.	10,24,26,47,89,100
Vandetanib[a] (Caprelsa)	VEGFR-1, -2, -3 EGFR PDGFR-β RET	HTN HF AF QT *Torsades de pointes* SCD	Postmortem human cardiac tissue;	Induced myocyte degeneration in the subendocardial zones and papillary muscles of the myocardium.	26,34,47,59

(continued on next page)

Table 1
(continued)

Agents	Receptor Target(s)	Cardiotoxicity	Preclinical Models	Proposed Cardiotoxic Signaling Mechanisms	Reference
Vemurafenib[b] (Zelboraf)	B-RAF	HTN QT CHF	HEK293 T; Isolated canine Purkinje fibers	Inhibition of B-RAF increases cAMP activity with subsequent increases in PKA. PKA phosphorylation of hERG channels and reduces their ability to open during, which prolongs the repolarization period and contributes to prolonged QT interval[b] and development of arrhythmias.	2,34,71

Abbreviations: AF, atrial fibrillation; AMPK, AMP-activated protein kinase; AT, arterial thromboembolism; ATP, adenosine triphosphate; Bcr-Abl, breakpoint cluster region-Abelson; BNP, brain natriuretic peptide; CaMKII, calcium/calmodulin-dependent protein kinase; cAMP, cyclic adenosine monophosphate; CDK, cyclin-dependent kinase; CHF, congestive heart failure; c-KIT, stem cell factor receptor; CSF-1R, colony-stimulating factor 1 receptor; DDR1/2, Discoidin domain receptor 1; 2, EGFR; epidermal growth factor receptor, EGFR; epidermal growth factor receptor, EPHA2; ephrin type-A receptor 2, ER; endoplasmic reticulum, ERK; extra-cellular-signal-regulated kinase, ET-1; endothelin-1, FGFR1/2; fibroblast growth factor receptor, FLT3; FMS-related tyrosine kinase 3, HEK293 T; human embryonic kidney cells 293 T, hERG; human ether-a-go-related gene, HF; heart failure, hiPSC; human induced pluripotent stem cells, HL1- HTN; hypertension, HO1; heme oxygenase 1, IHD; ischemic heart disease, I$_{Kr}$; potassium currents, LVEF; left ventricular ejection fraction, LVSD; left ventricular systolic dysfunction, MCSFR-1; macrophage colony-stimulating factor-1 receptor; MHC; myosin heavy chain, MI; myocardial ischemia/infarction, NO; nitric oxide, NRVMs; Neonatal rat ventricular myocytes, PDGFR; platelet derived growth factor receptors, PI3K; phosphoinositide 3-kinase, PKA; protein kinase A, QT; QT prolongation, RET; rearranged during transfection, ROS; reactive oxygen species, RSK; ribosomal S6 kinase, SCD; sudden cardiac death, Src; short for sarcoma-proto-oncogene, TKI; tyrosine kinase inhibitors, VEGFR; vascular endothelial growth factor receptors.

ª Note (s): All VEGFR-TKIs have the potential to cause hypertension via this molecular mechanism. Further, the mechanisms leading to VEGFR-TKIs is multifactorial and might be related to microvascular dysfunction, ATP depletion in the mitochondria, myocardial proapoptotic kinases, microvascular dysfunction, and profound vasoconstriction.

[b] All B-RAF inhibitors have the potential to promote QTc prolongation by this mechanism.[68] (NA) indicates that to the authors knowledge there are no preclinical studies, which directly evaluated these drugs on cardiomyocyte tissue.

The emerging cardiovascular side effects associated with TKIs warrant an increase in patient risk factor surveillance, further research into the mechanisms of these oncologic cardiovascular insults, and strategies to reduce TKI-induced cardiac-related morbidity. To date, concurrent treatment with clinically available drugs such as β-blockers, angiotensin-converting enzyme inhibitors (ACEIs), and angiotensin receptor blockers (ARBs) has been shown to reduce TKI-induced morbidity.[2,13,14] In addition, it is hypothesized that drugs such as statins, which possess systemic pleiotropic effects, can be used with TKIs to reduce cardiotoxicity.[15–18] In this review, we further assess tyrosine kinase signaling in cancer and discuss recent understandings of TKI-induced cardiotoxicity along with the intracellular signaling pathways by which these drugs disrupt cardiomyocyte function. We will also broadly discuss current and possible strategies to treat and prevent cardiovascular dysfunction associated with the use of these cancer therapies.

TYROSINE KINASE INHIBITORS AND MECHANISM OF ACTION

Tyrosine kinases are crucial for extracellular signal transduction in a variety of cellular processes that regulate signaling pathways impacting cell growth, differentiation, migration, motility, and death (**Fig. 2**).[2,19,20] The 2 major classes of tyrosine kinases are receptor tyrosine kinases (RTKs) and non-receptor tyrosine kinases (NRTKs). Tyrosine kinases are normally quiescent until activated by extracellular stimuli, growth factor ligands (eg, VEGF, PDGF, and c-KIT), or intracellular stimuli such as oxidative stress. Binding of tyrosine kinase receptors lead to the activation of tyrosine kinase in the cytoplasmic tail of the receptor, which transfers phosphate residues from adenosine triphosphate (ATP) to tyrosine residues on target protein substrates.[2,21,22] Some of these protein substrates are responsible for activating the canonical Ras/Raf/Mek/Erk signaling cascade, along with possible concurrent signaling via the phosphoinositide 3-kinase (PI3K)/protein kinase B (Akt) and adenosine 5′-monophosphate-activated protein kinase-mammalian target of rapamycin (AMPK-mTOR) pathways (see **Fig. 2**).[22–24] Under normal physiologic conditions, a balance between the activity of tyrosine kinases and dephosphorylation of tyrosine residues by tyrosine phosphatases is necessary to control the timing and duration of cell signaling.[19,20] As such, tight regulation of tyrosine kinase activity is critical for preserving normal cellular communication, growth, and maintenance of homeostasis.

Tyrosine kinase signaling is also required for tumorigenesis, tumor growth, angiogenesis, and metastasis.[19,22] In several cancers, dysregulation of tyrosine kinase signaling is responsible for the development and production of abnormal blood vessels essential to maintaining tumor growth.[19,20] Notably, about 60% of human cancers overexpress VEGF, promoting tumor progression and metastasis.[19] Cancer cells also express additional proangiogenic factors such as placental growth factor (PLGF), fibroblast growth factor (FGF), and PDGF, ligands of RTKs.[19] As tyrosine kinase receptor signaling is a fundamental converging point for angiogenesis and tumor growth, TKIs have emerged as a pharmacologic approach to interrupt cancer growth and metastases.

Tyrosine kinase receptors can be inhibited by small molecule inhibitors that predominantly target and block the evolutionary conserved ATP-binding pocket of both RTKs and NRTKs.[2,19,20] RTK inhibitors block the activity of the intracellular kinase domain, preventing trans-autophosphorylation and activation of the intracellular kinase receptor domains following ligand binding. This inhibits receptor dimerization, phosphorylation, and recruitment of downstream signaling proteins, terminating the signaling cascade.[19,20] Similarly, TKIs block NRTK signaling by gaining entry to the cell and targeting intracellular kinases, blocking signal transduction. Some TKIs target multiple receptors given the conserved residues for signaling, thus inhibiting growth factors or receptors involved in angiogenesis, as well as kinases involved in tumor cell proliferation. Examples of these multitargeted receptor TKIs include axitinib, cabozantinib, pazopanib, sunitinib, and vandetanib. Targeted inhibition of VEGFR/PDGFR/c-KIT receptor signaling by TKIs is not locally restricted to the tumor environment.[22,25] Owing to their lack of selectivity, TKIs also act systemically where they mediate their AEs. In this review, we focus on how dysregulation of VEGF, PDGF, and c-KIT receptor signaling by TKIs mediates cardiovascular toxicity.

RECEPTOR SIGNALING PATHWAYS AND CARDIOMYOPATHY

Several receptors targeted by TKIs, including VEGFR, PDGFR, and c-KIT, have been shown to mediate normal cardiac physiology and warrant investigation. In the following sections, we discuss the physiologic roles of these receptors and how the inhibition of these receptor signaling pathways contributes to the observed cardiac disturbances seen in patients receiving TKI therapy.

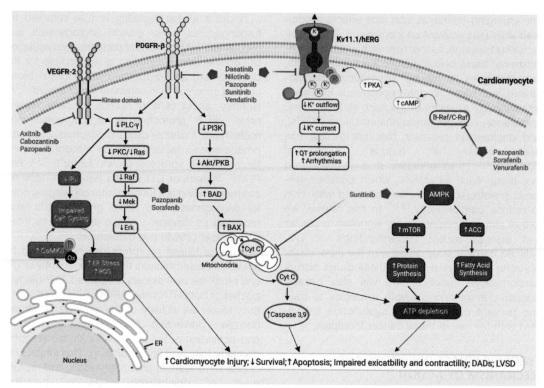

Fig. 2. Intracellular signaling pathways mediating tyrosine kinase inhibitor cardiotoxicity. TKI-mediated inhibition of VEGFR-2 results in the downregulation of PLC-γ, which alters IP3 and Ras/Raf/Mek/Erk signal transduction cascades. Reduced IP3 contributes LVSD and reduced myocardial contractility, which results from impaired calcium cycling and increased ER stress and ROS. Increased ROS is proposed to activate and increase CaMKII phosphorylation and further dysregulation in Ca²⁺ homeostasis. Reduced Ras/Raf/Mek/Erk signaling is also directly affected by PDGFR-β inhibition resulting in decreased cardiomyocyte survival, increased apoptosis, and LVSD. Inhibition of PDGFR-β reduces PI3K/Akt signaling and upregulates the proapoptotic proteins, BAD and BAX, leading to mitochondrial dysfunction, release of Cyt C, activation of caspase 3 and 9, ATP depletion, and cell death. AMPK inhibition by sunitinib also depletes ATP due to increased energy sink from mTOR and ACC-mediated protein and fatty acid synthesis, respectively. Loss of ATP contributes to cardiomyocyte injury and death. TKIs also directly inhibit myocyte Kv11.1/hERG channels disrupting K⁺ currents. Inhibition of cytoplasmic C-RAF/B-RAF enzymes increases cAMP promoting PKA phosphorylation and inhibition of hERG channels, leading to QT prolongation and the development of arrhythmias. ACC, acetyl-coenzyme A carboxylase; Akt, protein kinase B; AMPK, adenosine 5′-monophosphate-activated protein kinase; BAD, BCL2-antagonist of cell death; BAX, BCL2-associated X protein; CaMKII, Ca²⁺/calmodulin-dependent protein kinase II; cAMP, cyclic adenosine monophosphate; Cyt C, cytochrome c; hERG, human ether-à-go-go; IP3, inositol-trisphosphate-3 kinase; LVSD, left ventricular systolic dysfunction; mTOR, mammalian target of rapamycin; PI3K, phosphatidyl inositol-3 kinase; PLC- γ, phospholipase C gamma; PKA/C, protein kinase A/C; PDGFR-β, platelet-derived growth factor receptor; Raf-1, rapidly accelerated fibrosarcoma-1; ROS, reactive oxygen species. (Created with BioRender.com.)

Vascular Endothelial Growth Factor/Vascular Endothelial Growth Factor Receptor Signaling

The main regulator of angiogenesis requires VEGF ligand activation of its cognate tyrosine kinase receptors, VEGFR-1, -2, and -3.[19] ECs express all 3 VEGFRs, whereas VEGFR-1 and -2 are predominantly expressed within the vasculature and are activated by VEGF-A and -B. Cardiomyocytes only express VEGFR-1 and -2.[4] The Ras/Raf/Mek/Erk pathway and PI3K/Akt pathway are the 2 main signaling cascade pathways activated by VEGF/

VEGFR interaction (see **Fig. 2**).[26] The activation of these signaling pathways via VEGFR-2 on ECs triggers increased vascular permeability, cell migration, proliferation, and survival.[4] VEGF also plays an important role in the development, maintenance, and survival of myocardial ECs and cardiomyocytes.[4] In the context of cardiovascular disease, an increase in VEGF secretion and upregulation of VEGF signaling within cardiomyocytes is essential for responding to myocardial stress and injury.[4,19] *In vitro* and *in vivo* studies support this, showing that cardiomyocytes upregulate the expression of VEGFR-1 and -2, in response to hypoxia.[27] In transgenic mice lacking VEGFR-1 on ECs, an increase in angiogenesis was reported along with the development of cardiomyocyte hypertrophy, suggesting a role for paracrine signaling or cross talk between ECs and cardiomyocytes.[28] VEGF's role in myocardial remodeling occurs through balanced activation of VEGFR-1, which prevents cardiomyocyte hypertrophy, and activation of VEGFR-2, which has prohypertrophic effects.[29,30] Regardless of the mechanism, there are strong data suggesting that VEGF/VEGFR signaling is important for maintaining normal and adaptive function of ECs, vasculature, and cardiomyocytes.[19]

Platelet-Derived Growth Factor/Platelet-Derived Growth Factor Receptor Signaling

PDGF receptors (PDGFR-α/β) are ubiquitously expressed on the cell membranes of human and mouse cardiomyocytes and ECs, where they also play a role in angiogenesis and response to mechanically induced pressure overload.[4,19] Overexpression of PDGFRs is found in CML and gastrointestinal stromal tumors (GIST). It is hypothesized that nonspecific effects of TKIs including the inhibition of PDGFR are responsible for the cardiac effects of these drugs. In cultured tumor cells, pazopanib is a potent inhibitor of PDGFR-β signaling,[19,31] and sunitinib inhibits PDGFR-β phosphorylation in rodent tumor models (see **Fig. 2**).[4,32–34] PDGFR-β is also upregulated in mouse models of left ventricular pressure overload via transverse aortic constriction (TAC). Although PDGFR-β is not required for normal cardiac development or function in murine models, cardiac-specific PDGFR-β knockout is associated with dysregulated left ventricular function and reduced angiogenesis following TAC when compared with TAC wild-type mice.[35] In rat models, the administration of PDGF improved cardiac function following myocardial infarction (MI).[36] Together, the TAC data suggest that direct cardiotoxic effects by TKIs via PGDFR signaling in the myocardium may be inconsequential and may instead be potentiated and/or unmasked by concurrent systemic disease (eg, HTN).

c-KIT Signaling

The pathogenesis of several cancers including acute myeloid leukemia, GIST, and small cell lung cancer are mediated by mutations, overexpression, or deletions of portions of the tyrosine kinase c-KIT.[19,37] Although not expressed on the cardiomyocyte, a role for c-KIT in maintaining normal cardiac function was demonstrated in studies using the c-KIT$^{W/W-v}$ transgenic model, in which one c-KIT allele is deleted and the other encodes a protein with reduced kinase activity.[19,38,39] A reduction in the amount of functional c-KIT in the model led to impaired honing of bone marrow-derived proangiogenic stem/progenitor cells to regions of infarction. This impaired honing led to impaired cardiac recovery following MI and a decline in cardiac function with aging.[38,39] LV structural remodeling, including chamber dilatation and hypertrophy, and LV functional deficits such as reduced left ventricular ejection fraction (LVEF) have also been demonstrated in aging c-KIT mutant mice.[40] Last, constitutive activation of c-KIT receptors in mice is associated with an increased cardiac myogenic and vasculogenic reparative potential after injury, with a significant improvement of survival.[41] Given the totality of these findings, we postulate that the reduction of cardiomyocyte c-KIT activity may disrupt the normal cardiac response to stress or injury within human myocardium leading to increased remodeling.

Several TKIs target c-KIT in vivo[8] and in vitro.[42–45] Dasatinib and pazopanib are potent c-KIT inhibitors, which markedly disrupted hematopoietic progenitor cells in vivo and in vitro. On the other hand, imatinib, sunitinib, and sorafenib have shown moderate and negligible activity against c-KIT.[8,42–45] However, the development of an imatinib variant lacking activity for the tyrosine-protein kinase ABL, but retaining c-KIT inhibitor activity, did not result in cardiac dysfunction in a mouse model.[19,46] The reduced potential for cardiac toxicity was attributed to a loss of ABL kinase inhibition[4] and raises some questions about the role of c-KIT inhibition in the development of TKI-induced cardiotoxicity.

TYROSINE KINASE INHIBITOR-INDUCED CARDIOVASCULAR DYSFUNCTION
Hypertension

Hypertension has emerged as an important side effect common to all VEGF/VEGFR inhibitors with an incidence ranging from 16% to 80%, leading to dose reductions of therapy in clinical trials depending on the TKIs assessed.[4,26] A recent network meta-analysis study assessing the cardiotoxicity risks of VEGFR-TKIs revealed that vandetanib-treated patients have the highest risk for cardiotoxicity, followed by pazopanib, axitinib, sorafenib, and sunitinib.[47] In patients receiving sunitinib and axitinib, several studies suggest that HTN may serve as a predictive factor for more favorable patient response to TKIs and outcomes[48,49]; however, this has yet to be proved for other TKIs.[2] Most of the literature has associated TKI-induced HTN with increased endothelial and cardiomyocyte dysfunction.[2,50–52] One of the main mechanisms hypothesized to mediate TKI-induced HTN involves cross talk and/or paracrine signaling between ECs and cardiomyocytes.[28] Presumably, this mechanism may stem from the disruption of basal VEGFR-2 signaling necessary to maintain the balance of the vasodilator, NO, and vasoconstrictor, ET-1, through the PI3K/Akt pathway.[4,53] For example, pazopanib, cabozantinib, and vandetanib inhibit VEGFR-2 signaling, which normally suppresses production of ET-1, thus resulting in an increased concentration of ET-1 in blood plasma.[53] ET-1 is a potent vasoconstrictor, and increased plasma levels promote sustained vasoconstriction and HTN. The PI3K pathway also plays an important role in cell survival and vasodilation through downstream NO.[53] Inhibition of VEGFR-2 by pazopanib further diminishes production of NO, leading to impaired cardiomyocyte contractility.[54] Recently, Ren and colleagues[55] also showed that sunitinib-induced HTN is also mediated via regulation of AMPK-mTOR signaling (see **Fig. 2**) and warrants further investigation.

Last, it is suggested that HTN seen in patients treated with TKIs is mediated by renal impairment, which involves the activation of the renin-angiotensin-aldosterone system. Because VEGF signaling is vital to the proliferation of renal glomerular ECs, it is thought that inhibition of VEGF/VEGFR signaling could contribute to capillary rarefaction in renal glomeruli, with an increased secretion of renin from the juxtaglomerular apparatus; this leads to downstream production of angiotensin II and sustained systemic vasoconstriction. However, there is currently no experimental evidence to support this hypothesis because plasma renin levels were decreased with administration of sunitinib.[2,4,28] This inconsistency calls for further research into the mechanisms behind increased concentrations of ET-1 and decreased levels of NO.

Arrhythmias

The presence of arrhythmias is a primary cause of permanent discontinuation of TKIs. Patients taking TKIs that primarily inhibit VEGF/VEGFR signaling can develop QT prolongation and arrhythmias including atrial fibrillation (AF), bradycardia,[56] and supraventricular tachycardia (see **Fig. 1**). QT prolongation is a major concern because this could lead to other serious heart effects such as *torsades de pointes* and sudden cardiac death.[13] In clinical trials, the incidence of QT prolongation and arrhythmias is small compared to HTN.[26]

The incidence of QT prolongation and arrhythmias is most common with first and second generation TKIs such as sorafenib, sunitinib, and imatinib, in addition to vandetanib and nilotinib. Risk of death/serious impairment associated with arrhythmia increases greatly among patients with cancer due to older age, underlying cardiovascular disease, and use of concomitant medications.[57,58] For example, in a study of 39 patients with advanced hepatocellular cancer treated with sorafenib, the incidence of AF was 5.1% when used in conjunction with chemotherapy such as 5-fluorouracil.[4,12] For patients taking vandetanib, incidence of QT interval prolongation was between 8% and 11% versus 1.2% in controls[59] with an increased incidence in patients taking vandetanib plus chemotherapy (QT-related events; 22%).[59] Previous cardiac injury can also preclude and potentiate TKI-mediated QT prolongation and arrhythmia where underlying myocardial injury, such as LV contractile dysfunction, or HTN may provide an arrhythmogenic substrate (see **Fig. 1**).[4] In addition, patients treated with TKIs may also experience treatment-associated hepatic dysfunction that impedes drug clearance and metabolism.[2,5,60,61] Diarrhea, commonly seen in patients taking pazopanib, can contribute to electrolyte imbalances/derangements that promote QT interval prolongation.[13,22,62,63]

The reported incidence of AF in patients taking TKIs or other VEGF inhibitors (VEGFI) is limited to case reports, making it difficult to ascribe causation, which could be multifactorial in nature.[64,65] Although the PI3K/Akt pathway has been reported as a primary mechanism for HTN, it is also a potential mechanism for AF in patients taking TKIs or other VEGFI.[59,66] As previously outlined, VEGFR-2 signaling and activation of the PI3K-Akt pathway results in increased cell survival and migration. However, inhibition of PI3K-Akt signaling has been implicated in the development of AF in mouse models.[4,67–70] In another preclinical study, reduced PI3K activity led to the development of AF, whereas increasing PI3K activity led to reduced atrial fibrosis and improved conduction.[4,70] In support of this mechanism, reduced PI3K activation has been shown to increase the susceptibility of AF.[70] Activity of PI3K in human atrial appendages isolated from patients with AF is lower than in appendages from patients in sinus rhythm.[70] In another preclinical study, Lu and colleagues[67] demonstrated that TKI-mediated QT interval prolongation may be mediated through a reduction in PI3K signaling and alteration of multiple ion currents. In the study, suppression of PI3K signaling in canine cardiac myocytes by TKIs and mouse hearts lacking the PI3K p110α catalytic subunit resulted in prolonged action potentials and QT intervals.[67]

Tyrosine kinase inhibitor-mediated potassium ion channel dysfunction

Another possible mechanism for TKI-induced arrhythmias includes changes in the electrical activity of the heart. Specifically, the dysregulation of potassium (K^+) ion channels can cause preventricular contractions resulting in arrhythmias. TKI-induced arrhythmia is predominantly associated with direct ion channel inhibition of KCNH2 (Kv11.1) or the human ether-à-go-go (hERG) channel (see **Fig. 2**).[34] The hERG channel regulates K^+ efflux out of the cardiomyocyte during repolarization and comprises the "rapid" delayed rectifier K^+ current (I_{Kr}) in intact heart myofibers. The inhibition of hERG channels may promote the QT interval prolongation-associated increase in the risk of arrhythmias, including the life-threatening *torsades de pointes*.[34,71] Many of the marketed TKIs are potent direct inhibitors of the hERG channel, including dasatinib, sunitinib, and nilotinib.[34,71,72] Another mechanism of QT interval prolongation in patients occurs due to cytoplasmic inhibition of the cardioprotective enzymes B-RAF and C-RAF by TKIs like vemurafenib.[2,73] It has been proposed that B-RAF inhibition can lead to an increase in cyclic adenosine monophosphate (cAMP), which overactivates protein kinase A (PKA) (see **Fig. 2**). PKA then phosphorylates hERG channels and reduces their ability to open during action potentials, therefore decreasing I_{Kr}.[2,71,73] This hyperphosphorylation of the hERG channels can also block repolarization and contribute to QT prolongation. Pazopanib and sorafenib have been reported to inhibit the hERG channel through inhibition of B-RAF signaling.[2,71,73,74] This inhibition is believed to contribute to the QT prolongation reported in patients treated with these TKIs.

Tyrosine kinase inhibitor dysregulation of calcium-mediated signaling

Current research has demonstrated that TKI treatment results in dysregulation of calcium (Ca^{2+}) through the activity of Ca^{2+}/calmodulin-dependent protein kinase II (CaMKII). CaMKII is a multifunctional protein found in a wide array of locations throughout the body and plays an essential role in the heart (predominantly, CaMKII isoforms δ and γ). CaMKII contributes to multiple functions in the heart such as apoptosis, inflammation, and scar tissue formation.[67,75,76] In disease states, overexpression of CaMKII is involved with pathologic hypertrophy,[76] which promotes HF. CaMKII is vital for proper handling of Ca^{2+} levels and excitation-contraction coupling, and cardiomyocyte activation of CaMKII activation promotes Ca^{2+} waves and delayed afterdepolarizations[77] primarily through phosphorylation mechanisms. Furthermore, the phosphorylation of L-type Ca^{2+} channels (LTCC) and ryanodine receptor (RyR2) by CaMKII facilitates Ca^{2+} influx, sarcoplasmic reticulum (SR) Ca^{2+} release in cardiomyocytes,[78] and subsequent contraction.[79] Increased expression of CaMKII can cause hyperphosphorylation of the LTCC, which induces Ca^{2+} influx,[66,80] and activates RyR2 at serine 2814 to spark SR Ca^{2+} release events linked with HF and arrhythmias.[81] Increased CaMKII expression leads to the hyperphosphorylation of RyR2, causing Ca^{2+} leakage from the SR, leading to arrhythmias.

CaMKII is significantly expressed in response to TKIs such as imatinib, sunitinib, and sorafenib. Ma and colleagues[10] showed that rat ventricular cardiomyocytes treated with sorafenib caused a significant increase of CaMKII expression, particularly phosphorylated and oxidized CaMKII, leading to preventricular contractions and dysregulation in Ca^{2+} homeostasis. Fibroblasts treated with sunitinib and imatinib also showed increased expression of CaMKII.[82,83] It is suggested that TKI-induced upregulation in CaMKII expression and activity is mediated by increased reactive oxygen species (ROS) production. It is proposed that ROS can oxidize and activate CaMKII at the M281/282 (methionine) position analogous to autophosphorylation. Further research demonstrated that cardiac fibroblasts treated with imatinib and sunitinib showed increased mitochondrial superoxide production, supporting a role for ROS in CaMKII activation.[84] In cardiomyocytes, sorafenib treatment also caused a significant increase in cytosolic and mitochondrial ROS production,[10] suggesting that CaMKII and ROS could be potential targets for modulating TKI-induced cardiotoxicity.

TYROSINE KINASE INHIBITORS AND HEART FAILURE

Congestive heart failure (CHF) defined as a LVEF decrease of more than 10% or to less than 50% in clinical trials is among the most important heart-related functional changes that occur in response to TKI therapy (see **Fig. 1**).[13] Among the TKIs, sunitinib, axitinib, sorafenib, and vandetanib have been associated with a reduction in LVEF and symptomatic HF.[13,85] In a meta-analysis with a total of 10,647 patients from 16 randomized phase III and 5 phase II trials, the risk of CHF associated with all US Food and Drug Administration

(FDA) approved VEGFR2 TKIs was evaluated.[86] Ghatalia and colleagues[86] observed a significant 2.69-fold increase in the risk of all grades of CHF with TKIs that target VEGFR compared with control. Given that patients with severe cardiac comorbidities are excluded from therapeutic trials, the prevalence of CHF may be higher in real-world populations. Surprisingly, third generation VEGFR2-selective TKIs such as axitinib conferred similar relative risks for CHF compared with nonspecific multitargeted TKIs (eg, sunitinib, sorafenib, and pazopanib).[13,86] In a study exploring early subclinical cardiac chamber dysfunction in mRCC patients treated with TKIs, the right ventricle appeared more vulnerable to TKI therapy in the absence of pulmonary HTN, compared to the left ventricle. This observed right ventricle vulnerability is ascribed to its thinner myocardial wall.[87] However, these data are inconclusive because the incidence of right-sided HF is often underreported in clinical trials.[88]

Systolic dysfunction and subsequent HF are hypothesized to occur because the pathways that induce the pathologic survival and abnormal proliferation of cancer cells may also regulate the survival of normal cells, including cardiomyocytes. In rat and zebrafish cardiomyocytes, sorafenib induced cardiomyocyte apoptosis through direct inhibition of Raf/Mek/Erk signaling.[89,90] VEGFR-2 signaling blockade and downstream inhibition of the PI3K/Akt pathway is also implicated in cardiomyocyte apoptosis.[2,91] In mouse models, Akt activation at baseline is cardioprotective and prevents cardiomyocyte cell death through Akt-mediated inhibition of BCL-2 antagonist of cell death (BAD), a proapoptotic protein.[2,91–93] In a rat model of cardiac ischemia-reperfusion injury, constitutive activation of Akt reduced cardiomyocyte apoptosis and improved cardiac function postinjury.[94] In another study, the administration of exogenous VEGF prevented cardiomyocyte apoptosis and preserved cardiac function[92] possibly through improved VEGF/VEGFR2/PI3K/Akt-mediated inhibition of proapoptotic proteins.[2] Although it is unknown whether inhibition of the PI3K/Akt pathway by TKI-induced VEGFR-2 blockade contributes to cardiomyocyte apoptosis and HF in patients treated with TKIs, this potential pathway warrants investigation.[2,19] PI3K/Akt signaling in the heart is also modulated by several other receptor pathways not affected by TKIs. Thus, further research should be conducted to determine the exact mechanism by which TKIs induce cardiomyocyte apoptosis.

Recently, it was demonstrated that the AMPK-mTOR signaling pathway may also promote TKI-mediated LVSD and cardiomyocyte death. Reduced in vivo and in vitro AMPK phosphorylation in sunitinib treated cells and mice promote cardiomyocyte cytotoxicity[95] and cardiomyocyte autophagy along with impaired LVEF and LVSD in vivo.[55] A selective sodium-glucose cotransporter-2 (SGLT2) inhibitor empagliflozin ameliorated this sunitinib-induced cardiac dysfunction.[55] TKIs can also contribute to HF development through activation of the endoplasmic reticulum (ER) stress response[96,100], and oxidative stress pathways (ie, increased caspase-3, p53),[97] as well as mitochondrial dysfunction, increased ROS, and proapototic BCL-XS to BCL-XL proteins[26]; this may lead to ATP depletion, reduced cardiac contractility, and cardiac cell death.[98–100]

Cross talk between ECs and cardiomyocytes is crucial to maintain cardiac homeostasis and angiogenesis. Excessive angiogenesis may also result in cardiomyocyte hypertrophy and remodeling, which is mediated by VEGF-B and PLGF.[101] VEGF binding affinity to VEGFR-2 is increased when VEGF-B and PLGF bind to VEGFR-1. Inhibition of VEGFR-2 on cardiac ECs initiates a cascade of downstream signaling changes that result in cardiomyocyte apoptosis, hypertrophy, and HTN, which can lead to cardiomyopathy and end-stage HF. In addition to VEGF signaling inhibition, the effect of TKIs on systolic function may also be caused by inhibition of FGF receptor (FGFR)-1 and -2. In the heart, normal FGFR signaling is vital for cell proliferation, differentiation, survival, and angiogenesis.[2,102–104] In mice lacking FGFR-2, thrombocytosis, poor vascular function, and impaired cardiac response to ischemia[102] has been reported. In a separate study, loss of FGFR-2 resulted in impaired hypertrophic response to pressure overload.[105] Acute expression of FGFR-1 has also been shown to increase contractility of cardiomyocytes, whereas chronic expression leads to hypertrophy and preservation of systolic function.[106] In addition, inhibition of receptors such as PDGFR and c-KIT can also disrupt coronary microvasculature through disruption of stress-induced coronary angiogenesis leading to HF.[35]

CURRENT AND PROPOSED TREATMENTS FOR TYROSINE KINASE INHIBITOR -INDUCED TOXICITY

Current management strategies for TKI cardiotoxicity have focused on minimizing HTN with antihypertensives, TKI dose reduction, and/or drug discontinuation.[22] Among treatment options for systemic HTN are the classic agents such as ACEIs, ARBs, and non-dihydropyridine calcium channel blockers, whereas β-blockers such as carvedilol and nebivolol may be the preferred agents to reduce the risk of cardiotoxicity leading to LV dysfunction.[2,13,85] Patients cotreated with metoprolol or diltiazem prevented pazopanib-mediated QT interval prolongation.[2,107] As detailed earlier, there is evidence to suggest that TKI-induced HTN is mediated by reduction in VEGFR-induced NO production, disrupting ET-1 and NO balance. Exogenous NO-producing drugs such as isosorbide dinitrate or isosorbide mononitrate and ET-1 receptor blockers may have potential uses.[22,108] Kruzliak and colleagues[109] showed promising clinical efficacy; however, the effects of nitrates in preventing TKI-induced HTN still needs to be evaluated in larger clinical trials.[22] Therefore, it is suggested that blood pressure should be normalized before treatment and monitored throughout treatment.

A growing body of evidence has demonstrated that statins and SGLT2 inhibitors also exert cardioprotective effects in several cardiovascular diseases[55,110,111] and can protect the heart from chemotherapy-induced cardiac injury.[85] Namely, although the mechanisms of cardiotoxicity may be different from TKIs, it was demonstrated that statins reduced HF in patients receiving anthracycline chemotherapy,[112] and preserved LVEF in patients taking trastuzumab,[113] suggesting a role for statins in treating drug-related cardiotoxicity.[15,85] In cultured H9c2 cardiomyocytes, treatment with atorvastatin and dasatinib significantly enhanced cell survival through reduction in cell death and restoration of cardiomyocyte homeostasis.[18] Hung and colleagues[15] demonstrated that statins improve overall survival in patients treated with TKIs. However, a specific role for statins in reducing cardiovascular AEs was not reported and warrants further investigation.[15] SGLT2 inhibitor empagliflozin was recently shown to ameliorate sunitinib-induced cardiac dysfunction both in terms of systolic blood pressure and LVEF *in vivo* and cardiomyocyte death and cell viability *in vitro*.[55] These data suggest that SGLT2 inhibitor therapy could be a potential cardioprotective approach for cardiovascular complications mediated by sunitinib, but requires validation in clinical trials.[55]

Arrhythmias are common AEs reported in patients using TKIs (see **Table 1**), which are mediated by inhibition of hERG channels, leading to changes in K^+ balance, dysregulation of Ca^{2+} and Na^+ homeostasis, and diarrhea. To help minimize risk of arrhythmias, patient electrolytes should be optimized and monitored before and during treatment in conjunction with monthly electrocardiography.[2] Even further, diuretics and other electrolyte-depleting drugs should be avoided or used judiciously in these patients.[13,17,22] In some studies, administration of β-blockers in conjunction with hydralazine was used to manage TKI-induced HTN, especially for patients with left ventricular dysfunction or arrhythmia.[114,115] It is also important to address the drug interactions between antihypertensives and TKIs. For example, axitinib, cabozantinib, and pazopanib are metabolized by the CYP3A4 enzyme; hence antihypertensive drugs that inhibit CYP3A4 should be avoided to maintain the therapeutic doses and plasma clearance.[2,22]

Echocardiographic monitoring is an effective tool for detecting early signs of HF in patients taking TKIs.[2] In a retrospective study following 23 patients with mRCC treated with TKIs, echocardiograms demonstrated early changes in left ventricular strain, which may be a precursor of TKI-induced systolic dysfunction.[116,117] Moustafa and colleagues[87] used velocity vector imaging to identify early subclinical cardiac chamber dysfunction secondary to TKIs in patients with mRCC. Therefore, we recommend close echocardiographic surveillance of all patients receiving TKIs starting at baseline, and at interval durations during TKI therapy, and that any observed abnormalities should result in a dose reduction or termination of treatment.[2] In addition, an LVEF cutoff for TKI dose adjustment or discontinuation must be established.

Another important area of research should be the optimization of TKI drug delivery to minimize systemic AEs. The development of nanoscale drug delivery vehicles such as liposome and photoactivatable multi-inhibitor nanoliposome—which has already been developed for cabozantinib—may reduce "off"-target cardiac effects.[22,118] In a pancreatic cancer model, this construct successfully reduced tumor size and metastasis following injection and near-infrared irradiation of the tumor.[118] However, clinical trials are required to establish whether these delivery methods reduce cardiac adverse events.

SUMMARY AND FUTURE DIRECTIONS

The prevalence of TKI-mediated cardiovascular complications remains high and can lead to increased comorbidity with HTN as well as life-threatening cardiac effects including arrhythmias and HF. The intracellular signaling cascades that are associated with TKI cardiotoxicity are currently not well understood. Many TKIs systemically inhibit multiple signaling pathways, which makes the investigation of the pathophysiological mechanisms underlying their cardiotoxicity challenging. Furthermore, there are no proven strategies or biomarkers that predict TKI-induced cardiac dysfunction. A multipronged approach may be required to address this issue. First, a standardized mechanism of cardiac surveillance should be established for patients on TKI therapy, which may be possible through interdisciplinary partnerships between cardiologists and oncologists. Second, an understanding of the mechanisms that promote adverse cardiac effects of TKIs is necessary for the development of cardioprotective strategies. Clinical trials must also explore the utility of administering cardioprotective drugs concurrently with TKIs or include patients with cardiovascular comorbidities to better reflect a real-world population. In addition, the investigation of TKI-mediated disruption of cardiac ion channel function can provide insight into the mechanisms of arrhythmias and HF. Collectively, the data summarized in this review suggests that further research into the general role of tyrosine kinases in cardiac biology is essential for combating TKI-induced cardiotoxicity.

CLINICS CARE POINTS

For the pathophysiologic mechanism that promotes TKI-mediated cardiotoxicity, remember:

- To evaluate and manage coexisting comorbidities, risk factors, and previous patient exposure to other chemotherapies that promote cardiac injury because their underlying pathophysiology may promote or exacerbate TKI-mediated cardiac disease.

- More preclinical studies are warranted to illuminate other novel kinase pathways that are critical to cardiac physiology and the development of arrhythmia and HF.

- Although rodent and cultured cardiomyocyte models have provided insights into TKI-associated cardiovascular dysfunction, human translational studies will be critical to elucidate underlying mechanisms.

FUNDING

The authors report that this work was supported by the following grants T32HL134616 and R01 NIHMS1018036.

DISCLOSURE

The authors have no relevant affiliations or financial involvement with any organization or entity with a financial interest in or financial conflict with the subject matter or materials discussed in the article. This includes employment, consultancies, honoraria, stock ownership or options, expert testimony, grants, patents received or pending, or royalties.

REFERENCES

1. Sasaki K, Strom SS, O'Brien S, et al. Relative survival in patients with chronic-phase chronic myeloid leukaemia in the tyrosine-kinase inhibitor era: analysis of patient data from six prospective clinical trials. Lancet Haematol 2015;2(5):e186–93.
2. Justice CN, Derbala MH, Baich TM, et al. The impact of pazopanib on the cardiovascular system. J Cardiovasc Pharmacol Ther 2018;23(5):387–98.
3. Siegel RL, Miller KD, Fuchs HE, et al. Cancer statistics, 2021. CA Cancer J Clin 2021;71(1):7–33.
4. Dobbin SJH, Petrie MC, Myles RC, et al. Cardiotoxic effects of angiogenesis inhibitors. Clin Sci 2021;135(1):71–100.
5. Sternberg CN, Davis ID, Mardiak J, et al. Pazopanib in locally advanced or metastatic renal cell carcinoma: results of a randomized phase III Trial. J Clin Oncol 2010;28(6):1061–8.
6. Pinkhas D, Ho T, Smith S. Assessment of pazopanib-related hypertension, cardiac dysfunction and identification of clinical risk factors for their development. Cardiooncology 2017;3(1):5.
7. Assuncao BMBL, Handschumacher MD, Brunner AM, et al. Acute leukemia is associated with cardiac alterations before chemotherapy. J Am Soc Echocardiogr 2017;30(11):1111–8.
8. Galanis A, Mark L. Inhibition of c-Kit by tyrosine kinase inhibitors. Haematologica 2015;100(3):e77–9.
9. Kappers MHW, van Esch JHM, Sluiter W, et al. Hypertension induced by the tyrosine kinase inhibitor sunitinib is associated with increased circulating endothelin-1 levels. Hypertension 2010;56(4):675–81.
10. Ma W, Liu M, Liang F, et al. Cardiotoxicity of sorafenib is mediated through elevation of ROS level and CaMKII activity and dysregulation of calcium homoeostasis. Basic Clin Pharmacol Toxicol 2020;126(2):166–80.
11. Shah DR, Shah RR, Morganroth J. Tyrosine kinase inhibitors: their on-target toxicities as potential indicators of efficacy. Drug Saf 2013;36(6):413–26.
12. Petrini I, Lencioni M, Ricasoli M, et al. Phase II trial of sorafenib in combination with 5-fluorouracil infusion in advanced hepatocellular carcinoma. Cancer Chemother Pharmacol 2012;69(3):773–80.
13. Zamorano JL, Lancellotti P, Rodriguez Muñoz D, et al. 2016 ESC position paper on cancer treatments and cardiovascular toxicity developed under the auspices of the ESC committee for practice guidelines: the task force for cancer treatments and cardiovascular toxicity of the European

society of cardiology (ESC). Eur Heart J 2016; 37(36):2768–801.

14. Kalay N, Basar E, Ozdogru I, et al. Protective effects of carvedilol against anthracycline-induced cardiomyopathy. J Am Coll Cardiol 2006;48(11): 2258–62.

15. Hung MS, Chen IC, Lee CP, et al. Statin improves survival in patients with EGFR-TKI lung cancer: a nationwide population-based study. In: Souglakos J, editor. PLoS One 2017;12(2):e0171137.

16. Matusewicz L, Czogalla A, Sikorski AF. Attempts to use statins in cancer therapy: an update. Tumor Biol 2020;42(7). https://doi.org/10.1177/101042832 0941760.

17. Medeiros BC, Possick J, Fradley M. Cardiovascular, pulmonary, and metabolic toxicities complicating tyrosine kinase inhibitor therapy in chronic myeloid leukemia: Strategies for monitoring, detecting, and managing. Blood Rev 2018;32(4): 289–99.

18. Enoma E, Wei L, Chen H. The impact of statin on chemotherapy-induced cardiotoxicity. FASEB J 2019;33(S1). https://doi.org/10.1096/fasebj.2019. 33.1_supplement.833.12.

19. Chen MH, Kerkelä R, Force T. Mechanisms of cardiac dysfunction associated with tyrosine kinase inhibitor cancer therapeutics. Circulation 2008; 118(1):84–95.

20. Du Z, Lovly CM. Mechanisms of receptor tyrosine kinase activation in cancer. Mol Cancer 2018; 17(1):58.

21. Metibemu DS, Akinloye OA, Akamo AJ, et al. Exploring receptor tyrosine kinases-inhibitors in Cancer treatments. Egypt J Med Hum Genet 2019;20(1):35.

22. Milling RV, Grimm D, Krüger M, et al. Pazopanib, cabozantinib, and vandetanib in the treatment of progressive medullary thyroid cancer with a special focus on the adverse effects on hypertension. Int J Mol Sci 2018;19(10):3258.

23. Asnani A, Moslehi JJ, Adhikari BB, et al. Preclinical models of cancer therapy–associated cardiovascular toxicity: a scientific statement from the american heart association. Circ Res 2021; 129(1):e21–34.

24. Strumberg D, Clark JW, Awada A, et al. Safety, pharmacokinetics, and preliminary antitumor activity of sorafenib: a review of four phase I trials in patients with advanced refractory solid tumors. Oncologist 2007;12(4):426–37.

25. Buza V, Rajagopalan B, Curtis AB. Cancer treatment–induced arrhythmias: focus on chemotherapy and targeted therapies. Circ Arrhythm Electrophysiol 2017;10(8):e005443.

26. Bronte E, Galvano A, Novo G, et al. Cardiotoxic effects of anti-VEGFR tyrosine kinase inhibitors. Cardio-Oncol 2017;69–89.

27. Zentilin L, Puligadda U, Lionetti V, et al. Cardiomyocyte VEGFR-1 activation by VEGF-B induces compensatory hypertrophy and preserves cardiac function after myocardial infarction. FASEB J 2010;24(5):1467–78.

28. Lankhorst S, Saleh L, Danser AJ, et al. Etiology of angiogenesis inhibition-related hypertension. Curr Opin Pharmacol 2015;21:7–13.

29. Hiratsuka S, Minowa O, Kuno J, et al. Flt-1 lacking the tyrosine kinase domain is sufficient for normal development and angiogenesis in mice. Proc Natl Acad Sci 1998;95(16):9349–54.

30. Zhou Y, Bourcy K, Kang YJ. Copper-induced regression of cardiomyocyte hypertrophy is associated with enhanced vascular endothelial growth factor receptor-1 signalling pathway. Cardiovasc Res 2009;84(1):54–63.

31. Kumar R, Knick VB, Rudolph SK, et al. Pharmacokinetic-pharmacodynamic correlation from mouse to human with pazopanib, a multikinase angiogenesis inhibitor with potent antitumor and antiangiogenic activity. Mol Cancer Ther 2007;6(7): 2012–21.

32. Abrams TJ, Lee LB, Murray LJ, et al. SU11248 inhibits KIT and platelet-derived growth factor receptor ` in preclinical models of human small cell lung cancer. Mol Cancer Ther 2003;2:471–8.

33. Mendel DB, Laird AD, Xin X, et al. In Vivo antitumor activity of SU11248, a novel tyrosine kinase inhibitor targeting vascular endothelial growth factor and platelet-derived growth factor receptors: determination of a pharmacokinetic/pharmacodynamic relationship. Clin Cancer Res 2003;9:327–37.

34. Lamore SD, Kohnken RA, Peters MF, et al. Cardiovascular toxicity induced by kinase inhibitors: mechanisms and preclinical approaches. Chem Res Toxicol 2020;33(1):125–36.

35. Chintalgattu V, Ai D, Langley RR, et al. Cardiomyocyte PDGFR-β signaling is an essential component of the mouse cardiac response to load-induced stress. J Clin Invest 2010;120(2):472–84.

36. Hsieh PCH, MacGillivray C, Gannon J, et al. Local controlled intramyocardial delivery of platelet-derived growth factor improves postinfarction ventricular function without pulmonary toxicity. Circulation 2006;114(7):637–44.

37. Abbaspour Babaei M, Kamalidehghan B, Saleem M, et al. Receptor tyrosine kinase (c-Kit) inhibitors: a potential therapeutic target in cancer cells. Drug Des Devel Ther 2016;10:2443–59.

38. Ayach BB, Yoshimitsu M, Dawood F, et al. Stem cell factor receptor induces progenitor and natural killer cell-mediated cardiac survival and repair after myocardial infarction. Proc Natl Acad Sci 2006; 103(7):2304–9.

39. Fazel S. Cardioprotective c-kit+ cells are from the bone marrow and regulate the myocardial balance

of angiogenic cytokines. J Clin Invest 2006;116(7): 1865–77.

40. Ye L, Zhang EY, Xiong Q, et al. Aging kit mutant mice develop cardiomyopathy. In: Qin G, editor. PLoS One 2012;7(3):e33407.

41. Di Siena S, Gimmelli R, Nori SL, et al. Activated c-Kit receptor in the heart promotes cardiac repair and regeneration after injury. Cell Death Dis 2016; 7(7):e2317.

42. Talpaz M, Paquette R, Blackwood-Chirchir MA, et al. Dasatinib in imatinib-resistant philadelphia chromosome–positive leukemias. N Engl J Med 2006;354(24):2531–41.

43. Demetri GD, Lo Russo P, MacPherson IRJ, et al. Phase I dose-escalation and pharmacokinetic study of dasatinib in patients with advanced solid tumors. Clin Cancer Res 2009;15(19):6232–40.

44. Brazzelli V, Grasso V, Barbaccia V, et al. Hair depigmentation and vitiligo-like lesions in a leukaemic paediatric patient during chemotherapy with dasatinib. Acta Derm Venereol 2012;92(2):218–9.

45. Hurwitz HI, Dowlati A, Saini S, et al. Phase I trial of pazopanib in patients with advanced cancer. Clin Cancer Res 2009;15(12):4220–7.

46. Fernández A, Sanguino A, Peng Z, et al. An anti-cancer C-Kit kinase inhibitor is reengineered to make it more active and less cardiotoxic. J Clin Invest 2007;117(12):4044–54.

47. Hou W, Ding M, Li X, et al. Comparative evaluation of cardiovascular risks among nine FDA-approved VEGFR-TKIs in patients with solid tumors: a Bayesian network analysis of randomized controlled trials. J Cancer Res Clin Oncol 2021;147(8):2407–20.

48. Rini BI, Cohen DP, Lu DR, et al. Hypertension as a biomarker of efficacy in patients with metastatic renal cell carcinoma treated with sunitinib. J Natl Cancer Inst 2011;103(9):763–73.

49. Rixe O, Billemont B, Izzedine H. Hypertension as a predictive factor of Sunitinib activity. Ann Oncol 2007;18(6):1117.

50. Cameron AC, Touyz RM, Lang NN. Vascular complications of cancer chemotherapy. Can J Cardiol 2016;32(7):852–62.

51. Touyz RM, Lang NN, Herrmann J, et al. Recent advances in hypertension and cardiovascular toxicities with vascular endothelial growth factor inhibition. Hypertension 2017;70(2):220–6.

52. Touyz RM, Herrmann SMS, Herrmann J. Vascular toxicities with VEGF inhibitor therapies–focus on hypertension and arterial thrombotic events. J Am Soc Hypertens 2018;12(6):409–25.

53. Horowitz JR, Rivard A, van der Zee R, et al. Vascular endothelial growth factor/vascular permeability factor produces nitric oxide–dependent hypotension: evidence for a maintenance role in quiescent adult endothelium. Arterioscler Thromb Vasc Biol 1997;17(11):2793–800.

54. Colliva A, Braga L, Giacca M, et al. Endothelial cell–cardiomyocyte crosstalk in heart development and disease. J Physiol 2020;598(14):2923–39.

55. Ren C, Sun K, Zhang Y, et al. Sodium–glucose cotransporter-2 inhibitor empagliflozin ameliorates sunitinib-induced cardiac dysfunction via regulation of AMPK–mTOR signaling pathway–mediated autophagy. Front Pharmacol 2021;12:664181.

56. Shioyama W, Oka T, Kamada R, et al. Symptomatic sinus bradycardia in a patient with solitary fibrous tumor/hemangiopericytoma treated with pazopanib. Intern Med 2021;60(18):2973–7.

57. Lenihan DJ, Oliva S, Chow EJ, et al. Cardiac toxicity in cancer survivors: cardiac toxicity in cancer survivors. Cancer 2013;119:2131–42.

58. Leiva O, AbdelHameid D, Connors JM, et al. Common pathophysiology in cancer, atrial fibrillation, atherosclerosis, and thrombosis. JACC Cardiooncol 2021;3(5):619–34.

59. Morabito A, Piccirillo MC, Falasconi F, et al. Vandetanib (ZD6474), a dual inhibitor of vascular endothelial growth factor receptor (VEGFR) and epidermal growth factor receptor (EGFR) tyrosine kinases: current status and future directions. Oncologist 2009;14(4):378–90.

60. Brell JM. Prolonged QTc interval in cancer therapeutic drug development: defining arrhythmic risk in malignancy. Prog Cardiovasc Dis 2010;53(2): 164–72.

61. Ahmad K, Dorian P. Drug-induced QT prolongation and proarrhythmia: an inevitable link? Europace 2007;9(Supplement 4):iv16–22.

62. Dy GK, Adjei AA. Understanding, recognizing, and managing toxicities of targeted anticancer therapies: toxicities of targeted anticancer therapies. CA Cancer J Clin 2013;63(4):249–79.

63. Hutson TE, Davis ID, Machiels JPH, et al. Efficacy and safety of pazopanib in patients with metastatic renal cell carcinoma. J Clin Oncol 2010;28(3): 475–80.

64. Mego M, Reckova M, Obertova J, et al. Increased cardiotoxicity of sorafenib in sunitinib-pretreated patients with metastatic renal cell carcinoma. Ann Oncol 2007;18(11):1906–7.

65. O'Neal WT, Lakoski SG, Qureshi W, et al. Relation between cancer and atrial fibrillation (from the REasons for geographic and racial differences in stroke study). Am J Cardiol 2015;115(8):1090–4.

66. Holden SN, Eckhardt SG, Basser R, et al. Clinical evaluation of ZD6474, an orally active inhibitor of VEGF and EGF receptor signaling, in patients with solid, malignant tumors. Ann Oncol 2005; 16(8):1391–7.

67. Lu Z, Wu CYC, Jiang YP, et al. Suppression of phosphoinositide 3-kinase signaling and alteration of multiple ion currents in drug-induced long QT syndrome. Sci Transl Med 2012;4(131):131ra50.

68. Abedi H, Zachary I. Vascular endothelial growth factor stimulates tyrosine phosphorylation and recruitment to new focal adhesions of focal adhesion kinase and paxillin in endothelial cells. J Biol Chem 1997;272(24):15442–51.

69. Gerber HP, McMurtrey A, Kowalski J, et al. Vascular endothelial growth factor regulates endothelial cell survival through the phosphatidylinositol 3′-kinase/Akt signal transduction pathway. J Biol Chem 1998;273(46):30336–43.

70. Pretorius L, Du XJ, Woodcock EA, et al. Reduced phosphoinositide 3-kinase (p110α) activation increases the susceptibility to atrial Fibrillation. Am J Pathol 2009;175(3):998–1009.

71. Bronte E, Bronte G, Novo G, et al. What links BRAF to the heart function? new insights from the cardiotoxicity of BRAF inhibitors in cancer treatment. Oncotarget 2015;6(34):35589–601.

72. Xu Z, Cang S, Yang T, et al. Cardiotoxicity of tyrosine kinase inhibitors in chronic myelogenous leukemia therapy. Hematol Rep 2009;1(1):4.

73. Gril B, Palmieri D, Qian Y, et al. Pazopanib reveals a role for tumor cell B-Raf in the prevention of HER2 + breast cancer brain metastasis. Clin Cancer Res 2011;17(1):142–53.

74. Pakladok T, Hosseinzadeh Z, Almilaji A, et al. Up-Regulation of hERG K+ Channels by B-RAF. In: Barnes S, editor. PLoS One 2014;9(1):e87457.

75. Zhu WZ, Wang SQ, Chakir K, et al. Linkage of β1-adrenergic stimulation to apoptotic heart cell death through protein kinase A–independent activation of Ca2+/calmodulin kinase II. J Clin Invest 2003;111(5):617–25.

76. Anderson ME, Brown JH, Bers DM. CaMKII in myocardial hypertrophy and heart failure. J Mol Cell Cardiol 2011;51(4):468–73.

77. Pandey V, Xie LH, Qu Z, et al. Mitochondrial contributions in the genesis of delayed afterdepolarizations in ventricular myocytes. Front Physiol 2021;12:744023.

78. Wehrens XHT, Lehnart SE, Reiken SR, et al. Ca 2+/Calmodulin-dependent protein kinase ii phosphorylation regulates the cardiac ryanodine receptor. Circ Res 2004;94(6):e61–70.

79. Beckendorf J, van den Hoogenhof MMG, Backs J. Physiological and unappreciated roles of CaMKII in the heart. Basic Res Cardiol 2018;113(4):29.

80. Hudmon A, Schulman H. Structure–function of the multifunctional Ca2+/calmodulin-dependent protein kinase II. Biochem J 2002;364(3):593–611.

81. van Oort RJ, McCauley MD, Dixit SS, et al. Ryanodine receptor phosphorylation by calcium/calmodulin-dependent protein kinase II promotes life-threatening ventricular arrhythmias in mice with heart failure. Circulation 2010;122(25):2669–79.

82. Deininger M, Buchdunger E, Druker BJ. The development of imatinib as a therapeutic agent for chronic myeloid leukemia. Blood 2005;105(7):2640–53.

83. Lee WS, Kim J. Cardiotoxicity associated with tyrosine kinase-targeted anticancer therapy. Mol Cell Toxicol 2018;14(3):247–54.

84. McMullen CJ, Chalmers S, Wood R, et al. Sunitinib and imatinib display differential cardiotoxicity in adult rat cardiac fibroblasts that involves a role for calcium/calmodulin dependent protein kinase II. Front Cardiovasc Med 2021;7:630480.

85. Curigliano G, Lenihan D, Fradley M, et al. Management of cardiac disease in cancer patients throughout oncological treatment: ESMO consensus recommendations. Ann Oncol 2020;31(2):171–90.

86. Ghatalia P, Morgan CJ, Je Y, et al. Congestive heart failure with vascular endothelial growth factor receptor tyrosine kinase inhibitors. Crit Rev Oncol Hematol 2015;94(2):228–37.

87. Moustafa S, Ho TH, Shah P, et al. Predictors of incipient dysfunction of all cardiac chambers after treatment of metastatic renal cell carcinoma by tyrosine kinase inhibitors: cardiac chambers' dysfunction with TKIs. J Clin Ultrasound 2016;44(4):221–30.

88. Groarke JD, Choueiri TK, Slosky D, et al. Recognizing and managing left ventricular dysfunction associated with therapeutic inhibition of the vascular endothelial growth factor signaling pathway. Curr Treat Options Cardiovasc Med 2014;16(9):335.

89. Cheng H, Kari G, Dicker AP, et al. A novel preclinical strategy for identifying cardiotoxic kinase inhibitors and mechanisms of cardiotoxicity. Circ Res 2011;109(12):1401–9.

90. Grabowska ME, Chun B, Moya R, et al. Computational model of cardiomyocyte apoptosis identifies mechanisms of tyrosine kinase inhibitor-induced cardiotoxicity. J Mol Cell Cardiol 2021;155:66–77.

91. Datta SR, Dudek H, Tao X, et al. Akt Phosphorylation of BAD couples survival signals to the cell-intrinsic death machinery. Cell 1997;91(2):231–41.

92. Friehs I, Barillas R, Vasilyev NV. Vascular endothelial growth factor prevents apoptosis and preserves contractile function in hypertrophied infant heart. Circulation 2006;114(1_suppl). I-290–I-295.

93. del Peso L, Gonzalez-Garcia M, Page C, et al. Interleukin-3-induced phosphorylation of BAD through the protein kinase Akt. Science 1997;278(5338):687–9.

94. Matsui T, Tao J, del Monte F, et al. Akt activation preserves cardiac function and prevents injury after transient cardiac ischemia in vivo. Circulation 2001;104(3):330–5.

95. Kerkela R, Woulfe KC, Durand JB, et al. Sunitinib-induced cardiotoxicity is mediated by off-target inhibition of AMP-activated protein kinase. Clin Transl Sci 2009;2(1):15–25.

96. Freebern W, Fang H, Slade M, et al. In vitro cardiotoxicity potential comparative assessments of chronic myelogenous leukemia tyrosine kinase inhibitor therapies: dasatinib, imatinib and nilotinib. Blood 2007;110(11):4582.

97. Korashy HM, Attafi IM, Ansari MA, et al. Molecular mechanisms of cardiotoxicity of gefitinib in vivo and in vitro rat cardiomyocyte: Role of apoptosis and oxidative stress. Toxicol Lett 2016;252:50–61.

98. Kerkelä R, Grazette L, Yacobi R, et al. Cardiotoxicity of the cancer therapeutic agent imatinib mesylate. Nat Med 2006;12(8):908–16.

99. Chaar M, Kamta J, Ait-Oudhia S. Mechanisms, monitoring, and management of tyrosine kinase inhibitors-associated cardiovascular toxicities. Oncotargets Ther 2018;11:6227–37.

100. Force T, Krause DS, Van Etten RA. Molecular mechanisms of cardiotoxicity of tyrosine kinase inhibition. Nat Rev Cancer 2007;7(5):332–44.

101. Kivelä R, Hemanthakumar KA, Vaparanta K, et al. Endothelial cells regulate physiological cardiomyocyte growth via VEGFR2-mediated paracrine signaling. Circulation 2019;139(22):2570–84.

102. Virag JAI, Rolle ML, Reece J, et al. Fibroblast growth factor-2 regulates myocardial infarct repair. Am J Pathol 2007;171(5):1431–40.

103. Lieu C, Heymach J, Overman M, et al. Beyond VEGF: inhibition of the fibroblast growth factor pathway and antiangiogenesis. Clin Cancer Res 2011;17(19):6130–9.

104. Baird A, Esch F, Mormede P, et al. Molecular characterization of fibroblast growth factor: distribution and biological activities in various tissues. Recent Prog Horm Res 1986;42:143–205.

105. Schultz JEJ, Witt SA, Nieman ML, et al. Fibroblast growth factor-2 mediates pressure-induced hypertrophic response. J Clin Invest 1999;104(6):709–19.

106. Cilvik SN, Wang JI, Lavine KJ, et al. Fibroblast growth factor receptor 1 signaling in adult cardiomyocytes increases contractility and results in a hypertrophic cardiomyopathy. In: Lionetti V, editor. PLoS One 2013;8(12):e82979.

107. Akman T, Erbas O, Akman L, et al. Prevention of pazopanib-induced prolonged cardiac repolarization and proarrhythmic effects. Arq Bras Cardiol 2014;103(5):403–9.

108. Kappers MHW, de Beer VJ, Zhou Z, et al. Sunitinib-induced systemic vasoconstriction in swine is endothelin mediated and does not involve nitric oxide or oxidative stress. Hypertension 2012;59(1):151–7.

109. Kruzliak P, Novak J, Novak M. Vascular endothelial growth factor inhibitor–induced hypertension: from pathophysiology to prevention and treatment based on long-acting nitric oxide donors. Am J Hypertens 2014;27(1):3–13.

110. Cholesterol Treatment Trialists' (CTT) Collaborators. The effects of lowering LDL cholesterol with statin therapy in people at low risk of vascular disease: meta-analysis of individual data from 27 randomised trials. Lancet 2012;380(9841):581–90.

111. Mills EJ, Rachlis B, Wu P, et al. Primary prevention of cardiovascular mortality and events with statin treatments. J Am Coll Cardiol 2008;52(22):1769–81.

112. Seicean S, Seicean A, Plana JC, et al. Effect of statin therapy on the risk for incident heart failure in patients with breast cancer receiving anthracycline chemotherapy. J Am Coll Cardiol 2012;60(23):2384–90.

113. Calvillo-Argüelles O, Abdel-Qadir H, Michalowska M, et al. Cardioprotective effect of statins in patients with her2-positive breast cancer receiving trastuzumab therapy. Can J Cardiol 2019;35(2):153–9.

114. Maitland ML, Bakris GL, Black HR, et al. Initial assessment, surveillance, and management of blood pressure in patients receiving vascular endothelial growth factor signaling pathway inhibitors. J Natl Cancer Inst 2010;102(9):596–604.

115. Wasserstrum Y, Kornowski R, Raanani P, et al. Hypertension in cancer patients treated with anti-angiogenic based regimens. Cardio-Oncol 2015;1(1):6.

116. Thavendiranathan P, Poulin F, Lim KD, et al. Use of myocardial strain imaging by echocardiography for the early detection of cardiotoxicity in patients during and after cancer chemotherapy. J Am Coll Cardiol 2014;63(25):2751–68.

117. Geyer H, Caracciolo G, Abe H, et al. Assessment of myocardial mechanics using speckle tracking echocardiography: fundamentals and clinical applications. J Am Soc Echocardiogr 2010;23(4):351–69.

118. Spring BQ, Bryan Sears R, Zheng LZ, et al. A photoactivable multi-inhibitor nanoliposome for tumour control and simultaneous inhibition of treatment escape pathways. Nat Nanotechnol 2016;11(4):378–87.

T-cell Immunotherapy and Cardiovascular Disease
Chimeric Antigen Receptor T-cell and Bispecific T-cell Engager Therapies

Ashley F. Stein-Merlob, MD[a,b,1], Sarju Ganatra, MD[c,2,3,*],
Eric H. Yang, MD[a,b,2,4,*]

KEYWORDS

- Cardiotoxicity • Immunotherapy • Chimeric Antigen Receptor (CAR) T-cell therapy
- Bispecific T-cell engager (BiTE) therapy • Cardio-Oncology

KEY POINTS

- Chimeric antigen receptor (CAR) T-cell therapy and bispecific T-cell engager (BiTE) therapies are novel immunotherapies for the treatment of refractory or relapsed leukemia, lymphoma, and multiple myeloma.
- An adverse effect of CAR T-cell and BiTE therapy is the development of cytokine release syndrome (CRS), ranging from mild flu-like symptoms to severe hemodynamic collapse, and can be associated with cardiotoxicity.
- Cardiotoxic manifestations of CAR T-cell therapy include hypotension, cardiomyopathy, heart failure, arrhythmia, myocardial injury, circulatory collapse, and cardiac arrest.
- Cardiovascular evaluation before CAR T-cell therapy, particularly for patients at increased risk of adverse cardiovascular events, should include evaluating for coronary ischemia and/or significant structural heart disease, as well as the optimization of preexisting or suspected cardiovascular disease in the anticipation of potential hemodynamic changes with high-grade CRS.
- Treatment of cardiotoxicity and high-grade CRS includes supportive care, anti-IL-6 agent such as tocilizumab and possibly corticosteroids.

INTRODUCTION

T-cell-based immunotherapy, including chimeric antigen receptor (CAR) T-cell and bispecific T-cell engager (BiTE) therapies, has transformed the field of oncology and particularly the treatment of relapsed or refractory lymphoma and leukemia. Immunotherapies harness the antitumor properties of the patient's native immune system to treat a wide variety of malignancies. In CAR T-cell therapy, T-cells are engineered *in vitro* to express a tumor-targeted antigen and then infused to target malignant cells.[1] BiTE therapy uses an engineered antibody with 2 antigen-binding sites that targets both a tumor-cell specific antigen and a native T-cell specific antigen (CD3) to

[a] Division of Cardiology, Department of Medicine, University of California at Los Angeles, Los Angeles, CA, USA; [b] Division of Cardiology, Department of Medicine, UCLA-Cardio-Oncology Program, University of California at Los Angeles, Los Angeles, CA, USA; [c] Cardio-Oncology Program, Division of Cardiovascular Medicine, Department of Medicine, Lahey Hospital and Medical Center, Burlington, MA, USA
[1] Present address: 650 Charles E. Young Dr. South, A2-237 CHS, Los Angeles, CA 90095-1679.
[2] Authors have contributed equally.
[3] Present address: 41 Mall Road, Burlington, MA 01805, USA.
[4] Address: 100 Medical Plaza, Suite 630, Los Angeles, CA 90095.
* Corresponding authors.
E-mail addresses: sarju.ganatra@lahey.org (S.G.); ehyang@mednet.ucla.edu (E.H.Y.)
Twitter: @A_SteinMerlob (A.F.S.-M.); @SarjuGanatraMD (S.G.); @datsunian (E.H.Y.)

Heart Failure Clin 18 (2022) 443–454
https://doi.org/10.1016/j.hfc.2022.02.008
1551-7136/22/© 2022 Elsevier Inc. All rights reserved.

colocalize these cells.[2,3] Although early clinical trials did not reveal significantly associated cardiotoxicity, with the growing use of immunotherapy in real-world, high-risk populations there has been greater recognition of off-target adverse effects including cardiotoxicity.

The scientific basis of CAR T-cell therapy has been in development for 3 decades with the first CAR T-cells engineered in the early 1990s. The most widely studied, and first FDA-approved, CAR T-cell therapies are directed at the B-lymphocyte antigen CD19. There are now 4 FDA-approved CD19-directed CAR T-cell therapies, 2 of which have been approved since 2020. These therapies, axicabtagene ciloleucel,[4] brexucabtagene autoleucel,[5] tisagenlecleucel,[6] and lisocabtagene maraleucel,[7] are approved for the treatment of relapsed or refractory hematologic malignancies including B-cell acute lymphoblastic leukemia (ALL), diffuse large B-cell lymphoma (DLBCL), follicular lymphoma, and mantle cell lymphoma (**Fig. 1**). In early 2021, idecabtagene vicleucel was the first B-cell maturation antigen (BCMA) targeted CAR T-cell therapy approved for treatment-refractory multiple myeloma.[8] To date, there is only one FDA-approved BiTE therapy, blinatumomab, for B-cell precursor ALL in multiple populations (see **Fig. 1**).[9]

Production of these specialized cells requires first isolating T-cells from human blood originating from the patient themselves (autologous) or from a healthy donor (allogeneic). Leukocytes are isolated via leukapheresis and specific T-cells are expanded using IL-2 and anti-CD3 antibodies. Subsequently, the T-cells are purified and a gene that encodes an engineered CAR is transduced using a retroviral vector.[1] The patient receives lymphodepletion chemotherapy (ie, fludarabine, cyclophosphamide) before the infusion of the engineered CAR T-cells. Once infused, CAR T-cells proliferate and attack cells that contain the target antigen. However, this response can be accompanied by significant cytokine production and release, leading to cytokine release syndrome (CRS) which causes cardiotoxicity likely through direct and indirect mechanisms of cardiac injury.

Bispecific T-cell engager (BiTE) molecules are fusion proteins of linked single-chain variable fragments (scFv) with 2 different antigen-binding sites—one directed against the CD3 receptor, which leads to downstream activation of cytotoxic T lymphocytes, and another directed specifically at antigens of malignant cells. The linked BiTE protein colocalizes these cells, leading to cell linkage with cytolytic synapses to initiate selective cell lysis and death (**Fig. 2**, Panel B).[2,3]

MECHANISMS OF CHIMERIC ANTIGEN RECEPTOR T-CELL AND BISPECIFIC T-CELL ENGAGER THERAPIES

CAR T-cell immunotherapy uses genetically engineered cells to induce tumor-cell apoptosis by targeting tumor-specific antigens (**Fig. 2**, Panel A).

CYTOKINE RELEASE SYNDROME

The presentation of CRS ranges from mild flu-like symptoms, including fever, fatigue, headache, arthralgia, and myalgia, to severe, hemodynamically unstable presentations, including hypotension, systemic inflammatory response, coagulopathy,

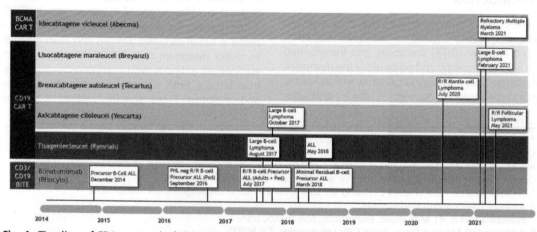

Fig. 1. Timeline of FDA-approval of chimeric antigen receptor (CAR) T-cell and bispecific T-cell engager (BiTE) therapies. Blinatumomab is the only FDA-approved BiTE therapy with multiple indications since 2014. There are 5 FDA-approved CAR T-cell therapies with 4 CD19-and one BCMA-targeted agent. There has been a significant increase in FDA approvals in 2020 to 2021. ALL = acute lymphoblastic leukemia; BCMA = B-cell maturation antigen; R/R = relapsed or refractory.

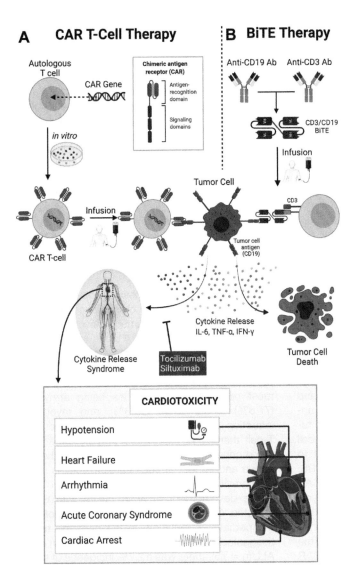

Fig. 2. Mechanism of chimeric antigen receptor (CAR) T-cell and bispecific T-cell engager (BiTE) therapies and cardiotoxicity. (*A*) Mechanism of CAR T-cell therapy. Autologous or allogenic T-cells are isolated and transfected *in vitro* with a gene encoding a chimeric antigen receptor that binds with an antigen expressed on tumor cells, most commonly the CD19. Engineered CAR T-cells are infused and then target antigen-positive tumor cells. Binding of the CAR and tumor cell antigen leads to tumor cell apoptosis. (*B*) Mechanism of BiTE therapy. The BiTE molecule links 2 scFv that bind a tumor antigen, such as CD19, and the T-cell antigen CD3. On binding these 2 antigens, the linked peptide brings the tumor and T-cell into close physical proximity. This activates the T-cell to cause tumor cell apoptosis. With both CAR T-cell and BiTE therapy, the T-cell activation that leads to tumor cell lysis initiates a cascade of cytokine release, including IL-1, IL-6, IFN-γ, and TNF-α. This inflammatory response can trigger CRS, a systemic disorder characterized by fever, hypotension, and multiorgan involvement. The most common treatment of CRS is tocilizumab, an anti-IL6 monoclonal antibody. CRS has been associated with cardiotoxicity including hypotension, heart failure, arrhythmia, acute coronary syndrome, and cardiac arrest. (Created with BioRender.com.)

multiorgan failure, and circulatory shock. CRS in CAR T-cell and BiTE therapy occurs through multiple mechanisms. Cytokines are released by infused CAR T-cells, activation of local "bystander" immune cells, and byproducts of CAR T-cell induced tumor cell apoptosis.[10] In particular, proliferation of CAR T-cells at the site of the targeted tumor cells leads to *in situ* cytokine production and systemic inflammatory response. It is thought that the release of cytokines changes the tumor microenvironment and provides additional antitumor effects beyond the direct cytotoxic effect of CAR T-cells of BiTE molecules.[3] Subsequent increases in vascular permeability and endothelial dysfunction causes hypotension, hypoxia, and multiorgan damage. Breakdown of the blood–brain barrier allows CAR T-cells, endogenous T-cells, and monocytes to translocate into the cerebrospinal fluid and central

nervous system, potentially leading to immune effector cell-associated neurotoxicity syndrome (ICANS).[10]

A variety of cytokines are implicated in the inflammatory cascade of CRS. The key mediator of CRS is thought to be IL-6 [11]. It was initially hypothesized that CAR T-cells directly increased IL-6 levels in CRS, but later studies found IL-6 production primarily by macrophages and monocytes. IL-6 antagonism has been the major focus for the treatment of CRS. Lymphodepletion therapy increases interleukin (IL)-2, IL-7, and IL-15, which synergistically leads to CAR T-cell proliferation and increased survival.[12] Macrophages, activated CAR T-cells, endothelial cells and fibroblasts produce high levels of IL-1β, IL-1, and granulocyte–macrophage colony-stimulating factor (GM-CSF) before the onset of CRS.[12] Tumor necrosis factor (TNF) exhibits direct tumoricidal activity while also mediating inflammation in CRS by activating T-cells, macrophages, and other immune cells. High levels of Interferon-γ, produced by activated T-cells, contribute to increased tissue permeability, including the blood–brain barrier, and have been associated with severe CRS.

The combination of sepsis-like stress of CRS and direct toxic effects of cytokines, particularly IL-6, is thought to contribute to myocardial dysfunction and subsequent cardiotoxicity.[13] Severe CRS also seems to trigger endothelial cell activation, including the upregulation of Ang-2 and von Willebrand factor, leading to clinical manifestations of capillary leakage, coagulopathy, and hypotension.[11,12]

MECHANISMS OF CARDIOTOXICITY

The mechanisms of cardiotoxicity from CAR T-cell and BiTE therapies are not well understood. Immunotherapy-related cardiotoxicities are thought to stem from several key mechanisms, including on-target, on-tumor effects (CRS), on-target, off-tumor effects (direct injury by T-cells of native tissue that share a common antigen with the tumor), and off-target, off-tumor effects (transduced T-cell unexpectedly attacks antigen other than intended tumor antigen).[14] The primary driver of CAR T-cell and BiTE-associated cardiotoxicity is thought to be "on-target, on-tumor" adverse effects of CRS, which is the most common adverse effect of CAR T-cell treatments. CRS stems from activated T lymphocytes, monocytes, macrophages, and endothelial cells releasing systemic inflammatory cytokines leading to multiorgan involvement. In contrast, the first investigational, patient-administered CAR T-cell therapy directed to melanoma-associated antigen 3 (MAGEA3) had significant "off-target, off-tumor" cardiotoxicity due to cross-reactivity of the MAGEA3 and myocyte titin protein.[15,16] This cross-reactivity led to fatal, fulminant acute myocarditis in 2 patients, limiting the clinical use of this agent. At this time, there have been no significant "off-target, off-tumor" effects specifically reported for CAR T-cell therapy.

CLINICAL EVIDENCE OF CARDIOTOXICITY

Early clinical trials of CAR T-cell therapy with highly selective patient enrollment reported significant rates of CRS, although the overall incidence of serious cardiovascular events was low. Initial Phase 2 trials showed a CRS incidence of up to 93% (**Table 1**) and with severe (greater than or equal to Grade 3) CRS in up to 46% of patients.[17–22] The notable exception,

however, was a pediatric study of relapsed and refractory acute lymphoblastic leukemia (ELIANA), which found an increased incidence of heart failure and cardiovascular death (2.7% and 4.0%, respectively).[17]

Subsequently, real-world institutional cohort studies have demonstrated significant incidences of cardiotoxicity not seen in Phase 2 trials despite similar rates of CRS. Cardiotoxicities include heart failure, arrhythmias, and myocardial infarction (see **Table 1**). In a single-center cohort study of 145 adult patients undergoing CD19-directed CAR T-cell therapy for DLBCL, ALL, and CLL, major adverse cardiac events (MACE) occurred in 21% of patients at a median of 11 days (interquartile range [IQR]: 6–151 days).[23] In the second study of 137 adult patients with DLBCL, transformed follicular lymphoma and multiple myeloma, there was a 12% incidence of MACE with median onset 21 days (IQR: 11–38 days).[24] The incidence of cardiovascular death was 4.3%,[24] the highest among clinical studies of cardiotoxicity (see **Table 1**). A cross-sectional analysis of the FDA Adverse Events Reporting System (FAERS), found that 19.7% of all adverse events reported to the FDA were cardiovascular related to the most reported cardiotoxicities being arrhythmia (77.6%), heart failure (14.3%), and myocardial infarction (0.5%). This may suggest that when CAR T-cell therapy is used more broadly under real-world conditions with higher risk patients, the incidence and impact of such cardiotoxicity is higher than previously estimated.

The development of heart failure with CD19-targeted CAR T-cell therapy was first noted in the pediatric population. In the pediatric trial of tisagenlecleucel in relapsed or refractory B-cell ALL (n = 75), there was a 2.7% incidence of symptomatic heart failure.[17] However, retrospectively, the incidence in the pediatric population has been as high as 10.8%, with reduced left ventricular ejection fraction (LVEF) in 41% of patients with hypotension requiring vasopressor support.[25] At time of discharge, 60% of these patients had persistent cardiac dysfunction. In the adult population, the incidence of symptomatic heart failure is as high as 15%.[23] Of 116 patients with relapsed or refractory non-Hodgkin's lymphoma with serial echocardiography during CD19-targeted CAR T-cell therapy, 10.3% (n = 12) developed new or worsening cardiomyopathy with an LVEF decline from 58% to 37% after a median duration of 12.5 days (range 2–24 days).[26] In long-term follow-up, LVEF improved in 75% of patients with reduced LVEF with normalization in half of the patients. In BiTE therapy, there are limited data on the incidence of heart failure. However, there is a case report of the development of fatal

Table 1
Major studies reporting chimeric antigen receptor (CAR) T-cell and bispecific T-cell engager (BiTE) cardiotoxicities

Study	Indication (n)	Therapy	CRS Any Grade (%)	CRS Grade 3–5 (%)	Adverse CV Event (%)									
					CV Death	Reduced LVEF	Symptomatic HF	ACS	Arrhythmia (all)	Atrial Fibrillation (all)	Hypotension (all)	Hypotension (Vasopressors)	Cardiac Arrest	Other
A. Institutional Cohort Studies of Cardiotoxicity														
Burstein et al,[25] *2018*	Pediatric ALL (2–27yo) (n = 93)	CD19-Directed CAR T	NA	25.8%	0	10.8						24	1.1	
Alvi et al,[24] *2019*	DLBCL, MM, Transf. Follicular, Other (n = 137)	CD19-Directed CAR T	59%	4%	4.3	5.8	4.3		5.1	2.2			2.2	
Lefebvre et al,[23] *2020*	DLBCL, ALL, CLL (n = 145)	CD19-Directed CAR T	72%	N/A	1.4		15.0	1.4	9.0	7.6		50.0	0.0	
Ganatra et al,[26] *2020*	R/R NHL (n = 187)	CD19-Directed CAR T	83%	5.3%		10.3	5.2		7.0			7.0	0	
Qi et al,[31] *2021*	MM, NHL, ALL (n = 126)	CD19-, CD20-, BCMA-Directed CAR T	81.7%	17.5%	1.6		11.9	7.1	5.6				0	
Brammer et al, 2021	R/R DLBCL, Mantle Cell or Follicular lymphoma (n = 90)	CD-19 Directed CAR T	88.9%	16.3%			1.1		12.2		87.8			Myocarditis (2.2%)
B. Single Therapy Investigational Phase 2 or 3 Studies														
TOWER Kantarjian, et al 2017	ALL (n = 271)	Blinatumomab, CD3/CD19 BiTE	14.2%	4.9%	0		0.4	0.4	0.8	0.4			0.4	HTN (6.4%)
ELIANA *Maude et al,*[17] *2018*	Pediatrics, Young Adults R/R B-ALL (n = 75)	Tisagenlecleucel (CD19)	77%	46%	4.0		2.7					25		

(continued on next page)

Table 1
(continued)

Study	Indication (n)	Therapy	CRS Any Grade (%)	CRS Grade 3–5 (%)	Adverse CV Event (%)									
					CV Death	Reduced LVEF	Symptomatic HF	ACS	Arrhythmia (all)	Atrial Fibrillation	Hypotension (all)	Hypotension (Vasopressors)	Cardiac Arrest	Other
ZUMA-1 Locke et al,[18] 2018	R/R B-ALL (n = 101)	Axicabtagene ciloleucel (CD19)	93%	11%	1.0						59	17	1.0	HTN (16%)
JULIET Schuster et al,[19] 2019	R/R DLBCL	Tisagenlecleucel (CD19)	58%	21.5%	0							26		
ZUMA-2 Wang et al,[20] 2020	R/R Mantle Cell lymphoma (n = 68)	Brexucabtagene autoleucel (CD19)	91%	15%							51	22		
Munshi et al,[21] 2021	Refractory MM (n = 128)	Idecabtagene vicleucel (BCMA)	84%	5%							16	1.0		
TRANSCEND Abramson et al,[22] 2021	R/R DLBCL (n = 269)	Lisocabtagene *maraleucel* (CD19)	42%	2%	0.3						22	3		HTN (14%)
C. Single Therapy Investigational Phase I Study														
Lee et al,[28] 2015	Pediatrics, ALL or r/r NHL (n = 21)	Investigational CD19-Directed CAR T	76%	29%		5					19.0		5	QTc (5%), HTN (5%)
Shalabi et al,[44] 2020	Pediatrics, Young Adults (R/R B-cell malignancies) (n = 52)	Investigational CD19-Directed CAR T	71%	17%		11.5						17.3	1.9	

(A) Retrospective single-institution cohort studies have provided the most detail regarding real-world cardiotoxicity of CAR T-cell therapies. Rates of heart failure, including reduced left ventricular ejection fraction (LVEF) and symptomatic heart failure, have been significantly higher than reported in early Phase 2 studies. (B) Important Phase 2 and Phase 3 single therapy CAR T-cell and BiTE therapy studies. The most commonly reported cardiotoxicity has been hypotension. ELIANA study was the notable exception for reporting significant rates of heart failure and cardiovascular death. (C) Phase I trials of investigation CAR T-cell therapies with reported cardiotoxicities. Colors indicate frequency of toxicity: red = greater than 10% incidence, yellow = 1 to 10% incidence, green = less than 1% incidence, gray = not reported heart failure due to Blinatumomab administration in a 5-year-old boy with ALL. Further studies of heart failure in BiTE therapy, particularly with serial echocardiographic monitoring, are needed.

Arrhythmias have been reported with an incidence ranging from 5.1% to 12.2% (see **Table 1**). The most common arrhythmia is atrial fibrillation, followed by supraventricular tachycardia and rare nonsustained ventricular tachycardia.[23,24,27] Additionally, there have been multiple reports of QTc prolongation.[24,28]

Cardiotoxicity is a potentially fatal adverse effect of CAR T-cell therapy. In retrospective cohort studies, the incidence of cardiovascular death in adults undergoing CAR T-cell therapy ranges from 1.4% to 4.3%.[23,24] Notable, in a FAERS study of cardiotoxicity, the mortality in patients with cardiovascular adverse events was 30.1%.

Dedicated studies of cardiotoxicity in BiTE therapy are lacking. In the Phase 3 TOWER trial of blinatumomab, CRS and acute coronary syndrome occurred in 2.6% and 2.2% of patients, respectively.[29] A subsequent real-world study of blinatumomab showed grade 3 to 4 CRS in up to 19% of patients. Ongoing surveillance for adverse cardiovascular effects is warranted for this evolving immunotherapy.[30]

RISK FACTORS FOR CARDIOTOXICITY

CAR T-cell therapy-associated cardiotoxicity is often accompanied by other systemic toxicities, particularly CRS, neurotoxicity, and graft versus host disease.[18,31] In Alvi and colleagues, all patients who developed MACE had at least Grade 2 CRS. In a retrospective analysis, Grade 3 and 4 CRS conferred a significantly increased risk of developing cardiotoxicity with hazard ratios of 3.31 (95% confidence interval 1.55–7.09) and 9.79 (95% CI: 3.96–24.21), respectively.[23] Additionally, early onset of CRS was associated with an increased risk of developing cardiotoxicity.[31] Although one recent retrospective study casts doubt on this theory, showing no association between cardiotoxicity and CRS Grade 3 and above,[32] the predominating theory continues to be that most of the cardiotoxicity is related to the inflammatory cascade of CRS. Neurotoxicity, particularly immune effector cell-associated encephalopathy (ICANS)—previously called CAR T-cell related encephalopathy syndrome—has also been associated with cardiotoxicity (odds ratio, 1.76; 95% confidence interval, 1.20–2.60; P = .004).[33]

The risk of developing cardiotoxicity due to baseline cardiovascular disease and prior cancer treatments is still unclear. Prior radiation, anthracycline dose and other cardiotoxic chemotherapy has not been found to be associated with the development of cardiotoxicity or hypotension.[25,26] However, a major predictor of severe CRS in both CAR T-cell or BiTE therapy is preexisting disease burden before treatment.[12] Prior use of insulin, statins and aspirin have been associated with MACE, likely indicating higher baseline cardiovascular risk.[34] Renal dysfunction is also associated with the development of MACE.[31,34] Development of heart failure has been associated with increased age, hyperlipidemia and coronary artery disease.[26] Elevated troponin has been associated with the development of cardiotoxicity and may be an important marker to identify patients at risk of cardiotoxicity.[24]

Currently, there are limited data on the 3 newest CAR T-cell therapies that have been FDA approved since 2020 as they have not yet been included in published retrospective cohort studies. The most recent CD-19 targeted CAR T-cell therapy, lisocabtagene maraleucel (Beryanzi) has a different 4-1BB costimulatory domain, which was designed to reduce the incidence of CRS.[22] In the clinical trial, the overall incidence of CRS was similar to prior agents at 84%, but the rate of Grade 3 to 4 CRS was decreased significantly to 5%.[22] Idecabtagene vicleucel has a unique target, BCMA, and had a lower overall rate of CRS.[21] Further studies will be required to evaluate if this reduction in severe CRS contributes to a different cardiotoxicity profile.

CLINICAL MANAGEMENT
Pre-chimeric antigen receptor T-cell therapy cardiovascular workup

Currently, there is no standardized protocol for pretherapy cardiovascular evaluation. However, the expert consensus recommendation is that each patient should undergo a detailed cardiovascular examination along with obtaining an ECG. An echocardiogram should also be performed in all patients at baseline given the associated risk of cardiomyopathy and to rule out any significant valvular or other structural heart diseases.[35] If the patient has a prior history of cardiovascular disease, any significant cardiovascular symptoms, impaired exercise capacity, or any abnormality noted on initial workup, further risk stratification with functional stress testing may need to be considered to evaluate for underlying obstructive coronary artery disease or other structural heart diseases to ensure that the patient will be able to withstand the hemodynamic changes associated with a high-grade CRS (**Fig. 3**).[35,36]

Many patients who need to undergo CAR T-cell therapy have one or multiple cardiovascular

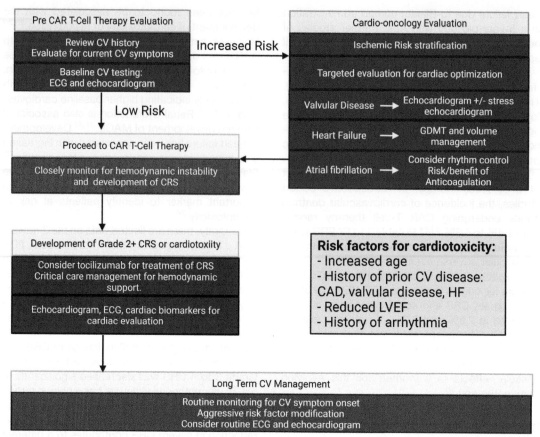

Fig. 3. Proposed algorithm for the management of cardiovascular risk and complications during chimeric antigen receptor (CAR) T-cell therapy. Before the initiation of CAR T-cell therapy all patients should undergo baseline evaluation to determine their level of cardiovascular risk. Patients with increased cardiovascular risk due to prior cardiovascular disease, current cardiovascular symptoms, or abnormal ECG or echocardiogram should be evaluated by a cardio-oncologist before the initiation of therapy. Ischemic evaluation should be pursued based on individual risk factors. Preexisting valvular heart disease, left ventricular dysfunction or arrhythmia should be medically optimized due to the potential for hemodynamic instability or cardiotoxicity during CAR T-cell therapy. Patients who develop CRS should be treated using the current standard of care with hemodynamic support and consideration of tocilizumab. Given the unknown long-term cardiovascular risks associated with CAR T-cell therapy, particular attention should be paid to aggressive risk factor modification and ongoing evaluation for the development of new cardiovascular toxicities after the completion of therapy. (Created with BioRender.com.)

comorbidities and are on medical therapies for those conditions.[26] Optimization of their preexisting cardiovascular conditions and their medications is crucial to minimize the CRS-associated adverse events. High-grade CRS is typically associated with hypotension, and hence it is important to consider either down titration or discontinuation of antihypertensive medications and diuretics.[35] Additionally, similar consideration should be given to antiplatelet and anticoagulation agents given the elevated risk of thrombocytopenia and, in turn bleeding events, on a case-by-case basis after weighing the risks and benefits.[35,37]

While the interaction between CAR T-cell therapy and preexisting cardiovascular conditions is not well established, patients with an uncorrected severe valvular disease or significant obstructive coronary artery disease are likely to suffer significant major adverse cardiovascular events even with transient hemodynamic changes associated with CRS. Although having a preexisting CVD may not be an absolute contraindication for receiving CAR T-cell therapy, such patients need to be identified, and their cardiovascular status should be optimized before CAR T-cell therapy so that they are able to withstand any potential hemodynamic instability during CRS.

Diagnosis

As the vast majority of adverse cardiovascular events with CAR T-cell therapy occur in the context of CRS, prompt recognition of CRS is crucial. A high degree of suspicion and close surveillance with close monitoring of vital signs [especially heart rate and blood pressure (BP)] are required to recognize the CRS promptly and also to classify the severity. While the markers of inflammation such as C-reactive protein, ferritin, and IL-6 are typically elevated with CRS, it is not specific and could be elevated due to other conditions. Similarly, cardiac troponin can be elevated in the context of an adverse cardiovascular event or high-grade CRS. However, routine surveillance with serial cardiac troponin may not be required or helpful. An echocardiogram should be repeated in patients with cardiovascular symptoms, hemodynamic instability, and/or grade ≥ 2 CRS. For patients with CRS-associated hemodynamic instability, while considering CRS and associated cardiotoxicity, other possible etiologies, such as sepsis, tumor lysis syndrome, pulmonary embolism, or primary cardiac events should also be ruled out.

Management

The cornerstones of the management are supportive hemodynamic care along with targeted anti-IL-6 therapy and, if required, broader immunosuppression with corticosteroids.[35] Intravenous fluid resuscitation should be considered as a first-line intervention for patients with tachycardia and hypotension secondary to CRS, weighing the risk of vascular leak and pulmonary congestion. If hypotension persists, vasopressors should be considered. In select, very high-risk patients, invasive pulmonary artery monitoring may be required. In a unique example, a patient with DLBCL and anthracycline-induced cardiomyopathy underwent invasive continuous pulmonary artery pressure monitoring with implantable CardioMEMS. Invasive monitoring tailored diuretic dosing during acute decompensated heart failure, noncardiogenic pulmonary edema, intubation, vasopressor use, and arrhythmia.[38]

Given the central mechanistic role of excessive IL-6 in causing CAR T-cell therapy associated CRS as well as myocardial depression,[13] anti-IL-6 therapy is considered first-line therapy for high-grade CRS along with supportive care.[39] Tocilizumab is a monoclonal anti-IL-6 receptor antibody used in the management of CRS-related toxicity. Typically, 8 mg/kg intravenously is given, and this dose could be repeated up to 3 times 8 hours apart.[39] Shorter time from CRS onset to tocilizumab is shown to be associated with a lower rate of adverse cardiovascular events.[24] However, there is also an unproven

concern that the anticancer efficacy of the CAR T-cell therapy may be reduced with the use of an anti-IL-6 agent. Hence, there is wide interinstitutional and interprovider variation in practice. While it is used generously with any grade CRS at some institutions, some experts believe that it should be reserved for patients with hemodynamic instability, such as hypotension requiring BP support for longer than 24 h, hypoxia, unstable arrhythmia, evidence of myocardial damage (increased troponin level), or new cardiomyopathy.

Siltuximab, another monoclonal antibody blocks IL-6 signaling by binding to IL-6 itself to prevent it from activating immune effector cells.[40] While it has not been studied extensively for the management of CRS, it has a higher affinity for IL-6 than tocilizumab. It can be considered in patients with refractory CRS to tocilizumab and corticosteroids. Unlike tocilizumab, siltuximab binds directly to IL-6 and not its receptors. Hence, it may decrease the IL-6 level in the central nervous system. In contrast, tocilizumab may potentially increase systemic and central nervous system IL-6 levels, which could precipitate or worsen neurotoxicity.[41]

Corticosteroids, by their broad immunosuppressive action, are effective in the treatment of CRS. However, given the concern of reduced CAR T-cell therapy efficacy with its use, they are often not used as a first-line agent and rather are considered second-line therapy for the management of CRS refractory to tocilizumab. Although corticosteroids are thought to potentially decrease CAR T-cell efficacy, this concern has been unfounded, and results from initial clinical trials did not show an association between the use of corticosteroids and cancer response rates.[41]

Prognosis

The long-term prognosis of patients who develop CAR T-cell therapy-associated adverse cardiovascular events remains unknown. A recent study of patients who developed CAR T-cell therapy-associated cardiomyopathy showed that LVEF recovered in 75% of patients with supportive care.[26] Long-term follow-up studies are needed to better understand cardiovascular effects of immune system modulation and continued circulation of CAR T-cells, particularly to assess if patients are at a higher risk of developing metabolic syndrome, hypertension, vascular disease, and cardiomyopathy after a latent period following CAR T-cell therapy.

In terms of patients cancer-related prognosis, there has been a theorized relationship between early immune-related toxicity and improved response to certain types of immunotherapy. In CAR T-cell therapy particularly, there has been a reported association between increased progression-free survival and moderate CRS. However, no specific association was noted with cardiotoxicity in particular.[32] Future, large-scale studies will be needed to determine the prognostic significance of cardiotoxicity.

NOVEL CARDIOVASCULAR TARGETED CHIMERIC ANTIGEN RECEPTOR T-CELL THERAPIES

In addition to the current oncologic applications of CAR T-cell therapy, preclinical studies have investigated the use of CAR T-cell therapy as a treatment of cardiovascular disease itself. In particular, antifibrotic CAR T-cells directed against fibroblast activated protein (FAP) have been used to target activated fibroblasts and prevent myocardial fibrosis in heart failure.[42,43] In addition to the traditional *in vitro* created FAP CAR T-cells, a novel method of *in vivo* CAR T-cell generation delivers mRNA packaged in CD5-targeted lipid nanoparticles (LNP)–different from the CD19 target used in cancer treatment—which can be intravenously injected. Using LNPs, mRNA is transported to lymphocyte cytoplasm and produces FAP CAR T-cells *in vivo*.[42] This method is based on the same technology as the LNP-mRNA COVID vaccines. Because mRNA is delivered to the cytoplasm, it does not integrate into the lymphocyte genome and thus creates a transient CAR T-cell. In a mouse model of pressure overload induced heart failure, FAP CAR T-cell treated mice using both methods of CAR T-cell production showed improvement in left ventricular systolic and diastolic function and left ventricular end-diastolic and end-systolic volumes. Histologic analysis showed a significant reduction in fibrosis. This promising and highly adaptable technology has the potential to target multiple traditional mechanisms and pathways of cardiovascular disease with the goal of translation to clinical care. In one preclinical study, FAP-targeted CAR T-cells were associated with cachexia and bone toxicity via effects on FAP mediated stromal cells in the bone marrow while having limited effects on the progression of various tumor types. Additionally, whether such FAP-directed CAR T-cell therapy is associated with CRS and cardiovascular complications similar to anti-CD-19 CAR T-cell therapy remain to be seen.

SUMMARY

Immunotherapy is a rapidly evolving field with frequent new applications of existing medications and a constant influx of novel, investigational therapies. Current CAR T-cell and BiTE therapies have been shown to cause infrequent, but potentially severe, cardiotoxicities that were not immediately apparent during initial clinical trials. As new immunotherapies enter the market, careful surveillance for emerging cardiotoxicities will be needed. Additionally, further studies and registry data are warranted to better understand the mechanisms, risk factors, and treatment of immunotherapy-associated cardiotoxicity.

CLINICS CARE POINTS

- All patients undergoing chimeric antigen receptor (CAR) T-cell or bispecific T-cell engager (BiTE) therapies should undergo baseline cardiovascular risk stratification and optimization of preexisting or suspected cardiovascular disease, particularly coronary artery disease, valvular disease, heart failure, and atrial fibrillation.

- Manifestations of CAR T-cell therapy-associated cardiotoxicity most commonly occur within the first few weeks after the initiation of therapy and can present as hypotension, cardiomyopathy, heart failure, arrhythmia, or myocardial injury.

- Patients undergoing CAR T-cell therapy who develop cytokine release syndrome (CRS) should be evaluated for cardiotoxicity with serum troponin levels, ECG, and echocardiogram.

- Cardiac biomarker elevation (ie, troponin) can be commonly seen in CAR T-cell therapy; however, in the presence of high-grade CRS, it can be associated with an increased risk of major adverse cardiovascular events.

- Early treatment of CRS with anti-IL-6 agents, such as tocilizumab, may lead to reduced rates of adverse cardiovascular events, but future research is needed.

DISCLOSURES

Dr E.H. Yang receives research funding from CSL Behring, Boehringer Ingelheim and Eli Lilly and Company (nonrelevant). Dr A.F. Stein-Merlob is supported by the National Institutes of Health Cardiovascular Scientist Training Program (T32 HL007895)

REFERENCES

1. Kalos M, Levine BL, Porter DL, et al. T cells with chimeric antigen receptors have potent antitumor effects and can establish memory in patients with

advanced leukemia. Sci translational Med 2011; 3(95). 95ra73-95ra73.

2. Sedykh S, Prinz V, Buneva V, et al. Bispecific antibodies: design, therapy, perspectives. Drug Des Development Ther 2018;ume 12:195–208.

3. Slaney CY, Wang P, Darcy PK, et al. CARs versus BiTEs: A Comparison between T Cell–Redirection Strategies for Cancer Treatment. Cancer Discov 2018;8(8):924–34.

4. YESCARTA (axicabtagene ciloleucel) FDA Approval. Available at: https://www.fda.gov/vaccines-blood-biologics/cellular-gene-therapy-products/yescarta-axicabtagene-ciloleucel. Accessed March 27, 2022.

5. TECARTUS (brexucabtagene autoleucel) FDA Approval. Available at: https://www.fda.gov/vaccines-blood-biologics/cellular-gene-therapy-products/tecartus-brexucabtagene-autoleucel. Accessed August 31 2021.

6. KYMRIAH (tisagenlecleucel) FDA Approval. 2021. Available at: https://www.fda.gov/vaccines-blood-biologics/cellular-gene-therapy-products/kymriah-tisagenlecleucel. Accessed August 31 2021.

7. BREYANZI (lisocabtagene maraleucel) FDA Approval. Available at: https://www.fda.gov/vaccines-blood-biologics/cellular-gene-therapy-products/breyanzi-lisocabtagene-maraleucel. Accessed August 31 2021.

8. ABECMA (idecabtagene vicleucel) FDA Approval. Available at: https://www.fda.gov/vaccines-blood-biologics/abecma-idecabtagene-vicleucel. Accessed August 31 2021.

9. FDA Approval letter for blinatumomab. Available at: *https://wwwaccessdatafdagov/drugsatfda_docs/nda/2014/125557Orig1s000Approvpdf.*

10. Morris EC, Neelapu SS, Giavridis T, et al. Cytokine release syndrome and associated neurotoxicity in cancer immunotherapy. Nat Rev Immunol 2022 Feb;22(2):85–96.

11. Khadka RH, Sakemura R, Kenderian SS, et al. Management of cytokine release syndrome: an update on emerging antigen-specific T cell engaging immunotherapies. Immunotherapy 2019;11(10):851–7.

12. Shimabukuro-Vornhagen A, Gödel P, Subklewe M, et al. Cytokine release syndrome. J ImmunoTherapy Cancer 2018;6(1).

13. Pathan N, Hemingway CA, Alizadeh AA, et al. Role of interleukin 6 in myocardial dysfunction of meningococcal septic shock. Lancet 2004;363(9404):203–9.

14. Baik AH, Oluwole OO, Johnson DB, et al. Mechanisms of Cardiovascular Toxicities Associated With Immunotherapies. Circ Res 2021;128(11):1780–801.

15. Cameron BJ, Gerry AB, Dukes J, et al. Identification of a Titin-Derived HLA-A1-Presented Peptide as a Cross-Reactive Target for Engineered MAGE A3-Directed T Cells. Sci Translational Med 2013; 5(197). 197ra103-197ra191.

16. Linette GP, Stadtmauer EA, Maus MV, et al. Cardiovascular toxicity and titin cross-reactivity of affinity-enhanced T cells in myeloma and melanoma. Blood 2013;122(6):863–71.

17. Maude SL, Laetsch TW, Buechner J, et al. Tisagenlecleucel in Children and Young Adults with B-Cell Lymphoblastic Leukemia. N Engl J Med 2018; 378(5):439–48.

18. Locke FL, Ghobadi A, Jacobson CA, et al. Long-term safety and activity of axicabtagene ciloleucel in refractory large B-cell lymphoma (ZUMA-1): a single-arm, multicentre, phase 1-2 trial. Lancet Oncol 2019;20(1):31–42.

19. Schuster SJ, Bishop MR, Tam CS, et al. Tisagenlecleucel in Adult Relapsed or Refractory Diffuse Large B-Cell Lymphoma. N Engl J Med 2019; 380(1):45–56.

20. Wang M, Munoz J, Goy A, et al. KTE-X19 CAR T-Cell Therapy in Relapsed or Refractory Mantle-Cell Lymphoma. N Engl J Med 2020;382(14):1331–42.

21. Munshi NC, Anderson LD Jr, Shah N, et al. Idecabtagene Vicleucel in Relapsed and Refractory Multiple Myeloma. N Engl J Med 2021;384(8): 705–16.

22. Abramson JS, Palomba ML, Gordon LI, et al. Lisocabtagene maraleucel for patients with relapsed or refractory large B-cell lymphomas (TRANSCEND NHL 001): a multicentre seamless design study. Lancet 2020;396(10254):839–52.

23. Lefebvre B, Kang Y, Smith AM, et al. Cardiovascular Effects of CAR T Cell Therapy. JACC: CardioOncology. 2020;2(2):193–203.

24. Alvi RM, Frigault MJ, Fradley MG, et al. Cardiovascular Events Among Adults Treated With Chimeric Antigen Receptor T-Cells (CAR-T). J Am Coll Cardiol 2019;74(25):3099–108.

25. Burstein DS, Maude S, Grupp S, et al. Cardiac Profile of Chimeric Antigen Receptor T Cell Therapy in Children: A Single-Institution Experience. Biol Blood Marrow Transplant 2018;24(8):1590–5.

26. Ganatra S, Redd R, Hayek SS, et al. Chimeric Antigen Receptor T-Cell Therapy-Associated Cardiomyopathy in Patients With Refractory or Relapsed Non-Hodgkin Lymphoma. Circulation 2020;142(17):1687–90.

27. Herrmann J. Adverse cardiac effects of cancer therapies: cardiotoxicity and arrhythmia. Nat Rev Cardiol 2020;17(8):474–502.

28. Lee DW, Kochenderfer JN, Stetler-Stevenson M, et al. T cells expressing CD19 chimeric antigen receptors for acute lymphoblastic leukaemia in children and young adults: a phase 1 dose-escalation trial. Lancet 2015;385(9967):517–28.

29. Kantarjian H, Stein A, Gökbuget N, et al. Blinatumomab versus Chemotherapy for Advanced Acute Lymphoblastic Leukemia. N Engl J Med 2017; 376(9):836–47.

30. Apel A, Ofran Y, Wolach O, et al. Safety and efficacy of blinatumomab: a real world data. Ann Hematol 2020;99(4):835–8.

31. Qi K, Yan Z, Cheng H, et al. An Analysis of Cardiac Disorders Associated With Chimeric Antigen Receptor T Cell Therapy in 126 Patients: A Single-Centre Retrospective Study. Front Oncol 2021;11(2264).

32. Brammer JE, Braunstein Z, Katapadi A, et al. Early toxicity and clinical outcomes after chimeric antigen receptor T-cell (CAR-T) therapy for lymphoma. J ImmunoTherapy Cancer 2021;9(8):e002303.

33. Guha A, Addison D, Jain P, et al. Cardiovascular Events Associated with Chimeric Antigen Receptor T Cell Therapy: Cross-Sectional FDA Adverse Events Reporting System Analysis. Biol Blood Marrow Transpl 2020;26(12):2211–6.

34. Khunger A, Battel L, Wadhawan A, et al. New Insights into Mechanisms of Immune Checkpoint Inhibitor-Induced Cardiovascular Toxicity. Curr Oncol Rep 2020;22(7).

35. Ganatra S, Carver JR, Hayek SS, et al. Chimeric Antigen Receptor T-Cell Therapy for Cancer and Heart: JACC Council Perspectives. J Am Coll Cardiol 2019; 74(25):3153–63.

36. Ganatra S, Parikh R, Neilan TG. Cardiotoxicity of Immune Therapy. Cardiol Clin 2019;37(4):385–97.

37. Dal'Bo N, Patel R, Parikh R, et al. Cardiotoxicity of Contemporary Anticancer Immunotherapy. Curr Treat Options Cardiovasc Med 2020;22(12).

38. Kanelidis AJ, Raikhelkar J, Kim G, et al. Cardio-MEMS-Guided CAR T Cell Therapy for Lymphoma in a Patient With Anthracycline-Induced Cardiomyopathy. JACC: CardioOncology 2020;2(3):515–8.

39. Le RQ, Li L, Yuan W, et al. FDA Approval Summary: Tocilizumab for Treatment of Chimeric Antigen Receptor T Cell-Induced Severe or Life-Threatening Cytokine Release Syndrome. Oncologist 2018; 23(8):943–7.

40. Riegler LL, Jones GP, Lee DW. Current approaches in the grading and management of cytokine release syndrome after chimeric antigen receptor T-cell therapy. Ther Clin Risk Manag 2019;15:323–35.

41. Locke FL, Neelapu SS, Bartlett NL, et al. Preliminary Results of Prophylactic Tocilizumab after Axicabtagene-neciloleucel (axi-cel; KTE-C19) Treatment for Patients with Refractory, Aggressive Non-Hodgkin Lymphoma (NHL). Blood 2017;130(Supplement 1):1547.

42. Rurik JG, Tombácz I, Yadegari A, et al. CAR T cells produced in vivo to treat cardiac injury. Science 2022;375(6576):91–6.

43. Aghajanian H, Kimura T, Rurik JG, et al. Targeting cardiac fibrosis with engineered T cells. Nature 2019;573(7774):430–3.

44. Shalabi H, Sachdev V, Kulshreshtha A, et al. Impact of cytokine release syndrome on cardiac function following CD19 CAR-T cell therapy in children and young adults with hematological malignancies. J Immunother Cancer 2020;8(2).

Cardiovascular Imaging in Cardio-Oncology

The Role of Echocardiography and Cardiac MRI in Modern Cardio-Oncology

John Alan Gambril, MD[a,b], Aaron Chum, BA[b,c], Akash Goyal, MD[b,c],
Patrick Ruz, BS[b,c], Katarzyna Mikrut, MD[b], Orlando Simonetti, PhD[b,c,d,e],
Hardeep Dholiya, MD[b,c], Brijesh Patel, DO[c,f], Daniel Addison, MD[b,g],*

KEYWORDS

- Cardio-oncology • Advanced imaging • Echocardiography • Cardiac MRI • Immunotherapy toxicity

KEY POINTS

- Echocardiography, the first-line imaging modality for cancer therapy-related cardiotoxicity (CTRCT) screening, should be obtained with signs or symptoms of cardiac involvement in patients with history of cardiotoxic cancer therapy.
- Echocardiographic strain imaging can detect subclinical cardiac dysfunction and is a promising tool for the prediction and prognostication of CTRCT.
- Cardiac MRI (CMR) should be obtained if echocardiography is insufficient or suboptimal, highly accurate volume assessments are needed, or myocarditis is suspected.
- Parametric T1 and T2 mapping should be included, when possible, in the CMR evaluation of cancer patients.
- CTRCT surveillance varies based on patient risk and cancer therapy. Baseline echocardiography should be obtained before therapy initiation in all intermediate and high-risk patients and considered in low-risk patients.

INTRODUCTION

The constant evolution of cancer treatment has led to improved outcomes in numerous malignancies.[1] With improved cancer survivorship and the introduction of novel therapies such as biologic agents and immunotherapeutics, the prevalence of systemic toxicities, in particular cardiotoxicity, has grown.[2] Because cardiovascular (CV) disease remains the leading noncancer cause of death in cancer survivors, cardio-oncology strives to understand and improve CV health in patients with cancer.[3,4]

[a] Department of Internal Medicine, Ohio State University Wexner Medical Center, Columbus, OH, USA; [b] Cardio-Oncology Program, Division of Cardiology, The Ohio State University Medical Center, Columbus, OH, USA; [c] Division of Cardiovascular Medicine, Davis Heart & Lung Research Institute, 473 West 12th Avenue, Suite 200, Columbus, OH 43210, USA; [d] Department of Internal Medicine, The Ohio State University Medical Center, Columbus, OH, USA; [e] Department of Radiology, The Ohio State University Medical Center, Columbus, OH, USA; [f] Cardio-Oncology Program, Heart and Vascular Institute, West Virginia University, Morgantown, WV, USA; [g] Division of Cancer Prevention and Control, Department of Internal Medicine, College of Medicine, The Ohio State University, Columbus, OH, USA

* Corresponding author. Division of Cardiovascular Medicine, Davis Heart & Lung Research Institute, 473 West 12th Avenue, Suite 200, Columbus, OH 43210.

E-mail address: daniel.addison@osumc.edu

Twitter: @GambrilAlan (J.A.G.); @agoyalMD (A.G.); @KatieMikrut (K.M.); @Hardeep_10 (H.D.)

Heart Failure Clin 18 (2022) 455–478
https://doi.org/10.1016/j.hfc.2022.02.007
1551-7136/22/© 2022 Elsevier Inc. All rights reserved.

CV imaging is crucial in recognizing, understanding, monitoring, and treating cancer treatment-related cardiotoxicities (CTRCT).[5] Structural and functional imaging modalities provide important information in the management of pathologic cardio-oncologic conditions. Echocardiography continues to be highly used for assessment of cardiac structure and function due to its low cost, accessibility, and effectiveness. Newer echocardiographic applications, such as strain imaging, are increasingly used in evaluation of CTRCT, especially to detect subclinical disease.[6,7] Similarly, cardiac magnetic resonance (CMR) has become a crucial imaging modality in cardio-oncology. Although less accessible, CMR offers accurate functional and structural assessment because of excellent reproducibility, high signal-to-noise ratio in addition to fine tissue characterization that is particularly helpful when echocardiography is insufficient or suboptimal.[6,8] This review will discuss current evidence for use of echocardiography and CMR in cardio-oncology and practical clinical uses for each.

Traditional 2D Echocardiography

Due to availability, low cost, short acquisition time, and safety, echocardiography is the first-line imaging modality for CTRCT screening by all published cardio-oncology guidelines and expert consensus statements.[5] **Fig. 1** illustrates the relative utility of echocardiography considering various parameters. Although left ventricular ejection fraction (LVEF) as measured by the Simpson biplane method is the most cited parameter in strict definitions of cardiotoxicity (definitions range from reduction in LVEF by 5%–10% to absolute LVEF of less than 50%–55%),[9] LVEF assessment via 2D echocardiography lacks the sensitivity and reproducibility for primary CTRCT screening.[10] Thus, newer echocardiographic applications such as strain imaging, 3D echocardiography, and contrast echocardiography have growing roles in screening for CTRCT.

Echocardiographic strain imaging
Myocardial strain, or deformation, is the measure of percent change in the length of a myocardial segment during a given timeframe. This parameter is helpful in quantifying myocardial function directly rather than indirectly via 2D LVEF with the Simpson biplane method. Speckle-tracking echocardiography (STE) is the preferred method of strain imaging. STE tracks the artifactual "speckles" created by reflected and scattered ultrasound beams through cardiac tissue. Strain can be calculated for the 3 major orientations of myocardial fibers (longitudinal, radial, and circumferential) and as global longitudinal strain (GLS), which uses data from multiple cardiac segments. All of these show promise in the early detection of CTRCT before changes in LVEF occur.[7,11] A decrease in GLS of less than or equal to 15% from baseline is considered abnormal and has been most extensively studied.[12]

Several studies have assessed the prognostic value of GLS in the early prediction of CTRCT before LVEF changes. A 2019 systematic review[13] evaluated 21 such studies of patients treated with anthracyclines with or without trastuzumab for a variety of cancers. Summary odds ratios (ORs) for the prediction of CTRCT based on threshold GLS values and percent change of GLS after treatment initiation were 12.27 and 15.82, respectively. Since the publication of this systematic review, newer studies have shown similar findings,[14–18] some incorporating several biomarkers for additional predictive value with mixed utility.[19–21] GLS has been studied in pediatric populations as well. Although less robust, the studies use strain-imaging to evaluate subclinical cardiac dysfunction in varying follow-up periods after anthracycline therapy or radiation.[22–27] As in adults, GLS in pediatric patients detects myocardial dysfunction before changes in LVEF. Future studies in all populations should focus on both early and long-term predictive value of strain imaging with and without biomarkers for the development of CTRCT.

Echocardiography in anthracyclines
Anthracyclines are antitumor antibiotics that play a major role in the treatment of a wide range of cancers. Both antitumor action and cardiotoxicity are thought to be due to activation of apoptotic pathways triggered by a combination of 3 separate mechanisms: direct DNA damage via intercalation into DNA strands, transcription interference via inhibition of topoisomerase enzymes, and DNA and cellular damage via generation of free radicals.[28,29] Cardiotoxicity manifests primarily in the form of myocardial dysfunction, usually within 1 year[30] of therapy initiation, and it can progress to irreversible heart failure, characterized by diffuse fibrosis.[31] Risk factors for cardiotoxicity include cumulative anthracycline exposure, age greater than 65 years or less than 18 years, female sex, preexisting cardiac risk factors, kidney disease, and exposure to other cardiotoxic therapies.[32] Patients can be categorized into low, intermediate, and high risk for cardiotoxicity based on these risk factors (**Table 1**). Echocardiography is the primary screening tool for anthracycline cardiotoxicity, with GLS emerging as the most sensitive measure of early myocardial dysfunction.[13]

Value of Echocardiography and Cardiac MRI	Echocardiography	Cardiac MRI
Cost Efficiency	●●●◐	●●●○
Availability	●●●◐	●●◐○
Reproducibility	●●◐○	●●●◐
Radiation Safety	●●●●	●●●●
Patient Tolerability	●●●◐	●●◐○
Pericardial Disease	●●○○	●●●◐
Tissue Characterization	●●○○	●●●●
Mass/Tumor Characterization	●●○○	●●●●
Inflammation	●○○○	●●●●
Perfusion/Ischemia	●○○○	●●●○
Myocardial Mass	●●◐○	●●●●
Volume	●●●○	●●●●
Functional Assessment	●●●○	●●●●
Valvular Disease	●●●●	●●●○

Fig. 1. Comparison of value of echocardiography and CMR. One filled in black circle represents minimal value, 2 represents limited value, 3 represents good value, and 4 represents gold standard.

Echocardiography in Her2/Neu therapy

Trastuzumab is a monoclonal antibody used mostly in the treatment of HER2-positive breast cancer that targets HER2/neu receptors, epidermal growth factor receptor tyrosine kinases (TKs) important in cell proliferation. Cardiotoxicity is the major adverse effect attributed to trastuzumab, primarily manifesting as potentially severe, reversible left ventricular (LV) dysfunction while on therapy[33] as well as right ventricular (RV) dysfunction.[34] Myocardial dysfunction has been reported in up to 30% of patients[19] with a 3% risk of severe cardiotoxicity.[35] Women treated with both anthracyclines and trastuzumab are at higher risk of cardiotoxicity than those treated with either alone.[36] Toxicity is thought to be due to inhibition of cardioprotective mechanisms (sarcomere maintenance, proapoptotic molecule scavenging) initiated by neuregulin-1-mediated activation of HER2. Subsequent oxidative stress and upregulation of angiotensin II is thought to further promote toxicity.[33] As with anthracyclines, GLS detects subclinical myocardial dysfunction before LVEF changes and should be implemented in any echocardiographic assessment of patients treated with trastuzumab.[13,18]

Echocardiography in targeted therapies and immunotherapy

Although anthracyclines and trastuzumab represent the classic culprits of CTRCT, emerging therapies also cause cardiotoxicities that can be assessed via echocardiography and strain imaging. These include targeted therapies (eg, proteasome inhibitors [PIs], vascular endothelial growth factor inhibitors [VEGF-Is], tyrosine kinase inhibitors [TKIs]) and immunotherapies (eg, immune checkpoint inhibitors [ICIs], chimeric antigen receptor T cell [CAR-T] therapy).

Echocardiography in proteasome inhibitors

Proteasome inhibitors (PI), such as bortezomib and carfilzomib, are used in the treatment of multiple myeloma and are known to cause cardiotoxicity in the form of myocardial dysfunction and heart failure.[37] Proposed mechanisms include interference of production of nitric oxide in the endothelium leading to vasoconstriction and

Table 1
Low, intermediate, and high-risk features for development of CTRCT. A patient should be grouped with their highest individual risk factor

Risk Factor Categories for CTRCT	
Low Risk	• Age 18–50 y • Cumulative dose <200 mg/m2 doxorubicin (or equivalent) • No preexisting or new CVD risk factors[a] • Cumulative RT dose <30 Gy without chest involvement
Intermediate Risk	• Age 50–65 y • Cumulative dose 200–400 mg/m2 doxorubicin (or equivalent) • 1–2 preexisting or new CVD risk factors[a] • Cumulative RT dose >30 Gy without chest involvement • Single-agent targeted therapy or immunotherapy
High Risk	• Age <18 or >65 y • Cumulative dose >400 mg/m2 doxorubicin (or equivalent) • Any RT involving the chest • Any combination of cardiotoxic cancer therapies, even within same class • >2 preexisting or new CVD risk factors[a] • Underlying CVD (CAD, HF, PAD, and so forth) • History of CTRCT

Abbreviations: CAD, coronary artery disease; CTRCT, cancer therapy-related cardiotoxicity; CVD, cardiovascular disease; Gy, Gray unit(s); HF, heart failure; PAD, peripheral artery disease; RT, radiation therapy.
[a] CVD risk factors include, but are not limited to, hypertension, insulin resistance, diabetes mellitus, smoking, obesity, and dyslipidemia.

inhibition of the ubiquitin-proteasome system leading to protein misfolding and cell death. Cardiomyocytes are particularly vulnerable to this second mechanism because they are nonproliferative and express elevated proteasome levels.[38] Meta-analyses of carfilzomib and bortezomib showed ORs of 2.03 and 1.74, respectively, for the development of cardiotoxicity and a cumulative incidence of cardiotoxicity in nearly 10% of those on carfilzomib.[39,40] PI use is associated with decreased GLS without change in LVEF, indicating subclinical cardiac dysfunction[41] and early detection of CTRCT,[38] but the amount of published data is minimal.

Echocardiography in vascular endothelial growth factor inhibitors

VEGF-Is are used to treat a variety of malignancies by inhibiting tumor angiogenesis. Numerous VEGF-Is are cardiotoxic, causing hypertension and myocardial dysfunction.[42] Hypertension is thought to be driven via inhibition of endothelial nitric oxide production. The myocardial dysfunction is less well understood but thought to include a multitude of effects leading to inhibition of cardioprotective cellular mechanisms, coronary microvasculature destabilization, and decreased density of myocardial capillaries.[43] Although LVEF effects have been inconsistent, STE monitoring in patients receiving various VEGF-Is

showed significant decrease in GLS from baseline both during treatment[44] and up to 6 months following treatment.[45,46]

Echocardiography in tyrosine kinase inhibitors

TKIs are a diverse group of agents that target TK molecules in various cellular functions. By targeting specific pathways, TKIs can be tailored for specific types of malignancies. Because TKs are so widely used in cellular biology, there is much cross-reactivity with other TKs leading to "off target" effects, including cardiotoxicity in the form of cardiomyopathy and heart failure.[47,48] Sunitinib and pazopanib, VEGF-Is acting via the TKI mechanism, are associated with myocardial dysfunction and demonstrate significant decrease in GLS.[45] Newer generation Bcr-abl-targeting TKIs cause significantly lower GLS compared with first generation, but the absolute value difference is minimal with no comparison to baseline, limiting the clinical relevance of this finding.[49] Another subset of TKIs, B-Raf proto-oncogene (BRAF), and mitogen-activated protein kinase kinase (MEK) inhibitors, are used in the treatment of melanoma and are known to be cardiotoxic, most commonly in the form of LVEF reduction (seen in 13% of patients[50]) and hypertension. Combination BRAF/MEK therapy poses higher risk for LVEF reduction, hypertension, and thromboembolic phenomena compared with BRAF therapy alone.[51,52] In TKI CTRCT, heart failure tends to present in the first 6 months of therapy. However, no published studies address predictive value of GLS or other parameters.

Echocardiography in immunotherapies

Immunotherapies such as ICIs and CAR-T therapy are used in a wide range of cancers. ICIs work by targeting molecules that inhibit immune destruction by T-cells. Not surprisingly, this general approach can lead to unintended inflammatory cascade throughout the body, including cardiac manifestations[53] such as myocarditis, pericarditis, arrhythmia, cardiomyopathy, or myocardial ischemia. The most apparent risk factor for ICI-cardiotoxicity is combination therapy with another cardiotoxic agent (including another ICI).[54] With increasing recognition of the immune phenomena associated with immunotherapy, retrospective studies estimate myocarditis occurs in up to 1% of patients taking ICIs.[55–57] In patients that develop ICI myocarditis, GLS is reduced even if LVEF is not and is associated with future major adverse cardiac events (MACE).[58] There is evidence of STE-detected RV dysfunction that correlates with duration of ICI use, suggesting a role in CTRCT monitoring.[59]

In contrast to ICIs, CAR-T therapy works by using T cells that have been harvested from the host, reprogramming them to target tumor cells, and reintroducing them into the host. CAR-T cardiotoxicity manifests primarily as arrhythmia, cardiomyopathy, or ischemic events. LVEF reduction has been demonstrated in 5% to 10% of patients on CAR-T therapy.[60–62] To our knowledge, there are no published studies evaluating strain imaging in patients receiving CAR-T therapy. Thus, the rate of cardiac toxicity is likely underestimated.

Echocardiography in radiation therapy

Radiation has long been used as a cancer therapy. Cardiotoxicity arises from direct cellular damage of the myocardium and endothelial tissue of the heart and vasculature within the field of radiation. Cardiotoxicity can manifest as hypertension, coronary artery disease (CAD), valvular disease, pericarditis, myocarditis, cardiomyopathy, or arrhythmia.[63] Cardiotoxicity risk is increased in patients with total exposure of greater than 15 Gy and increases with increasing doses.[64] Strain imaging, GLS mostly, has been used to evaluate CTRCT following radiotherapy (RT) to the chest. Numerous studies show subclinical cardiac dysfunction after initiation of chest RT (in the absence of other cardiotoxic therapies) for the treatment of breast cancer in both acute and follow-up periods of up to 3 years.[65–71] Higher radiation doses[66–68,70,71] and left-sided breast radiation[67,68] are associated with larger decreases in GLS. The apical region[72] and subendocardial region of the heart receiving the most radiation[65] have demonstrated earlier detection of strain reduction, suggesting higher sensitivity for the detection of CTRCT by assessing these regions.

3D Echocardiography

3D echocardiography is a modality that has emerging potential in cardio-oncology. Although not as ubiquitous as 2D echocardiography, it offers superior capability in the assessment of LVEF,[4,73] providing values that agree with CMR.[74] Compared with 2D echocardiography, 3D echocardiography offers more reproducible LVEF,[10] faster and earlier strain assessment,[75,76] and more detailed structural and anatomic characteristics of cardiac masses.

Echocardiography and Cardiac Masses

Echocardiography plays a pivotal role in the detection and diagnosis of cardiac masses. Although rare, neoplastic cardiac masses carry significant morbidity and mortality.[77] Benign cardiac tumors are more common than malignant ones. Metastatic cardiac tumors, seen in 10% to 12% of patients with a known primary cancer,[78] are more common than primary cardiac malignancy. 2D echocardiography can delineate cardiac masses and certain characteristics (size, shape, mobility, relative density, associated effusions) quite well for initial evaluation (**Fig. 2**, Panel A). However, there is limited ability to distinguish right-sided masses, left atrial (LA) appendage masses, extracardiac masses, tissue characteristics, and type of mass.[79] 3D echocardiography better evaluates size and anatomic associations of cardiac masses, adding benefit in surgical planning.[76] Perfusion contrast with 2D echocardiography enhances diagnostic utility and has sensitivity and specificity of 93% to 100% in differentiating thrombi versus benign tumor versus malignant tumor.[80–82] Transesophageal echocardiography (TEE) has shown high diagnostic accuracy[82] with better anatomic resolution of right-sided and posterior structures,[83] but it is an invasive procedure associated with risks including those of sedation and expense.

Echocardiography in Tamponade and Pericardiocentesis

Pericardial effusions can be due to infection, autoimmune inflammation, direct effect of malignancy, adverse effect of cancer therapy (radiation-induced pericardial disease, ICI inflammation, volume overload), postsurgical, or idiopathic.

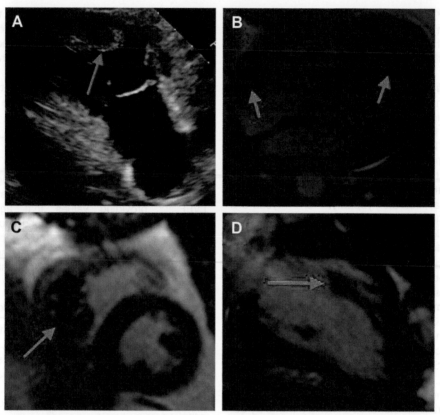

Fig. 2. (*A*) Mass identified in the RV outflow tract on echocardiography. Suspected to be a metastatic lesion from an unknown primary source. (*B*) Two masses identified on CMR (horizontal long axis view). The LV mass is a metastatic melanoma. The RA mass is a thrombus. (*C*) One RV mass on CMR (short axis view), diagnosed as metastatic melanoma with surrounding thrombus. (*D*) One LV mass identified on CMR (vertical long axis view), diagnosed as a poorly differentiated synovial sarcoma.

Pericardial effusions are readily identified on traditional 2D echocardiography, although may require multiple views if the effusion is loculated. If posterior, TEE may be required to adequately view the effusion. Pericardiocentesis, drainage of a pericardial effusion, is generally indicated for asymptomatic and large effusions, hemodynamically significant effusions (ie, impending or active tamponade), or fluid biopsy to aid diagnosis. Although overt tamponade implies active hemodynamic consequences such as hypotension, tachycardia, dyspnea, or pulsus paradoxus from compression of the heart, effusions at high risk for developing tamponade cannot be readily identified on physical examination alone. Echocardiography, viewed as the gold-standard for diagnosis, can identify signs of compression before the presence of symptoms. These include RA or RV collapse during diastole, abnormal septal motion indicating interventricular dependence, dilated inferior vena cava without inspiratory collapse, swinging heart,

or decreased mitral early filling velocity on doppler.[84] Echocardiography-guided pericardiocentesis, which has been used for decades, is safe and effective in patients with cancer and should be used before surgical drainage when possible.[85–87]

Echocardiography in Cardiac Amyloidosis

Cardiac amyloidosis is a group of conditions that result in the infiltration and expansion of myocardial extracellular space with amyloid protein deposits. Although various proteins can misfold and deposit, amyloid from transthyretin (ATTR) and amyloid from immunoglobulin light chains (AL) account for 95% of cases. Cardiac amyloidosis usually manifests clinically as heart failure (preserved ejection fraction more often than reduced ejection fraction), restrictive cardiomyopathy, and dysrhythmias. Typical 2D echocardiographic findings include ventricular wall hypertrophy (concentric more common in AL, asymmetric more common in ATTR), diastolic and/or systolic dysfunction, restrictive LV filling, biatrial enlargement, valvular thickening, and a "sparkling" texture of the myocardium.[9,88] Two-dimensional STE often reveals a characteristic pattern of reduced GLS with apical sparing, due to segmental differences in total amyloid mass distribution,[89] with a reported sensitivity of 93% and specificity of 82% for cardiac amyloidosis when compared with LV hypertrophy controls.[90] The combination of GLS values with apical sparing and serum T-troponin offers better sensitivity and specificity.[91] One recent study[92] found a GLS/Ejection Fraction (EF) ratio greater than 4.1 to be a strong predictor of cardiac amyloidosis, with an OR of 35.57. Although echocardiography is the universal initial imaging modality when suspicious for cardiac amyloidosis, it cannot reliably distinguish between amyloidosis and other causes of hypertrophy. Thus, echocardiography alone is not sufficient for diagnosis.

Practical Use of Echocardiography in Everyday Clinical Practice

Each institution and case will have varying protocols for which views and data are obtained on echocardiogram. The following has been suggested for comprehensive initial echocardiographic assessment in screening for CTRCT: 2D LVEF via Simpson biplane method or 3D LVEF, 2D or 3D GLS, 2D or 3D LV systolic volume, RV function markers (such as tricuspid annular plane systolic excursion, RV fractional area change, RV ejection fraction [RVEF], RV free wall strain), velocity of tricuspid regurgitation.[9] Suggested echocardiographic surveillance protocols for patients on anthracycline therapy and trastuzumab therapy can be found in **Fig. 3** and **Fig. 4**, respectively. Suggested echocardiographic surveillance protocols for patients on radiation therapy, targeted therapy, or immunotherapy can be found in **Table 2**. Recommendations for targeted therapies and immunotherapy are less defined due to the relative dearth of data in novel agents. Individual risk assessment and joint decision making is paramount in developing a patient-centered screening plan. Regardless of therapy, baseline echocardiography before initiation of therapy should be obtained in all intermediate and high-risk patients and can be considered in low-risk patients. Additionally, any time there are signs or symptoms of cardiotoxicity, echocardiography should be obtained, and referral to a cardio-oncologist should be considered.

Cardiac MRI

Cardiac MRI and left ventricular ejection fraction

Although CMR is not deployed for routine screening in cardio-oncology, it offers superior imaging in tissue characterization, volume assessments, spatial resolution, and potentially strain imaging. **Fig. 1** illustrates the relative utility of CMR in various parameters. CMR can investigate most adverse cardiac effects from cancer therapies and allows the specific assessment of RV and LV function, ventricular and atrial volumes, ventricular and LA deformation, myocardial mass, pericardial disease, fibrosis, infiltrative tissue, edema, and inflammation.[9,93] Measurement of LVEF is considered the gold standard due to excellent accuracy and precision.[6,94] CMR is used for LVEF measurement when there are poor echocardiographic windows or echocardiography is equivocal or unreliable. Given the poor agreement of 2D echocardiography with CMR-derived LVEF, CMR should be used any time highly accurate LVEF quantification is needed, especially if 3D echocardiography is not available.[5,95]

Cardiac MRI strain imaging

Similar to echocardiography, CMR-derived LVEF lacks the sensitivity to detect early myocardial dysfunction in CTRCT. Cardiac deformation quantification via strain imaging techniques is available in some clinical CMR laboratories and is useful in detection of subclinical myocardial dysfunction. Techniques include CMR reference tagging, phase velocity mapping, displacement encoding with stimulated echoes, strain encoded (SENC) imaging (**Fig. 5**), and feature tracking (FT). CMR reference tagging is the most validated and considered gold standard for CMR strain imaging; however, CMR-FT is gaining traction due to ease of clinical use.[93,96,97] Analogous to STE but with better resolution,[98] CMR-FT is a postacquisition processing method that can be applied to images obtained for LVEF assessment, requiring no additional scanner time.[96] CMR-FT shows good reproducibility in global strain measurements, provided the same software package is used.[99,100] The potential for early detection and prognostication in CTRCT by CMR strain has been demonstrated in patients receiving various cardiotoxic chemotherapies,[101,102] and is discussed further below. CMR-FT has even shown promise in evaluation of LA strain, which, along with MRI measured LA volume, could represent an important marker for potential development of atrial arrhythmias and clot formation.[98,103]

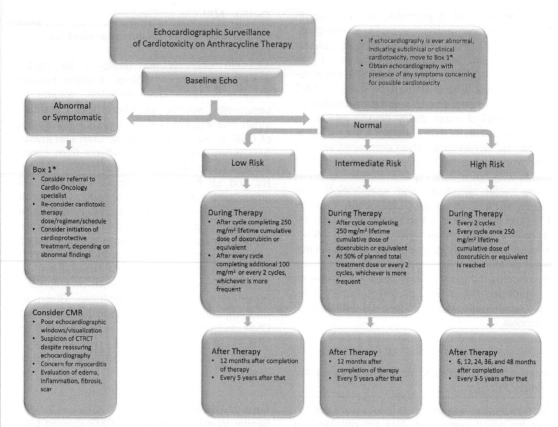

Fig. 3. Suggested echocardiographic surveillance protocol of cardiotoxicity in patients on anthracycline therapy. Low risk features include age 18 to 50 years, cumulative dose less than 200 mg/m² doxorubicin (or equivalent), no preexisting or new CVD risk factors. Intermediate features include age 50 to 65 years, cumulative dose 200 to 400 mg/m² doxorubicin (or equivalent), 1 to 2 preexisting or new CVD risk factors. High-risk features include age less than 18 or greater than 65 years, cumulative dose greater than 400 mg/m² doxorubicin (or equivalent), any combination of cardiotoxic cancer therapies, underlying CVD, history of CTRCT. CAD, coronary artery disease; CMR, cardiovascular magnetic resonance imaging; CTRCT, cancer therapy-related cardiotoxicity; CVD, cardiovascular disease; Echo, echocardiography; mo, month.

Cardiac MRI T1 and T2 mapping

T1-weighted imaging (**Fig. 6**) reflects the inherent intracellular and extracellular makeup of tissue. Unitless values of intensity (compared with a reference "region of interest" within the same image) are assigned to each pixel but are only comparable within the same image. T1 is lengthened (brightened) by water, edema, and inflammation; it is shortened (darkened) by iron, fat, and contrast.[104] T1 mapping is a relatively new CMR application that allows for creation of color maps, where each colored pixel represents a quantified, parametric, tissue-specific T1 value of the corresponding voxel that is comparable across images.[105] This allows sensitive detection of subtle T1 changes within the myocardium, often representing early stages of disease. T1 mapping reliably distinguishes regional and diffuse fibrosis

(scar),[106] edema,[107] and infarction.[108] It has shown promise in detecting numerous cardiac disease states.[98,109,110] Late gadolinium enhancement (LGE; see **Fig. 6**), conversely, only visualizes regional fibrosis well.[98] T1 mapping solves this limitation while providing a contrast-free alternative for fibrosis detection. T1 mapping is primarily used for evaluation of the LV, but there are sequences that can evaluate fibrosis of the LA, with possible application in cancer therapies causing atrial arrhythmias.[111] Contrast T1 imaging is useful, however, in quantifying extracellular volume (ECV), which correlates histologically[112] with the excess collagen deposition of fibrosis.

T2-weighted imaging (see **Fig. 6**), like T1, is reflective of the intracellular and extracellular makeup of tissue. T2 time is increased by free water and most helpful in distinguishing edema and

Table 2
Suggested echocardiographic and CMR surveillance protocols of cardiotoxicity for patients undergoing targeted therapy, immunotherapy, or radiation therapy

Suggested Clinical Imaging Surveillance Protocols for CTRCT in Various Cancer Therapies		
Class	Echocardiography	Cardiac MRI
All classes	• Consider baseline for all intermediate and high risk patients before initiation of therapy • Any time there are signs or symptoms concerning for possible CTRCT	• Consider with abnormal echo or poor visualization • Consider if clinical suspicion for CTRCT persists despite normal/equivocal echo • Unexplained CVD
PI	• Periodically if history of other cardiotoxic cancer therapy, personal CVD or risk factors, or specifically taking carfilzomib	• Consider with abnormal echo or poor windows/visualization • Unexplained CVD
VEGF-I and TKI (including BRAF, MEK, and VEGF inhibitors with TKI mechanism)	• High risk patients on TKI: consider screening Echo every 1–3 mo during therapy • Intermediate risk patients on TKI: consider every 6–12 mo during therapy • Intermediate or greater risk of CAD before initiation of TKI: consider stress echo • All patients on VEGF-I, high risk in particular: consider echo every 3–6 mo during therapy • High-risk patients on combination BRAF/MEK therapy: consider echo every 1–3 mo during therapy • Low or intermediate risk patients on BRAF or BRAF/MEK therapy: consider echo at 6 mo, then every 6–12 mo while on therapy	• Low threshold to move to CMR after echo • With any cardiac symptoms, suspicious elevation in troponin, or ECG change • Consider if concern for ischemic cardiotoxicity • Unexplained CVD
Immunotherapies (ex. ICIs, CAR-T cell therapies, allogeneic stem transplantation)	• High risk or taking other cardiotoxic therapy (including 2nd ICI): serial echo reasonable • In high risk patients, first echo should be obtained within 1-2 months after initiation of therapy • If LV function abnormal prior to initiation of ICI, every 3-6 months for duration of therapy • Consider anytime screening ECG or serum biomarkers are abnormal	• Low threshold to move to CMR after echo • With any cardiac symptoms, suspicious elevation in troponin, or ECG change • Consider if concern for ischemic cardiotoxicity • Unexplained CVD

(continued on next page)

Table 2
(continued)

Suggested Clinical Imaging Surveillance Protocols for CTRCT in Various Cancer Therapies		
Class	Echocardiography	Cardiac MRI
RT	• High-risk patients: 1–2 y after completion of therapy and every 5–10 y following • Intermediate risk or lower: every 5–10 y after therapy completion	• If concern for radiation-induced myocardial or pericardial disease despite normal or equivocal echo • Unexplained CVD

Abbreviations: BRAF, B-Raf proto-oncogene; CAD, coronary artery disease; CAR-T, chimeric antigen T-cell therapy; CMR, cardiovascular magnetic resonance imaging; CTRCT, cancer therapy-related cardiotoxicity; CVD, cardiovascular disease; ECG, electrocardiogram; Echo, echocardiography; ICI, immune checkpoint inhibitor; LV, left ventricular; MEK, mitogen-activated protein kinase kinase; mo, month; RV, right ventricular; TKI, tyrosine kinase inhibitor; VEGF-I, vascular endothelial growth factor inhibitor; y, year.

inflammation, proving to be comparable to Lake Louise criteria for diagnosis of myocarditis.[113] T2 mapping can now be created, just as T1 mapping can,[104] with good reproducibility.[114] However, it has not been as thoroughly studied in CTRCT as has T1 mapping.

Cardiac MRI in anthracyclines
Anthracycline cardiotoxicity is characterized by myocardial dysfunction that in its most severe presentation manifests as heart failure with reduced ejection.[28] Although CMR is more sensitive and accurate in LVEF assessment than echocardiography,

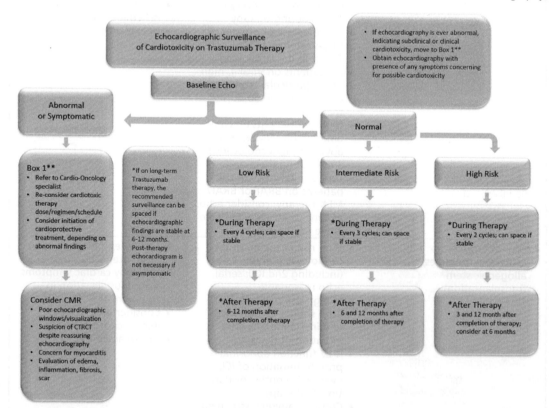

Fig. 4. Suggested echocardiographic surveillance protocol of cardiotoxicity in patients on trastuzumab therapy. Low risk features include age 18 to 50 years, no preexisting or new CVD risk factors. Intermediate features include age 50 to 65 years, 1 to 2 preexisting or new CVD risk factors. High-risk features include age less than 18 or greater than 65 years, any combination of cardiotoxic cancer therapies, underlying CVD, history of CTRCT. CAD, coronary artery disease; CMR, cardiovascular magnetic resonance imaging; CTRCT, cancer therapy-related cardiotoxicity; CVD, cardiovascular disease; Echo, echocardiography; mo, month.

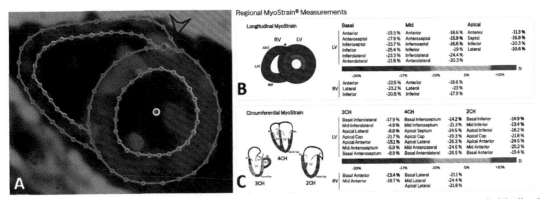

Fig. 5. (*A*) Representative screenshot of CMR (SENC) image in short axis view with overlying endocardial (yellow) and epicardial (green) borders. (*B*) MyoStrain LV and RV longitudinal strain with corresponding heat map, and absolute values of each individual segment. (*C*) MyoStrain LV and RV circumferential strain with corresponding heat map, and absolute values of each individual segment. CMR, cardiovascular magnetic resonance imaging; LV, left ventricular; RV, right ventricular; SENC, strain encoded.

it is not sensitive enough for CTRCT screening.[109] CMR strain imaging, while not as extensively studied or as readily available as echocardiographic strain imaging, shows a similar promise in early detection and prediction of CTRCT[96] via both systolic[115–119] and diastolic[120] measurements. Because anthracycline CTRCT is characterized by diffuse fibrosis,[31] LGE is seen in just 6% of patients.[121] Numerous studies have demonstrated that T1 mapping and ECV quantification detect fibrosis after anthracycline therapy, representing an avenue for early diagnosis of CTRCT.[118,122–125] One prospective study[118] showed elevated T1 and T2 mapping values in patients on anthracycline therapy compared with controls 3 months after therapy initiation but only elevated T1 more than 12 months after therapy initiation. This suggests that initial edema/inflammation eventually progresses to fibrosis. The authors created criteria for detection of cardiotoxicity in these patients, which led to

diagnostic accuracy of 84% for detection of CTRCT, outperforming both GLS and troponin alone. More studies are needed to elucidate ideal threshold values for optimum diagnostic and prognostic ability. Published data on T2 mapping in anthracyclines, although minimal, shows early edema and inflammation[118,126] after administration, indicating early signs of CTRCT, with excellent sensitivity.[127] There is encouraging data for the utility of T2 mapping in CTRCT in various animal models,[128–130] but human studies remain relatively sparse. Other CMR-derived measurements have been studied in anthracycline use. LA enlargement has been associated with increasing anthracycline doses, potentially offering a marker of diastolic dysfunction.[131] Decrease in myocardial mass after anthracycline therapy has been repeatedly demonstrated,[95,121,132,133] which is associated with increased risk of MACE[121] and HF symptoms.[133]

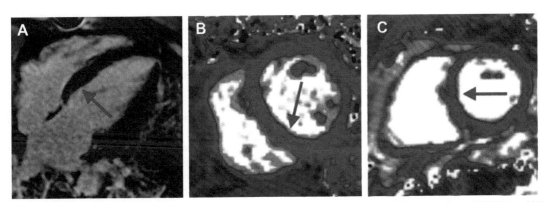

Fig. 6. Representative images of (*A*) late gadolinium enhancement, and elevated (*B*) myocardial native T1, and (*C*) myocardial native T2 in a patient with suspected targeted cancer therapy (TKI) cardiotoxicity, as visualized by cardiac magnetic resonance imaging. Red arrows in panels (*B*) and (*C*) indicate areas of elevated T1 and T2, respectively; the pink outline in panel (*B*) denotes a region of interest (ROI) in the septum.

Cardiac MRI in HER2/Neu therapy

CMR strain parameters have shown promising ability to predict the development of CTRCT in patients on trastuzumab therapy. One prospective study demonstrated that a 15% relative decrease in tagged-CMR GLS, tagged-CMR global circumferential strain (GCS), and CMR-FT correspond to increased odds of CTRCT of 47%, 50%, and 87%, respectively.[134] Multiple other studies have shown a decrease in various CMR-measured strain parameters, often with persistence up to 12 months. Recovery by 18 months is frequently seen, highlighting the reversibility of trastuzumab cardiotoxicity.[135–137] Diastolic function has been assessed with both strain and LV diastolic filling rates, but these data are inconsistent.[137,138] CMR evaluation of LGE highlights a key difference in the pathogenesis of trastuzumab from anthracyclines. Although LGE is uncommon in anthracycline cardiotoxicity due to diffuse fibrosis, LV lateral wall LGE enhancement is seen in 94% to 100%[139,140] of patients treated with trastuzumab who had reduced LVEF. This parallels the knowledge that trastuzumab cardiotoxicity primarily affects the LV. There is CMR evidence to add to echocardiographic evidence[34] that RV myocardial dysfunction is also seen, although more subtle than LV dysfunction.[141] Animal studies show increased T1 and T2 values in subjects receiving trastuzumab with eventual recovery.[142–144] Human data show similar findings,[145] but clinical utility in early detection and prediction of CTRCT is limited due to temporal variability.[101,146]

Cardiac MRI in proteasome inhibitors

Case reports represent the bulk of literature covering the heterogeneous CMR findings in PI cardiotoxicity. Fibrosis indicated by LGE is the most common finding, seen mostly at the basal and inferior portions of the septum.[147–149] Conversely, 2 patients receiving both carfilzomib and bortezomib developed significant but reversible LVEF reduction with wall motion abnormalities without LGE.[37] The only prospective study we are aware of studied 11 patients with CV risk factors but no preexisting CV disease for up to 6 months after bortezomib therapy with echocardiography and CMR. All imaging parameters, including echocardiographic GLS and CMR LGE, were normal.[150] More data is needed for proper understanding of CMR findings in PI-associated CTRCT.

Cardiac MRI in tyrosine kinase inhibitors and vascular endothelial growth factor inhibitors

There is scant published data on CMR findings in VEGF-Is and TKIs, mostly in the form of case reports. Many overlap as they involve TKIs that inhibit VEGF pathways. One prospective study evaluated cardiotoxicity of 90 patients in phase I trials of a VEGF-I monoclonal antibody, VEGF-I TKI, or a kinesin inhibitor.[151] Out of 90 patients, 10 developed cardiotoxicity. Of these 10 patients, 2 were taking the VEGF-I TKI and 6 were taking the VEGF-I monoclonal antibody. The only patient with a reduced EF was taking the VEGF-I TKI. None of the 10 patients had LGE on CMR. One case report of sunitinib-induced cardiomyopathy included CMR evaluation that showed no LGE or resting perfusion defects.[152] We are not aware of any published data pertaining to CMR strain, T1 mapping, or T2 mapping in relation to cardiotoxicity of TKIs or VEGF-Is. Because of the propensity of some TKIs to invoke atrial arrhythmias, such as ibrutinib, LA evaluation with LGE, T1 and T2 mapping, and CMR strain could be beneficial and warrants further study. Hypertension and vascular effects of therapies that inhibit VEGF pathways make CAD and myocardial ischemia an important adverse effect to monitor for. Along with stress and perfusion imaging, CMR offers techniques with the ability to quantify myocardial viability.[6,98]

Cardiac MRI in immunotherapy

CMR is the gold-standard noninvasive diagnostic tool for myocarditis, the most important cardiotoxic effect of immunotherapy. The Lake Louise Criteria (LLC), introduced in 2009 for the diagnosis of non-ICI myocarditis, require clinical suspicion of myocarditis plus 2 of the following: regional or global myocardial increase in T2-weighted images, increased global myocardial early T1 gadolinium enhancement, or ≥ 1 focal lesion with nonischemic regional LGE.[153] The emergence of T1 and T2 mapping and ECV quantification has outdated the original criteria, leading some groups to use modified LLC to incorporate these parameters to increase diagnostic accuracy.[55,154,155] One study found 100% of ICI myocarditis cases met original LLC or had abnormal T1 or T2 imaging.[155] A meta-analysis of non-ICI myocarditis patients found native T1 and T2 mapping and ECV provide comparable diagnostic performance to LLC with native T1 having higher sensitivity than LLC for non-ICI myocarditis. It is important to note the underlying inflammatory mechanisms of ICI myocarditis are not necessarily comparable to non-ICI myocarditis. Additionally, diagnostic specificity is challenging in ICI myocarditis due to inherent heterogeneity, stemming from varying levels of inflammation in varying cardiac structures.[156] This heterogeneity is reflected in the literature in both clinical presentations and imaging findings.[157–159]

Reduced LVEF on CMR is not a sensitive finding for ICI myocarditis, reported in just 39%

to 50% of patients.[155,158–160] Strain imaging via CMR-FT has demonstrated significant reduction of LV-GLS in all ICI myocarditis patients, with even larger reduction in those with reduced LVEF.[158] Although LA strain has demonstrated additional prognostic value when combined with LV strain and LLC[161] in non-ICI myocarditis, this was not seen in ICI myocarditis. In ICI myocarditis, LGE has been reported in 48% to 80% of patients.[56,157–159] LGE occurs in noncoronary distributions, but location varies by case.[159] Presence of LGE is an independent predictor of mortality in ICI myocarditis[158] but has not been associated with MACE.[159] Interestingly, in one study,[159] LGE was seen in 21.6% of patients when CMR was obtained before day 4 of admission and 72% when obtained on or after that. Thus, LGE prognostic value might differ depending on the timing of CMR acquisition.

Qualitative T1 and T2 lack adequate sensitivity compared with quantitative mapping.[155,158,162] A retrospective[155] study that evaluated T1 and T2 mapping in patients with ICI myocarditis found elevated values compared with controls in 78% and 43% of the patients, respectively. Elevated T1 values were independently associated with MACE and lower MACE-free survival. No patients with normal T1 values had MACE, suggesting a clinically important negative predictive value. Although abnormal T2-mapping has been associated with MACE in non-ICI myocarditis,[163] this is not reflected in ICI myocarditis.[155,159] Increased ECV is also associated with MACE and death in non-ICI myocarditis,[164,165] although no published data addresses this in ICI myocarditis.

Cardiac MRI in radiation therapy

Cardiotoxicity from RT has a wide spectrum of manifestations, all stemming from direct macrovascular and microvascular damage. Literature surrounding radiation can be difficult to interpret, as most studies involve patients who, in addition to RT, have received anthracyclines and/or trastuzumab. Radiation cardiotoxicity can lead to reduction in LVEF detectable by CMR. This is seen transiently at 6 months with resolution at 2 years,[166] and, in survivors, many years after therapy.[167] LA volume assessment reveals an association between LA size and radiation dose, suggesting a possible early marker of diastolic dysfunction.[131] CMR strain imaging for the detection of subclinical cardiac dysfunction in patients who received radiation is not as well studied. In one study, there is a transient decrease in CMR-derived strain at 6 and 12 months that recovers by 24 months.[166] Other studies in humans and rats have similar findings, but it is unclear if there

is a correlation between GLS reduction and radiation dose.[168,169] Fibrosis indicated by LGE has been well-documented following RT; however, studies are vastly heterogeneous, reporting LGE incidence of 0% to 100%.[168,170–173] Multiple studies demonstrate LGE presence in areas that received the highest radiation doses.[170,172,173] Studies of T1 mapping post-RT are sparse and inconsistent. Some show elevated T1 mapping values in areas of higher radiation,[172,174] whereas others found either no elevation of T1 values[168] or no correlation with radiation dose.[171] There is minimal published data on T2 mapping post-RT.

CMR offers sensitive and detailed structural and tissue characterization of pericardial toxicity and its associated hemodynamic consequences. LGE of the pericardium indicates active pericarditis, whereas chronic constrictive pericarditis will not enhance. CMR tagging can identify pericardial adhesions. Real-time cine imaging during respiration can reveal hemodynamic consequences of constrictive pericarditis, such as ventricular interdependence. Real-time phase contrast imaging can be useful in detecting effects of respiration on flow through the mitral and tricuspid valves.[6,63,104] CMR can also be helpful in evaluation of valvular pathologic conditions induced by radiation toxicity, generally not seen for 10 to 20 years after therapy. CMR is particularly useful in visualizing the pulmonary valve, which can be challenging via echocardiography. CAD and ischemic heart disease secondary to radiation therapy are also assessable by CMR via perfusion imaging and coronary artery visualization.[6,63,98,104] CMR can even play a role in prevention of cardiotoxicity. Through various techniques under investigation, CMR shows promise in preparatory and real-time imaging to improve safety and precision of RT[175] and radiosurgery,[176] reducing total radiation exposure.

Potential Role of Stress Perfusion and Other Cardiac MRI Imaging Techniques

Numerous cancer therapies increase risk of vascular disease, as does malignancy itself. Contrast-enhanced myocardial stress perfusion has excellent diagnostic performance in the detection of ischemic disease.[177] However, screening via stress-perfusion CMR without symptoms does not provide additional benefit in cardiotoxicity diagnosis or management.[178] Pulse wave velocity, an MRI method of quantifying arterial stiffness, is elevated during and after breast cancer treatment with various anticancer therapies[179,180] and could represent a method of risk stratification. Four-dimensional flow MRI can provide flow and pressure parameters of the vasculature. Its role in risk stratification is still under exploration.[181] Real-time CMR has shown benefit in enhancing precision of radiation targeting to reduce total radiation exposure[175,176] and increasing diagnostic yield of endomyocardial biopsy.[182]

Cardiac MRI and Cardiac Masses

The superior tissue characterization and spatial resolution of CMR makes it the preferred method of imaging for intracardiac and pericardial masses (see **Fig. 2**, Panels B-D). CMR is particularly helpful in confirmation and further characterization when echocardiography is not sufficient.[183] Balanced steady-state free precession (SSFP) is the primary method for detailed anatomic description. T1-weighted or T2-weighted double inversion recovery imaging with or without fat saturation is useful in tissue characterization of masses. Gadolinium enhancement is helpful in assessing tumor vascularity and associated myocardial fibrosis.[184] CMR performs well at distinguishing nontumors from tumors and benign tumors from malignant ones.[185,186] With a wider field of view, CMR can catch pericardial and extracardiac masses missed by echocardiography. Additionally, CMR outperforms echocardiography in predicting ultimate tumor diagnosis as confirmed by pathology. CMR has fewer false positives and can eliminate the need for biopsy by ruling out a mass seen on echocardiography.[183]

Cardiac MRI in Tamponade and Pericardiocentesis

Although echocardiography is generally sufficient to diagnose pericardial effusion and tamponade, CMR can offer further details in the assessment of pericardial disease. CMR can identify loculated or posterior effusions, pericardial thickening, and pericardial masses where echocardiography often cannot. As described above, CMR is certainly capable of detecting signs of tamponade[6,63,104]; however, it is generally unnecessary unless echocardiography is unavailable or CMR is to be obtained for another reason. One of the more helpful applications of CMR in pericardial disease is the ability to distinguish constrictive pericarditis (thickened pericardium, interventricular dependence) from restrictive cardiomyopathy (diastolic dysfunction, large but normally contoured atria, thickened myocardium, normal pericardium).[187,188] CMR does not play a role in percutaneous pericardiocentesis but can aid in planning for surgical drainage of a pericardial effusion.

Cardiac MRI in Cardiac Amyloidosis

CMR, with its fine tissue characterization, plays an important role in cardiac amyloidosis screening,

diagnosis, and surveillance of disease burden. LGE is almost invariably seen in cardiac amyloidosis, with the typical patterns being diffuse subendocardial (representing earlier stages) and diffuse transmural (representing later stages). RV LGE is also seen in greater than 90% of patients. Transmural LGE is more common in ATTR than AL[189] and also carries prognostic value.[190] Native T1 values are markedly elevated in cardiac amyloid, and T1 mapping is particularly helpful when amyloid renal disease precludes the use of gadolinium.[162] ECV quantification is a valuable tool given the underlying pathologic mechanisms of amyloidosis.[191] ECV values are markedly elevated in cardiac amyloidosis, often indicating greater than 40% ECV. Serial measurement of ECV is reliable,[192] prognostic,[193] and indicates disease progression or response to therapy.[194–196] T2 mapping, of which there is little published data in regards to amyloid, shows higher values in amyloidosis compared with controls. However, there is little difference in AL and ATTR.[197] Although LGE, T1 mapping, and ECV all provide valuable roles in cardiac amyloidosis, a recent meta-analysis suggests that ECV provides the highest diagnostic and prognostic capability of the 3.[198] Regardless, all should be included in any cardiac amyloidosis evaluation.

Practical Use of Cardiac MRI in Everyday Clinical Practice

Guidelines do not recommend routine screening for CTRCT via CMR unless echocardiography is not feasible due to poor windows or CMR is needed for other indications.[5] Additionally, if echocardiography is normal or equivocal, but clinical suspicion for cardiotoxicity remains high, CMR should be obtained. CMR protocols for CTRCT evaluation differ between institutions and individual cases. Commonly used sequences include cine balanced SSFP, strain imaging through myocardial tagging or other methods, phase contrast flow, native T1 and T2 sequences with respective parametric mapping, postcontrast T1 ECV mapping, first pass arterial perfusion, inversion recovery, and 4D flow.[93,199] Suggested CMR surveillance protocols for patients on anthracyclines and trastuzumab can be found in **Figs. 3** and **4**, respectively. Suggested CMR surveillance protocols for patients on radiation therapy, targeted therapy, and immunotherapy can be found in **Table 2**. Again, individual risk assessment and joint decision-making is a crucial part in developing a patient-centered surveillance plan. Patients should be referred to a cardio-oncologist any time there are signs or symptoms of cardiotoxicity.

Future Directions and Ongoing Clinical Trials

Cardio-oncology has seen a boom in research during the past 10 years. The more we learn, the more our gaps in knowledge become evident. Strain imaging via echocardiography represents our best early imaging biomarker for CTRCT, and the addition of serum biomarkers can increase diagnostic and prognostic value. Most of the available data, however, are in observational studies of patients exposed to anthracyclines, trastuzumab, or radiation. More prospective studies with larger cohorts are needed in patients exposed to all groups of cardiotoxic cancer therapies, especially novel therapies. The LATER CARDS study will provide a large prospective dataset of echocardiographic findings and serum biomarkers in the understudied pediatric population.[200]

CMR, although offering better imaging sensitivity and specificity for most cardiac pathologic conditions, is more difficult to clinically implement and has not been as robustly studied as echocardiography. Future research should aim for larger, prospective studies evaluating traditional and emerging CMR protocols. Patients on targeted and immunotherapies are understudied compared with anthracyclines, trastuzumab, and radiation and should be a major focus of research as well. The CARTIER study is a prospective study of elderly patients on cardiotoxic chemotherapy who will receive serial CMR before each cycle of treatment and with follow-up after treatment completion.[127] The CareBest prospective study, currently underway, will enroll greater than 2000 patients with breast cancer and study various CMR parameters in a short CMR protocol[201]. Similarly, other CMR-based trials across various cancer drug-classes are underway, which should illuminate the role of trackable subclinical disease in the development of limiting CVD.

Machine learning is a growing research tool with much potential in cardio-oncology. It allows for identification of similar groups buried within the noise of highly heterogenous populations. Machine learning has been used to identify potentially cardioprotective variants in cardiac injury pathway genes among pediatric cancer survivors with anthracycline-induced CTRCT[202]. It has also been used to identify unique asymptomatic diastolic dysfunction phenotypes based on echocardiographic parameters, each with distinct long-term outcome risks.[203] It is natural to foresee the incredible value of machine learning to sift and organize the vast amount of hard data collected with echocardiography and CMR into clinically useful CTRCT prediction tools[6]. Some combination of serum biomarkers and echocardiographic strain parameters is the intuitive place to start given our current knowledge.

Finally, research should also focus on our ability to implement CTRCT screening protocols. Only 30% to 40% of patients receive optimal screening via echocardiography.[204] Implementing user-friendly guidelines and clinical tools, development of dedicated cardio-oncology programs and multidisciplinary clinics, improved patient and provider education of CTRCT, and development of quicker and cheaper imaging protocols could increase patient participation in CTRCT screening. Continued improvement of CTRCT screening protocols has the potential to positively impact survival and outcomes in the ever-growing population of patients with cancer.

CLINICS CARE POINTS

- When using echocardiography to measure LVEF, remember there is limited precision. Values can vary up to 10% between studies.

- A normal EF does not rule out the possibility of CTRCT.

- When interpreting deformation values, remember that threshold numbers and strict normal ranges have not been widely agreed upon. Relative change from baseline is a better datapoint to follow.

- Multidisciplinary clinics can minimize patient stress, enhance communication, and increase patient access to guideline and evidence-based screening/treatment.

- Echocardiography alone is not sufficient to diagnose myocarditis. CMR should be obtained anytime there is a question of myocarditis.

- Normal EF and lack of LGE do not rule out myocarditis.

- Although appropriate surveillance practices allow us to catch and treat CTRCT early, optimizing modifiable risk factors (diet, exercise, smoking, hypertension, and so forth) is equally important.

- Educating patients on signs and symptoms of CTRCT is important for patient empowerment and home monitoring of symptoms.

- Consult with an imaging or cardio-oncology specialist before obtaining echocardiography and/or CMR to ensure all needed parameters/sequences are acquired. This can prevent repeated scans and optimize available clinical data.

DISCLOSURE

The Authors have nothing to disclose.

FUNDING

This study was supported in part by an NIH P50-CA140158 grant. The funder had no role in the following: design and conduct; collection, management, and interpretation of the data; in the preparation, review, or approval of the article; and the decision to submit the article for publication. Dr. Addison is supported by NIH grant number K23-HL155890, and an American Heart Association-Robert Wood Johnson Foundation Faculty Development Program grant. All other authors have reported that they have no relationships relevant to the contents of this article to disclose.

ACKNOWLEDGMENTS

The article's content is solely the responsibility of the authors and does not necessarily represent the official views of the National Institutes of Health.

REFERENCES

1. Siegel RL, Miller KD, Jemal A. Cancer statistics, 2020. CA Cancer J Clin 2020;70(1):7–30.
2. Shahrokni A, Wu AJ, Carter J, et al. Long-term toxicity of cancer treatment in older patients. Clin Geriatr Med 2016;32(1):63–80.
3. Campia U, Moslehi JJ, Amiri-Kordestani L, et al. Cardio-oncology: vascular and metabolic perspectives: a scientific statement from the american heart association. Circulation 2019;139(13): e579–602.
4. Zamorano JL, Lancellotti P, Rodriguez Muñoz D, et al. ESC position paper on cancer treatments and cardiovascular toxicity developed under the auspices of the ESC committee for practice guidelines: the task force for cancer treatments and cardiovascular toxicity of the European Society of Cardiology (ESC). Eur Heart J 2016;37(36): 2768–801.
5. Biersmith MA, Tong MS, Guha A, et al. Multimodality cardiac imaging in the era of emerging cancer therapies. J Am Heart Assoc 2020;9(2):e013755.
6. Seraphim A, Westwood M, Bhuva AN, et al. Advanced imaging modalities to monitor for cardiotoxicity. Curr Treat Options Oncol 2019;20(9):73.
7. Fava AM, Meredith D, Desai MY. Clinical applications of echo strain imaging: a current appraisal. Curr Treat Options Cardiovasc Med 2019;21(10):50.
8. Bottinor W, Trankle CR, Hundley WG. The role of cardiovascular MRI in cardio-oncology. Heart Fail Clin 2021;17(1):121–33.
9. Čelutkienė J, Pudil R, López-Fernández T, et al. Role of cardiovascular imaging in cancer patients receiving cardiotoxic therapies: a position statement on behalf of th##on (HFA), the european association of cardiovascular imaging (EACVI) and the Cardio-oncology council of the european society of cardiology (ESC). Eur J Heart Fail 2020; 22(9):1504–24.
10. Thavendiranathan P, Grant AD, Negishi T, et al. Reproducibility of echocardiographic techniques for sequential assessment of left ventricular ejection fraction and volumes: application to patients undergoing cancer chemotherapy. J Am Coll Cardiol 2013;61(1):77–84.
11. Bansal M, Kasliwal RR. How do I do it? Speckle-tracking echocardiography. Indian Heart J 2013; 65(1):117–23.
12. Liu JE, Barac A, Thavendiranathan P, et al. Strain imaging in cardio-oncology. JACC CardioOncol 2020;2(5):677–89.
13. Oikonomou EK, Kokkinidis DG, Kampaktsis PN, et al. Assessment of prognostic value of left ventricular global longitudinal strain for early prediction of chemotherapy-induced cardiotoxicity: a systematic review and meta-analysis. JAMA Cardiol 2019; 4(10):1007–18.
14. Cascino GJ, Voss WB, Canaani J, et al. Two-dimensional speckle-tracking strain detects subclinical cardiotoxicity in older patients treated for acute myeloid leukemia. Echocardiography. 2019; 36(11):2033–40.
15. Keramida K, Farmakis D, López Fernández T, et al. Focused echocardiography in cardio-oncology. Echocardiography 2020;37(8):1149–58.
16. Wang B, Yu Y, Zhang Y, et al. Speckle tracking echocardiography in the early detection and prediction of anthracycline cardiotoxicity in diffuse large B-cell lymphoma treated with (R)-CHOP regimen. Echocardiography 2020;37(3):421–8.
17. Laufer-Perl M, Arnold JH, Mor L, et al. The association of reduced global longitudinal strain with cancer therapy-related cardiac dysfunction among patients receiving cancer therapy. Clin Res Cardiol 2020;109(2):255–62.
18. McGregor PC, Moura FA, Banchs J, et al. Role of myocardial strain imaging in surveillance and management of cancer therapeutics-related cardiac dysfunction: a systematic review. Echocardiography. 2021;38(2):314–28.
19. El-Sherbeny WS, Sabry NM, Sharbay RM. Prediction of trastuzumab-induced cardiotoxicity in breast cancer patients receiving anthracycline-based chemotherapy. J Echocardiogr 2019;17(2): 76–83.
20. Chen J, Wang L, Wu FF, et al. Early detection of cardiotoxicity by 3D speckle tracking imaging of area strain in breast cancer patients receiving

chemotherapy. *Echocardiography* 2019;36(9): 1682–8.

21. Mahjoob MP, Sheikholeslami SA, Dadras M, et al. Prognostic value of cardiac biomarkers assessment in combination with myocardial 2D strain echocardiography for early detection of anthracycline-related cardiac toxicity. Cardiovasc Hematol Disord Drug Targets 2020;20(1):74–83.

22. Khairat I, Khalfallah M, Shaban A, et al. Right ventricular 2D speckle-tracking echocardiography in children with osteosarcoma under chemotherapy. Egypt Heart J 2019;71(1):23.

23. Slieker MG, Fackoury C, Slorach C, et al. Echocardiographic assessment of cardiac function in pediatric survivors of anthracycline-treated childhood cancer. Circ Cardiovasc Imaging 2019;12(12): e008869.

24. Wolf CM, Reiner B, Kühn A, et al. Subclinical cardiac dysfunction in childhood cancer survivors on 10-years follow-up correlates with cumulative anthracycline dose and is best detected by cardiopulmonary exercise testing, circulating serum biomarker, speckle tracking echocardiography, and tissue doppler imaging. Front Pediatr 2020;8:123.

25. Martinez HR, Salloum R, Wright E, et al. Echocardiographic myocardial strain analysis describes subclinical cardiac dysfunction after craniospinal irradiation in pediatric and young adult patients with central nervous system tumors. Cardiooncology 2021;7(1):5.

26. Sitte V, Burkhardt B, Weber R, et al. Advanced imaging and new cardiac biomarkers in long-term follow-up after childhood cancer. J Pediatr Hematol Oncol 2021;44(2):e374–80.

27. Yu HK, Yu W, Cheuk DK, et al. New three-dimensional speckle-tracking echocardiography identifies global impairment of left ventricular mechanics with a high sensitivity in childhood cancer survivors. J Am Soc Echocardiogr 2013;26(8): 846–52.

28. Bhagat A, Kleinerman ES. Anthracycline-induced cardiotoxicity: causes, mechanisms, and prevention. Adv Exp Med Biol 2020;1257:181–92.

29. Cappetta D, De Angelis A, Sapio L, et al. Oxidative stress and cellular response to doxorubicin: a common factor in the complex milieu of anthracycline cardiotoxicity. Oxid Med Cell Longev 2017;2017: 1521020.

30. Cardinale D, Colombo A, Bacchiani G, et al. Early detection of anthracycline cardiotoxicity and improvement with heart failure therapy. Circulation 2015;131(22):1981–8.

31. Bernaba BN, Chan JB, Lai CK, et al. Pathology of late-onset anthracycline cardiomyopathy. Cardiovasc Pathol 2010;19(5):308–11.

32. Saleh Y, Abdelkarim O, Herzallah K, et al. Anthracycline-induced cardiotoxicity: mechanisms of action, incidence, risk factors, prevention, and treatment. Heart Fail Rev 2020;26(5):1159–73.

33. Nicolazzi MA, Carnicelli A, Fuorlo M, et al. Anthracycline and trastuzumab-induced cardiotoxicity in breast cancer. Eur Rev Med Pharmacol Sci 2018; 22(7):2175–85.

34. Keramida K, Farmakis D, Bingcang J, et al. Longitudinal changes of right ventricular deformation mechanics during trastuzumab therapy in breast cancer patients. Eur J Heart Fail 2019;21(4):529–35.

35. Mantarro S, Rossi M, Bonifazi M, et al. Risk of severe cardiotoxicity following treatment with trastuzumab: a meta-analysis of randomized and cohort studies of 29,000 women with breast cancer. Intern Emerg Med 2016;11(1):123–40.

36. Balduzzi S, Mantarro S, Guarneri V, et al. Trastuzumab-containing regimens for metastatic breast cancer. Cochrane Database Syst Rev 2014;6. https://doi.org/10.1002/14651858.CD006242.pub2.

37. Grandin EW, Ky B, Cornell RF, et al. Patterns of cardiac toxicity associated with irreversible proteasome inhibition in the treatment of multiple myeloma. J Card Fail 2015;21(2):138–44.

38. Wu P, Oren O, Gertz MA, et al. Proteasome inhibitor-related cardiotoxicity: mechanisms, diagnosis, and management. Curr Oncol Rep 2020; 22(7):66.

39. Shah C, Bishnoi R, Jain A, et al. Cardiotoxicity associated with carfilzomib: systematic review and meta-analysis. Leuk Lymphoma 2018;59(11):2557–69.

40. Scott K, Hayden PJ, Will A, et al. Bortezomib for the treatment of multiple myeloma. Cochrane Database Syst Rev 2016;4. https://doi.org/10.1002/14651858.CD010816.pub2.

41. Iannaccone A, Bruno G, Ravera A, et al. Evaluation of cardiovascular toxicity associated with treatments containing proteasome inhibitors in multiple myeloma therapy. High Blood Press Cardiovasc Prev 2018;25(2):209–18.

42. Abdel-Qadir H, Ethier JL, Lee DS, et al. Cardiovascular toxicity of angiogenesis inhibitors in treatment of malignancy: A systematic review and meta-analysis. Cancer Treat Rev 2017;53:120–7.

43. Touyz RM, Herrmann J. Cardiotoxicity with vascular endothelial growth factor inhibitor therapy. NPJ Precis Oncol 2018;2:13.

44. Moreo A, Vallerio P, Ricotta R, et al. Effects of cancer therapy targeting vascular endothelial growth factor receptor on central blood pressure and cardiovascular system. Am J Hypertens 2016;29(2): 158–62.

45. Nhola LF, Abdelmoneim SS, Villarraga HR, et al. Echocardiographic assessment for the detection of cardiotoxicity due to vascular endothelial growth factor inhibitor therapy in metastatic renal cell and colorectal cancers. J Am Soc Echocardiogr 2019; 32(2):267–76.

46. Sonaglioni A, Albini A, Fossile E, et al. Speckle-tracking echocardiography for cardioncological evaluation in bevacizumab-treated colorectal cancer patients. Cardiovasc Toxicol 2020;20(6):581–92.

47. Chaar M, Kamta J, Ait-Oudhia S. Mechanisms, monitoring, and management of tyrosine kinase inhibitors-associated cardiovascular toxicities. Onco Targets Ther 2018;11:6227–37.

48. Brown SA, Ray JC, Herrmann J. Precision cardio-oncology: a systems-based perspective on cardiotoxicity of tyrosine kinase inhibitors and immune checkpoint inhibitors. J Cardiovasc Transl Res 2020;13(3):402–16.

49. Novo G, Di Lisi D, Bronte E, et al. Cardiovascular toxicity in cancer patients treated with tyrosine kinase inhibitors: a real-world single-center experience. Oncology 2020;98(7):445–51.

50. Berger M, Amini-Adlé M, Maucort-Boulch D, et al. Left ventricular ejection fraction decrease related to BRAF and/or MEK inhibitors in metastatic melanoma patients: a retrospective analysis. Cancer Med 2020;9(8):2611–20.

51. Mincu RI, Mahabadi AA, Michel L, et al. Cardiovascular Adverse Events Associated With BRAF and MEK Inhibitors: A Systematic Review and Meta-analysis. JAMA Netw Open 2019;2(8):e198890.

52. Guha A, Jain P, Fradley MG, et al. Cardiovascular adverse events associated with BRAF versus BRAF/MEK inhibitor: Cross-sectional and longitudinal analysis using two large national registries. Cancer Med 2021;10(12):3862–72.

53. Waheed N, Fradley MG, DeRemer DL, et al. Newly diagnosed cardiovascular disease in patients treated with immune checkpoint inhibitors: a retrospective analysis of patients at an academic tertiary care center. Cardiooncology. 2021;7(1):10.

54. Lyon AR, Yousaf N, Battisti NML, et al. Immune checkpoint inhibitors and cardiovascular toxicity. Lancet Oncol 2018;19(9):e447–58.

55. Bonaca MP, Olenchock BA, Salem JE, et al. Myocarditis in the setting of cancer therapeutics: proposed case definitions for emerging clinical syndromes in cardio-oncology. Circulation 2019; 140(2):80–91.

56. Mahmood SS, Fradley MG, Cohen JV, et al. Myocarditis in patients treated with immune checkpoint inhibitors. J Am Coll Cardiol 2018;71(16):1755–64.

57. Ganatra S, Neilan TG. Immune checkpoint inhibitor-associated myocarditis. Oncologist 2018; 23(8):879–86.

58. Awadalla M, Mahmood SS, Groarke JD, et al. Global longitudinal strain and cardiac events in patients with immune checkpoint inhibitor-related myocarditis. J Am Coll Cardiol 2020;75(5):467–78.

59. Mylvaganam R, Avery R, Goldberg I, et al. Adverse effects of immune checkpoint inhibitor therapies on right ventricular function and pulmonary arterial dilatation. Pulm Circ 2021; 11(1). 2045894021992236.

60. Stein-Merlob AF, Rothberg MV, Holman P, et al. Immunotherapy-associated cardiotoxicity of immune checkpoint inhibitors and chimeric antigen receptor t cell therapy: diagnostic and management challenges and strategies. Curr Cardiol Rep 2021;23(3):11.

61. Alvi RM, Frigault MJ, Fradley MG, et al. Cardiovascular events among adults treated with chimeric antigen receptor T-cells (CAR-T). J Am Coll Cardiol 2019;74(25):3099–108.

62. Ganatra S, Redd R, Hayek SS, et al. Chimeric antigen receptor T-cell therapy-associated cardiomyopathy in patients with refractory or relapsed non-hodgkin lymphoma. Circulation 2020;142(17): 1687–90.

63. Lancellotti P, Nkomo VT, Badano LP, et al. Expert consensus for multi-modality imaging evaluation of cardiovascular complications of radiotherapy in adults: a report from the european association of cardiovascular imaging and the american society of echocardiography. Eur Heart J Cardiovasc Imaging 2013;14(8):721–40.

64. Darby SC, Cutter DJ, Boerma M, et al. Radiation-related heart disease: current knowledge and future prospects. Int J Radiat Oncol Biol Phys 2010;76(3):656–65.

65. Walker V, Lairez O, Fondard O, et al. Myocardial deformation after radiotherapy: a layer-specific and territorial longitudinal strain analysis in a cohort of left-sided breast cancer patients (BACCARAT study). Radiat Oncol 2020;15(1):201.

66. van den Bogaard VAB, van Luijk P, Hummel YM, et al. Cardiac function after radiation therapy for breast cancer. Int J Radiat Oncol Biol Phys 2019;104(2): 392–400.

67. Skyttä T, Tuohinen S, Luukkaala T, et al. Adjuvant radiotherapy-induced cardiac changes among patients with early breast cancer: a three-year follow-up study. Acta Oncol 2019;58(9):1250–8.

68. Erven K, Jurcut R, Weltens C, et al. Acute radiation effects on cardiac function detected by strain rate imaging in breast cancer patients. Int J Radiat Oncol Biol Phys 2011;79(5):1444–51.

69. Tuohinen SS, Skyttä T, Poutanen T, et al. Radiotherapy-induced global and regional differences in early-stage left-sided versus right-sided breast cancer patients: speckle tracking echocardiography study. Int J Cardiovasc Imaging 2017;33(4): 463–72.

70. Lo Q, Hee L, Batumalai V, et al. Strain imaging detects dose-dependent segmental cardiac dysfunction in the acute phase after breast irradiation. Int J Radiat Oncol Biol Phys 2017;99(1):182–90.

71. Lo Q, Hee L, Batumalai V, et al. Subclinical cardiac dysfunction detected by strain imaging during

breast irradiation with persistent changes 6 weeks after treatment. Int J Radiat Oncol Biol Phys 2015; 92(2):268–76.

72. Tuohinen SS, Skyttä T, Huhtala H, et al. 3-year follow-up of radiation-associated changes in diastolic function by speckle tracking echocardiography. JACC CardioOncol 2021;3(2):277–89.

73. Jenkins C, Bricknell K, Hanekom L, et al. Reproducibility and accuracy of echocardiographic measurements of left ventricular parameters using real-time three-dimensional echocardiography. J Am Coll Cardiol 2004;44(4):878–86.

74. Habeeb NM, Youssef OI, Elguindy WM, et al. Three dimensional (3D) echocardiography as a tool of left ventricular assessment in children with dilated cardiomyopathy: comparison to cardiac MRI. J Med Sci 2018;6(12):2310–5. Open Access Maced.

75. Altman M, Bergerot C, Aussoleil A, et al. Assessment of left ventricular systolic function by deformation imaging derived from speckle tracking: a comparison between 2D and 3D echo modalities. Eur Heart J Cardiovasc Imaging 2014;15(3): 316–23.

76. Song FY, Shi J, Guo Y, et al. Assessment of biventricular systolic strain derived from the two-dimensional and three-dimensional speckle tracking echocardiography in lymphoma patients after anthracycline therapy. Int J Cardiovasc Imaging 2017;33(6):857–68.

77. Poterucha TJ, Kochav J, O'Connor DS, et al. Cardiac tumors: clinical presentation, diagnosis, and management. Curr Treat Options Oncol 2019; 20(8):66.

78. Abraham KP, Reddy V, Gattuso P. Neoplasms metastatic to the heart: review of 3314 consecutive autopsies. Am J Cardiovasc Pathol 1990; 3(3):195–8.

79. Patel R, Lim RP, Saric M, et al. Diagnostic performance of cardiac magnetic resonance imaging and echocardiography in evaluation of cardiac and paracardiac masses. Am J Cardiol 2016; 117(1):135–40.

80. Mansencal N, Revault-d'Allonnes L, Pelage JP, et al. Usefulness of contrast echocardiography for assessment of intracardiac masses. Arch Cardiovasc Dis 2009;102(3):177–83.

81. Tang QY, Guo LD, Wang WX, et al. Usefulness of contrast perfusion echocardiography for differential diagnosis of cardiac masses. Ultrasound Med Biol 2015;41(9):2382–90.

82. Xia H, Gan L, Jiang Y, et al. Use of transesophageal echocardiography and contrast echocardiography in the evaluation of cardiac masses. Int J Cardiol 2017;236:466–72.

83. Mügge A, Daniel WG, Haverich A, et al. Diagnosis of noninfective cardiac mass lesions by two-dimensional echocardiography. Comparison of the transthoracic and transesophageal approaches. Circulation 1991;83(1):70–8.

84. Tsang TS, Oh JK, Seward JB, et al. Diagnostic value of echocardiography in cardiac tamponade. Herz 2000;25(8):734–40.

85. Tsang TS, Seward JB, Barnes ME, et al. Outcomes of primary and secondary treatment of pericardial effusion in patients with malignancy. Mayo Clin Proc 2000;75(3):248–53.

86. Tsang TS. Echocardiography-guided pericardiocentesis for effusions in patients with cancer revisited. J Am Coll Cardiol 2015;66(10):1129–31.

87. El Haddad D, Iliescu C, Yusuf SW, et al. Outcomes of cancer patients undergoing percutaneous pericardiocentesis for pericardial effusion. J Am Coll Cardiol 2015;66(10):1119–28.

88. Addison D, Slivnick JA, Campbell CM, et al. Recent advances and current dilemmas in the diagnosis and management of transthyretin cardiac amyloidosis. J Am Heart Assoc 2021;10(9):e019840.

89. Bravo PE, Fujikura K, Kijewski MF, et al. Relative apical sparing of myocardial longitudinal strain is explained by regional differences in total amyloid mass rather than the proportion of amyloid deposits. JACC Cardiovasc Imaging 2019;12(7 Pt 1):1165–73.

90. Phelan D, Collier P, Thavendiranathan P, et al. Relative apical sparing of longitudinal strain using two-dimensional speckle-tracking echocardiography is both sensitive and specific for the diagnosis of cardiac amyloidosis. Heart 2012;98(19): 1442–8.

91. Nicol M, Baudet M, Brun S, et al. Diagnostic score of cardiac involvement in AL amyloidosis. Eur Heart J Cardiovasc Imaging 2020;21(5):542–8.

92. Kyrouac D, Schiffer W, Lennep B, et al. Echocardiographic and clinical predictors of cardiac amyloidosis: limitations of apical sparing. ESC Heart Fail 2022;9(1):385–97.

93. Harries I, Liang K, Williams M, et al. Magnetic resonance imaging to detect cardiovascular effects of cancer therapy: JACC CardioOncology state-of-the-art review. JACC CardioOncol. 2020;2(2): 270–92.

94. Moody WE, Edwards NC, Chue CD, et al. Variability in cardiac MR measurement of left ventricular ejection fraction, volumes and mass in healthy adults: defining a significant change at 1 year. Br J Radiol 2015;88(1049):20140831.

95. Armstrong GT, Plana JC, Zhang N, et al. Screening adult survivors of childhood cancer for cardiomyopathy: comparison of echocardiography and cardiac magnetic resonance imaging. J Clin Oncol 2012;30(23):2876–84.

96. Scatteia A, Baritussio A, Bucciarelli-Ducci C. Strain imaging using cardiac magnetic resonance. Heart Fail Rev 2017;22(4):465–76.

97. Amzulescu MS, Langet H, Saloux E, et al. Head-to-head comparison of global and regional two-dimensional speckle tracking strain versus cardiac magnetic resonance tagging in a multicenter validation study. Circ Cardiovasc Imaging 2017;10(11).

98. Soufer A, Baldassarre LA. The role of cardiac magnetic resonance imaging to detect cardiac toxicity from cancer therapeutics. Curr Treat Options Cardiovasc Med 2019;21(6):28.

99. Barreiro-Pérez M, Curione D, Symons R, et al. Left ventricular global myocardial strain assessment comparing the reproducibility of four commercially available CMR-feature tracking algorithms. Eur Radiol 2018;28(12):5137–47.

100. Ananthapadmanabhan S, Deng E, Femia G, et al. Intra- and inter-observer reproducibility of multi-layer cardiac magnetic resonance feature tracking derived longitudinal and circumferential strain. Cardiovasc Diagn Ther 2020;10(2):173–82.

101. Lambert J, Lamacie M, Thampinathan B, et al. Variability in echocardiography and MRI for detection of cancer therapy cardiotoxicity. *Heart.* 2020; 106(11):817–23.

102. Suerken CK, D'Agostino RB Jr, Jordan JH, et al. Simultaneous left ventricular volume and strain changes during chemotherapy associate with 2-year postchemotherapy measures of left ventricular ejection fraction. J Am Heart Assoc 2020;9(2): e015400.

103. Evin M, Cluzel P, Lamy J, et al. Assessment of left atrial function by MRI myocardial feature tracking. J Magn Reson Imaging 2015;42(2):379–89.

104. Burrage MK, Ferreira VM. The use of cardiovascular magnetic resonance as an early non-invasive biomarker for cardiotoxicity in cardio-oncology. Cardiovasc Diagn Ther 2020;10(3):610–24.

105. Taylor AJ, Salerno M, Dharmakumar R, et al. T1 mapping: basic techniques and clinical applications. JACC Cardiovasc Imaging 2016;9(1):67–81.

106. Karamitsos TD, Arvanitaki A, Karvounis H, et al. Myocardial Tissue characterization and fibrosis by imaging. JACC Cardiovasc Imaging 2020; 13(5):1221–34.

107. Ferreira VM, Piechnik SK, Dall'Armellina E, et al. Non-contrast T1-mapping detects acute myocardial edema with high diagnostic accuracy: a comparison to T2-weighted cardiovascular magnetic resonance. J Cardiovasc Magn Reson 2012;14(1):42.

108. h-Ici DO, Jeuthe S, Al-Wakeel N, et al. T1 mapping in ischaemic heart disease. Eur Heart J Cardiovasc Imaging 2014;15(6):597–602.

109. Löffler AI, Salerno M. Cardiac MRI for the evaluation of oncologic cardiotoxicity. J Nucl Cardiol 2018;25(6):2148–58.

110. Nakamori S, Dohi K, Ishida M, et al. Native T1 mapping and extracellular volume mapping for the assessment of diffuse myocardial fibrosis in dilated cardiomyopathy. JACC Cardiovasc Imaging 2018; 11(1):48–59.

111. Hu C, Sinusas AJ, Huber S, et al. T1-refBlochi: high resolution 3D post-contrast T1 myocardial mapping based on a single 3D late gadolinium enhancement volume, Bloch equations, and a reference T1. J Cardiovasc Magn Reson 2017; 19(1):63.

112. Sibley CT, Noureldin RA, Gai N, et al. T1 mapping in cardiomyopathy at cardiac MR: comparison with endomyocardial biopsy. Radiology 2012; 265(3):724–32.

113. Pan JA, Lee YJ, Salerno M. Diagnostic performance of extracellular volume, native T1, and T2 mapping versus lake louise criteria by cardiac magnetic resonance for detection of acute myocarditis: a meta-analysis. Circ Cardiovasc Imaging 2018;11(7):e007598.

114. Yu AF, Chan AT, Steingart RM. Cardiac magnetic resonance and cardio-oncology: does t(2) signal the end of anthracycline cardiotoxicity? J Am Coll Cardiol 2019;73(7):792–4.

115. Lunning MA, Kutty S, Rome ET, et al. Cardiac magnetic resonance imaging for the assessment of the myocardium after doxorubicin-based chemotherapy. Am J Clin Oncol 2015;38(4):377–81.

116. Toro-Salazar OH, Lee JH, Zellars KN, et al. Use of integrated imaging and serum biomarker profiles to identify subclinical dysfunction in pediatric cancer patients treated with anthracyclines. Cardiooncology 2018;4. https://doi.org/10.1186/s40959-018-0030-5.

117. Jolly MP, Jordan JH, Meléndez GC, et al. Automated assessments of circumferential strain from cine CMR correlate with LVEF declines in cancer patients early after receipt of cardio-toxic chemotherapy. J Cardiovasc Magn Reson 2017;19(1):59.

118. Haslbauer JD, Lindner S, Valbuena-Lopez S, et al. CMR imaging biosignature of cardiac involvement due to cancer-related treatment by T1 and T2 mapping. Int J Cardiol 2019;275:179–86.

119. Safaei AM, Kamangar TM, Asadian S, et al. Detection of the early cardiotoxic effects of doxorubicin-containing chemotherapy regimens in patients with breast cancer through novel cardiac magnetic resonance imaging: a short-term follow-up. J Clin Imaging Sci 2021;11:33.

120. Barbosa MF, Fusco DR, Gaiolla RD, et al. Characterization of subclinical diastolic dysfunction by cardiac magnetic resonance feature-tracking in adult survivors of non-Hodgkin lymphoma treated with anthracyclines. BMC Cardiovasc Disord 2021;21(1):170.

121. Neilan TG, Coelho-Filho OR, Pena-Herrera D, et al. Left ventricular mass in patients with a cardiomyopathy after treatment with anthracyclines. Am J Cardiol 2012;110(11):1679–86.

122. Neilan TG, Coelho-Filho OR, Shah RV, et al. Myocardial extracellular volume by cardiac magnetic resonance imaging in patients treated with anthracycline-based chemotherapy. Am J Cardiol 2013;111(5):717–22.

123. Tham EB, Haykowsky MJ, Chow K, et al. Diffuse myocardial fibrosis by T1-mapping in children with subclinical anthracycline cardiotoxicity: relationship to exercise capacity, cumulative dose and remodeling. J Cardiovasc Magn Reson 2013;15(1):48.

124. Jordan JH, Vasu S, Morgan TM, et al. Anthracycline-associated T1 mapping characteristics are elevated independent of the presence of cardiovascular comorbidities in cancer survivors. Circ Cardiovasc Imaging 2016;9(8). https://doi.org/10.1161/circimaging.115.004325.

125. Wassmuth R, Lentzsch S, Erdbruegger U, et al. Subclinical cardiotoxic effects of anthracyclines as assessed by magnetic resonance imaging-a pilot study. Am Heart J 2001;141(6):1007–13.

126. Lustberg MB, Reinbolt R, Addison D, et al. Early detection of anthracycline-induced cardiotoxicity in breast cancer survivors with T2 cardiac magnetic resonance. Circ Cardiovasc Imaging 2019;12(5):e008777.

127. Martin-Garcia A, Diaz-Pelaez E, Lopez-Corral L, et al. T2 mapping identifies early anthracycline-induced cardiotoxicity in elderly patients with cancer. JACC Cardiovasc Imaging 2020;13(7):1630–2.

128. Park HS, Hong YJ, Han K, et al. Ultrahigh-field cardiovascular magnetic resonance T1 and T2 mapping for the assessment of anthracycline-induced cardiotoxicity in rat models: validation against histopathologic changes. J Cardiovasc Magn Reson 2021;23(1):76.

129. Galán-Arriola C, Lobo M, Vílchez-Tschischke JP, et al. Serial magnetic resonance imaging to identify early stages of anthracycline-induced cardiotoxicity. J Am Coll Cardiol 2019;73(7):779–91.

130. Noel CV, Rainusso N, Robertson M, et al. Early detection of myocardial changes with and without dexrazoxane using serial magnetic resonance imaging in a pre-clinical mouse model. Cardiooncology 2021;7(1):23.

131. de Ville de Goyet M, Brichard B, Robert A, et al. Prospective cardiac MRI for the analysis of biventricular function in children undergoing cancer treatments. Pediatr Blood Cancer 2015;62(5):867–74.

132. Drafts BC, Twomley KM, D'Agostino R Jr, et al. Low to moderate dose anthracycline-based chemotherapy is associated with early noninvasive imaging evidence of subclinical cardiovascular disease. JACC Cardiovasc Imaging 2013;6(8):877–85.

133. Jordan JH, Castellino SM, Meléndez GC, et al. Left ventricular mass change after anthracycline chemotherapy. Circ Heart Fail 2018;11(7):e004560.

134. Houbois CP, Nolan M, Somerset E, et al. Serial cardiovascular magnetic resonance strain measurements to identify cardiotoxicity in breast cancer: comparison with echocardiography. JACC Cardiovasc Imaging 2021;14(5):962–74.

135. Nakano S, Takahashi M, Kimura F, et al. Cardiac magnetic resonance imaging-based myocardial strain study for evaluation of cardiotoxicity in breast cancer patients treated with trastuzumab: a pilot study to evaluate the feasibility of the method. Cardiol J 2016;23(3):270–80.

136. Ong G, Brezden-Masley C, Dhir V, et al. Myocardial strain imaging by cardiac magnetic resonance for detection of subclinical myocardial dysfunction in breast cancer patients receiving trastuzumab and chemotherapy. Int J Cardiol 2018;261:228–33.

137. Gong IY, Ong G, Brezden-Masley C, et al. Early diastolic strain rate measurements by cardiac MRI in breast cancer patients treated with trastuzumab: a longitudinal study. Int J Cardiovasc Imaging 2019;35(4):653–62.

138. Song L, Brezden-Masley C, Ramanan V, et al. Serial measurements of left ventricular systolic and diastolic function by cardiac magnetic resonance imaging in patients with early stage breast cancer on trastuzumab. Am J Cardiol 2019;123(7):1173–9.

139. Fallah-Rad N, Lytwyn M, Fang T, et al. Delayed contrast enhancement cardiac magnetic resonance imaging in trastuzumab induced cardiomyopathy. J Cardiovasc Magn Reson 2008;10(1):5.

140. Wadhwa D, Fallah-Rad N, Grenier D, et al. Trastuzumab mediated cardiotoxicity in the setting of adjuvant chemotherapy for breast cancer: a retrospective study. Breast Cancer Res Treat 2009;117(2):357–64.

141. Barthur A, Brezden-Masley C, Connelly KA, et al. Longitudinal assessment of right ventricular structure and function by cardiovascular magnetic resonance in breast cancer patients treated with trastuzumab: a prospective observational study. J Cardiovasc Magn Reson 2017;19(1):44.

142. Naresh NK, Misener S, Zhang Z, et al. Cardiac MRI myocardial functional and tissue characterization detects early cardiac dysfunction in a mouse model of chemotherapy-induced cardiotoxicity. NMR Biomed 2020;33(9):e4327.

143. Cottin Y, Ribuot C, Maupoil V, et al. Early incidence of adriamycin treatment on cardiac parameters in the rat. Can J Physiol Pharmacol 1994;72(2):140–5.

144. Lightfoot JC, D'Agostino RB Jr, Hamilton CA, et al. Novel approach to early detection of doxorubicin cardiotoxicity by gadolinium-enhanced cardiovascular magnetic resonance imaging in an experimental model. Circ Cardiovasc Imaging 2010;3(5):550–8.

145. Thavendiranathan P, Walls M, Giri S, et al. Improved detection of myocardial involvement in

acute inflammatory cardiomyopathies using T2 mapping. Circ Cardiovasc Imaging 2012;5(1):102–10.

146. Altaha MA, Nolan M, Marwick TH, et al. Can quantitative CMR Tissue characterization adequately identify cardiotoxicity during chemotherapy?: impact of temporal and observer variability. JACC Cardiovasc Imaging 2020;13(4):951–62.

147. Foley PW, Hamilton MS, Leyva F. Myocardial scarring following chemotherapy for multiple myeloma detected using late gadolinium hyperenhancement cardiovascular magnetic resonance. J Cardiovasc Med (Hagerstown) 2010;11(5):386–8.

148. Jouni H, Aubry MC, Lacy MQ, et al. Ixazomib cardiotoxicity: a possible class effect of proteasome inhibitors. Am J Hematol 2017;92(2):220–1.

149. Diwadkar S, Patel AA, Fradley MG. Bortezomib-Induced complete heart block and myocardial scar: the potential role of cardiac biomarkers in monitoring cardiotoxicity. Case Rep Cardiol 2016;2016:3456287.

150. Heitner SB, Minnier J, Naher A, et al. Bortezomib-based chemotherapy for multiple myeloma patients without comorbid cardiovascular disease shows no cardiotoxicity. Clin Lymphoma Myeloma Leuk 2018;18(12):796–802.

151. Ederhy S, Massard C, Dufaitre G, et al. Frequency and management of troponin I elevation in patients treated with molecular targeted therapies in phase I trials. Invest New Drugs 2012;30(2):611–5.

152. Wu CF, Chuang WP, Li AH, et al. Cardiac magnetic resonance imaging in sunitinib malate-related cardiomyopathy: no late gadolinium enhancement. J Chin Med Assoc 2009;72(6):323–7.

153. Friedrich MG, Sechtem U, Schulz-Menger J, et al. Cardiovascular magnetic resonance in myocarditis: a JACC white paper. J Am Coll Cardiol 2009;53(17):1475–87.

154. Ferreira VM, Piechnik SK, Dall'Armellina E, et al. T(1) mapping for the diagnosis of acute myocarditis using CMR: comparison to T2-weighted and late gadolinium enhanced imaging. JACC Cardiovasc Imaging 2013;6(10):1048–58.

155. Thavendiranathan P, Zhang L, Zafar A, et al. Myocardial T1 and T2 mapping by magnetic resonance in patients with immune checkpoint inhibitor-associated myocarditis. J Am Coll Cardiol 2021;77(12):1503–16.

156. Friedrich MG. Immune checkpoint inhibitor cardiotoxicity: what can we learn from real life data on CMR as a diagnostic tool? Eur Heart J 2020;18:1744–6.

157. Guo CW, Alexander M, Dib Y, et al. A closer look at immune-mediated myocarditis in the era of combined checkpoint blockade and targeted therapies. Eur J Cancer 2020;124:15–24.

158. Higgins AY, Arbune A, Soufer A, et al. Left ventricular myocardial strain and tissue characterization by cardiac magnetic resonance imaging in immune checkpoint inhibitor associated cardiotoxicity. PLoS One 2021;16(2):e0246764.

159. Zhang L, Awadalla M, Mahmood SS, et al. Cardiovascular magnetic resonance in immune checkpoint inhibitor-associated myocarditis. Eur Heart J 2020;41(18):1733–43.

160. Touat M, Maisonobe T, Knauss S, et al. Immune checkpoint inhibitor-related myositis and myocarditis in patients with cancer. Neurology 2018;91(10):e985–94.

161. Doerner J, Bunck AC, Michels G, et al. Incremental value of cardiovascular magnetic resonance feature tracking derived atrial and ventricular strain parameters in a comprehensive approach for the diagnosis of acute myocarditis. Eur J Radiol 2018;104:120–8.

162. Messroghli DR, Moon JC, Ferreira VM, et al. Clinical recommendations for cardiovascular magnetic resonance mapping of T1, T2, T2* and extracellular volume: a consensus statement by the society for cardiovascular magnetic resonance (SCMR) endorsed by the european association for cardiovascular imaging (EACVI). J Cardiovasc Magn Reson 2017;19(1):75.

163. Spieker M, Haberkorn S, Gastl M, et al. Abnormal T2 mapping cardiovascular magnetic resonance correlates with adverse clinical outcome in patients with suspected acute myocarditis. J Cardiovasc Magn Reson 2017;19(1):38.

164. Gräni C, Bière L, Eichhorn C, et al. Incremental value of extracellular volume assessment by cardiovascular magnetic resonance imaging in risk stratifying patients with suspected myocarditis. Int J Cardiovasc Imaging 2019;35(6):1067–78.

165. Gräni C, Eichhorn C, Bière L, et al. Prognostic value of cardiac magnetic resonance tissue characterization in risk stratifying patients with suspected myocarditis. J Am Coll Cardiol 2017;70(16):1964–76.

166. Heggemann F, Grotz H, Welzel G, et al. Cardiac Function after multimodal breast cancer therapy assessed with functional magnetic resonance imaging and echocardiography imaging. Int J Radiat Oncol Biol Phys 2015;93(4):836–44.

167. Ylänen K, Eerola A, Vettenranta K, et al. Three-dimensional echocardiography and cardiac magnetic resonance imaging in the screening of long-term survivors of childhood cancer after cardiotoxic therapy. Am J Cardiol 2014;113(11):1886–92.

168. Bergom C, Rubenstein J, Wilson JF, et al. A pilot study of cardiac mri in breast cancer survivors after cardiotoxic chemotherapy and three-dimensional conformal radiotherapy. Front Oncol 2020;10:506739.

169. Ibrahim EH, Baruah D, Croisille P, et al. Cardiac magnetic resonance for early detection of radiation therapy-induced cardiotoxicity in a small animal model. *JACC CardioOncol.* 2021;3(1):113–30.

170. Huang YJ, Harrison A, Sarkar V, et al. Detection of late radiation damage on left atrial fibrosis using cardiac late gadolinium enhancement magnetic resonance imaging. Adv Radiat Oncol 2016;1(2):106–14.

171. Ricco A, Slade A, Canada JM, et al. Cardiac MRI utilizing late gadolinium enhancement (LGE) and T1 mapping in the detection of radiation induced heart disease. Cardiooncology 2020;6:6.

172. Takagi H, Ota H, Umezawa R, et al. Left ventricular T1 mapping during chemotherapy-radiation therapy: serial assessment of participants with esophageal cancer. Radiology 2018;289(2):347–54.

173. Umezawa R, Ota H, Takanami K, et al. MRI findings of radiation-induced myocardial damage in patients with oesophageal cancer. Clin Radiol 2014;69(12):1273–9.

174. Tuohinen S, Skytta T, Virtanen V, et al. 30Radiotherapy-induced changes in breast cancer patients in extra cellular volume and T1 mapping in cardiac magnetic resonance imaging and in ECG six years after radiotherapy treatment. Eur Heart J - Cardiovasc Imaging 2019;20(2).

175. Lee SL, Mahler P, Olson S, et al. Reduction of cardiac dose using respiratory-gated MR-linac plans for gastro-esophageal junction cancer. Med Dosim 2021;46(2):152–6.

176. Ipsen S, Blanck O, Oborn B, et al. Radiotherapy beyond cancer: target localization in real-time MRI and treatment planning for cardiac radiosurgery. Med Phys 2014;41(12):120702.

177. Danad I, Szymonifka J, Twisk JWR, et al. Diagnostic performance of cardiac imaging methods to diagnose ischaemia-causing coronary artery disease when directly compared with fractional flow reserve as a reference standard: a meta-analysis. Eur Heart J 2017;38(13):991–8.

178. Kirkham AA, Virani SA, Campbell KL. The utility of cardiac stress testing for detection of cardiovascular disease in breast cancer survivors: a systematic review. Int J Womens Health 2015;7:127–40.

179. Di Lisi D, Madonna R, Zito C, et al. Anticancer therapy-induced vascular toxicity: VEGF inhibition and beyond. Int J Cardiol 2017;227:11–7.

180. Grover S, Lou PW, Bradbrook C, et al. Early and late changes in markers of aortic stiffness with breast cancer therapy. Intern Med J 2015;45(2):140–7.

181. Sierra-Galan LM, François CJ. Clinical applications of MRA 4D-flow. Curr Treat Options Cardiovasc Med 2019;21(10):58.

182. Unterberg-Buchwald C, Ritter CO, Reupke V, et al. Targeted endomyocardial biopsy guided by real-time cardiovascular magnetic resonance. J Cardiovasc Magn Reson 2017;19(1):45.

183. Rathi VK, Czajka AT, Thompson DV, et al. Can cardiovascular MRI be used to more definitively characterize cardiac masses initially identified using echocardiography? Echocardiography 2018;35(5):735–42.

184. Lichtenberger JP 3rd, Dulberger AR, Gonzales PE, et al. MR imaging of cardiac masses. Top Magn Reson Imaging 2018;27(2):103–11.

185. Tumma R, Dong W, Wang J, et al. Evaluation of cardiac masses by CMR-strengths and pitfalls: a tertiary center experience. Int J Cardiovasc Imaging 2016;32(6):913–20.

186. Slonimsky E, Konen O, Di Segni E, et al. Cardiac MRI: a useful tool for differentiating cardiac thrombi from tumors. Isr Med Assoc J 2018;20(8):472–5.

187. Gupta A, Singh Gulati G, Seth S, et al. Cardiac MRI in restrictive cardiomyopathy. Clin Radiol 2012;67(2):95–105.

188. Adler Y, Charron P, Imazio M, et al. ESC Guidelines for the diagnosis and management of pericardial diseases: the task force for the diagnosis and management of pericardial diseases of the european society of cardiology (ESC)endorsed by: the european association for cardio-thoracic surgery (EACTS). Eur Heart J 2015;36(42):2921–64.

189. Martinez-Naharro A, Treibel TA, Abdel-Gadir A, et al. Magnetic resonance in transthyretin cardiac amyloidosis. J Am Coll Cardiol 2017;70(4):466–77.

190. Fontana M, Pica S, Reant P, et al. Prognostic value of late gadolinium enhancement cardiovascular magnetic resonance in cardiac amyloidosis. Circulation 2015;132(16):1570–9.

191. Dorbala S, Cuddy S, Falk RH. How to image cardiac amyloidosis: a practical approach. JACC Cardiovasc Imaging 2020;13(6):1368–83.

192. Fontana M, White SK, Banypersad SM, et al. Comparison of T1 mapping techniques for ECV quantification. Histological validation and reproducibility of ShMOLLI versus multibreath-hold T1 quantification equilibrium contrast CMR. J Cardiovasc Magn Reson 2012;14(1):88.

193. Wan K, Li W, Sun J, et al. Regional amyloid distribution and impact on mortality in light-chain amyloidosis: a T1 mapping cardiac magnetic resonance study. *Amyloid.* 2019;26(1):45–51.

194. Martinez-Naharro A, Abdel-Gadir A, Treibel TA, et al. CMR-verified regression of cardiac al amyloid after chemotherapy. JACC Cardiovasc Imaging 2018;11(1):152–4.

195. Richards DB, Cookson LM, Berges AC, et al. Therapeutic clearance of amyloid by antibodies to serum amyloid P component. N Engl J Med 2015;373(12):1106–14.

196. Fontana M, Martinez-Naharro A, Chacko L, et al. Reduction in CMR derived extracellular volume

with patisiran indicates cardiac amyloid regression. JACC Cardiovasc Imaging 2021;14(1):189–99.

197. Kotecha T, Martinez-Naharro A, Treibel TA, et al. Myocardial edema and prognosis in amyloidosis. J Am Coll Cardiol 2018;71(25):2919–31.

198. Pan JA, Kerwin MJ, Salerno M. Native T1 mapping, extracellular volume mapping, and late gadolinium enhancement in cardiac amyloidosis: a meta-analysis. JACC Cardiovasc Imaging 2020;13(6): 1299–310.

199. Jeong D, Gladish G, Chitiboi T, et al. MRI in cardio-oncology: a review of cardiac complications in oncologic care. J Magn Reson Imaging 2019; 50(5):1349–66.

200. Leerink JM, Feijen E, van der Pal HJH, et al. Diagnostic tools for early detection of cardiac dysfunction in childhood cancer survivors: Methodological aspects of the Dutch late effects after childhood cancer (LATER) cardiology study. Am Heart J 2020;219:89–98.

201. Hong YJ, Kim GM, Han K, et al. Cardiotoxicity evaluation using magnetic resonance imaging in breast Cancer patients (CareBest): study protocol for a prospective trial. BMC Cardiovasc Disord 2020; 20(1):264.

202. Chaix MA, Parmar N, Kinnear C, et al. Machine learning identifies clinical and genetic factors associated with anthracycline cardiotoxicity in pediatric cancer survivors. JACC CardioOncol. 2020;2(5): 690–706.

203. Kobayashi M, Huttin O, Magnusson M, et al. Machine learning-derived echocardiographic phenotypes predict heart failure incidence in asymptomatic individuals. JACC Cardiovasc Imaging 2021;15(2):193–208.

204. McDonald JP, MacNamara JP, Zaha VG. Challenges in implementing optimal echocardiographic screening in cardio-oncology. Curr Treat Options Cardiovasc Med 2019;21(8):39.

Cardiac Amyloidosis

Morie A. Gertz, MD, MACP

KEYWORDS

- Amyloidosis • Stem cell transplantation • Chemotherapy • Cardiac transplantation
- Amyloid echocardiography • Light chains • Transthyretin

KEY POINTS

- Amyloidosis is a common cause of heart failure with preserved ejection fraction (HFpEF) and a high index of suspicion is required to confirm this diagnosis
- The major types of cardiac amyloidosis are amyloid light-chain (AL) or light chain amyloidosis and transthyretin (TTR) or transthyretin amyloidosis (senile cardiac amyloidosis)
- The diagnosis can be suspected by simple screening blood tests and simple imaging studies
- Endomyocardial biopsy is not required to make the diagnosis
- All forms of cardiac amyloidosis have FDA-approved therapies that result in improved outcomes

INTRODUCTION

Amyloid deposits are defined by their tinctorial properties. Under the light microscope amyloid deposits are eosinophilic and amorphous when stained with hematoxylin and eosin. With Congo red staining the deposits are positive and under polarized light will exhibit green birefringence. Sixty years later electron microscopy demonstrated that all deposits were fibrillar. All amyloid deposits are protein derived. The clinical characteristics will be driven by the nature of the protein subunit. In cardiology, the 2 most common subunits accounting for well more than 90% of cardiac amyloidosis are either immunoglobulin light chain, amyloid light-chain (AL) amyloidosis, or transthyretin; transthyretin (TTR) amyloidosis. Although 70% of patients with systemic amyloidosis have cardiac involvement the diagnosis is made by cardiologists only 20% of the time,[1] suggesting significant gaps in knowledge in how to establish a workflow to arrive at a diagnosis in everyday practice (**Fig. 1**).

One of the problems with the early recognition of cardiac amyloidosis is its ability to mimic a host of other disorders. There is no one diagnostic test, except for magnetic resonance imaging with gadolinium that is specific for amyloidosis.[2] If stains for amyloid are not requested on biopsy tissue the diagnosis may be overlooked. Bowel amyloidosis has been misdiagnosed as collagenous colitis, glomerular amyloid has been misdiagnosed as hyaline destruction and patients with a history of hereditary cardiomyopathy have been misdiagnosed as hypertrophic cardiomyopathy.[3] The lack of higher reported mortality rates in states with a greater number of black residents suggests under-diagnosis of amyloidosis.[4]

Clinical Presentation

The classic presentation of amyloid cardiomyopathy is heart failure with preserved ejection fraction (HFpEF).[5] The symptoms are typical include dyspnea on exertion, lower extremity edema due to high right-sided filling pressures, small pleural effusions with conspicuous absence of ischemic symptomatology. Standard echocardiography will show thickened walls which without Doppler studies can be interpreted as demonstrating hypertrophy either related to hypertension or hypertrophic cardiomyopathy.[6] As amyloidosis is a disease of diastole the rapid rise of filling pressure leads to a very low end-diastolic volume with a resultant reduction in stroke volume and consequent reduced cardiac output. Compensatory tachycardia is typical and often necessary to sustain cardiac output. Most patients will note the

Permission has been obtained from Mayo Foundation for publication of copy righted figures used in the central illustration.

Department of Medicine, Mayo Clinic Rochester, 200 Southwest First Street, W10, Rochester, MN 55905, USA

E-mail address: gertz.morie@mayo.edu

Heart Failure Clin 18 (2022) 479–488
https://doi.org/10.1016/j.hfc.2022.02.005
1551-7136/22/Published by Elsevier Inc.

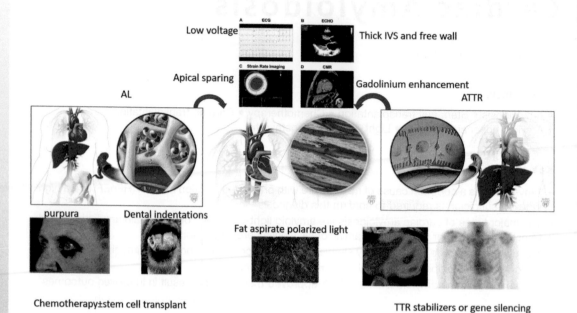

Low voltage

Thick IVS and free wall

Apical sparing

Gadolinium enhancement

AL

ATTR

purpura   Dental indentations

Fat aspirate polarized light

Chemotherapy±stem cell transplant

TTR stabilizers or gene silencing

Fig. 1. Pathopysiology and clinical features of cardiac amyloidosis. (*Used with permission* of Mayo Foundation for MedicalEducation and Research. All rights reserved.)

decline in systolic blood pressure over time. Systolic pressures of less than 100 mm Hg are common at diagnosis. The median age at diagnosis is 66 years. The estimated incidence is 12.1 cases per million person-years and the median survival is 2.45 years.[7] In Olmsted county Minnesota, however, the median age at diagnosis was 76 years with an anticipated 3852 new cases of AL amyloidosis in the United States each year.[8]

Conduction system amyloid is common leading to atrial fibrillation and is a common presentation, particularly in TTR cardiac amyloidosis. One of the important clues that lead to the correct diagnosis in practice is the common association of extra-cardiac amyloid organ dysfunction. Although 70% of patients with amyloidosis have cardiac involvement, 3/4 of the patient with cardiac amyloid will also have evidence of amyloid in other organs. The clinician should be particularly alert to the presence of proteinuria reflecting kidney involvement. Among 1000 patients with AL amyloidosis 318 had combined cardiac and renal involvement. Fifty or 16% of patients required renal replacement therapy the median survival was 18.5 months an independent predictor of death and dialysis were NT proBNP greater than 8500 ng/L and eGFR less than 30 mL/min[9]

20% of patients will have simultaneous peripheral neuropathy which is uncommon in other forms of HFpEF. One patient in 6 will have bilateral carpal tunnel syndrome in light chain amyloidosis but almost half of patients with TTR cardiac amyloid will have bilateral carpal tunnel syndrome antedating the diagnosis by as much as a decade.[10] (**Table 1**) Hepatomegaly with the elevation of the blood alkaline phosphatase out of proportion to the degree of right-sided filling pressure elevation may reflect simultaneous liver involvement with amyloid. In TTR cardiac amyloidosis lumbar spinal stenosis causing pseudoclaudication and biceps tendon rupture are quite specific findings.[11] when technetium pyrophosphate scanning was performed in patients referred for transaortic valve replacement TTR cardiac amyloidosis was found in 10%. Today all patients referred for[12] TAVR at Mayo clinic are required to have pyrophosphate scanning to ensure amyloid is not contributing to cardiac symptomatology. The association of aortic stenosis with ATTR cardiac amyloidosis is seen in both ATTRwt and ATTRv.[13] Periorbital purpura is seen in approximately 1 patient in 6 with light chain amyloidosis (**Fig. 2**)

Diagnosis

The electrocardiogram can be quite useful in a patient with thickened walls by echocardiography. Patients with prolonged QTc (≥483 msec) had significantly poorer survival. One would anticipate hypertensive cardiomyopathy patients to have increased voltage across the precordium. The finding of low voltage in the limb leads or a pseudoinfarction pattern in a patient with no evidence of ischemic symptomatology should raise the

Table 1
Signs and symptoms associated with cardiac amyloidosis

	AL	ATTR
Carpal Tunnel Syndrome	+	++
Purpura	+	
Pseudoclaudication		+
Paresthesia/neuropathy	+	+
Proteinuria	++	
Biceps Rupture		+
Glossomeagaly	+	

suspicion of amyloidosis.[14] Like echocardiography magnetic resonance imaging will demonstrate wall thickening, however, after gadolinium late enhancement is seen with myocardial nulling and is considered diagnostic for amyloidosis.[15] magnetic resonance imaging also allows the assessment of extracellular volume which is significantly increased in cardiac amyloidosis and is prognostic for survival.[16] ECV is independently predictive of prognosis.[16] PET imaging has also been applied for the detection of cardiac amyloidosis. In a meta-analysis the pooled sensitivity of PET for amyloidosis was 0.97 and the specificity was 0.98 the pooled sensitivity of combined amyloid and sodium fluoride PET was 0.88 with a specificity of 0.98. Further studies are required to substantiate the diagnostic role of PET imaging for the detection of cardiac amyloidosis.[17] Using florbetapir[^{18}F] PET-CT Retention index in a cohort of patients not felt to have cardiac amyloidosis by conventional methods such as echocardiography, changes consistent with cardiac involvement was seen in 50% of subjects manifest by increased retention. The same "noncardiac" amyloid patients had late gadolinium enhancement in 20% by magnetic resonance imaging and elevated extracellular volume in 20%. This suggests that amyloid infiltration does occur in a preclinical phase and that these patients are at risk of developing symptomatic cardiac amyloidosis.[18]

When a patient is seen with heart failure and preserved ejection fraction and the echocardiogram demonstrates wall thickening (**Fig. 3**) of any degree the 2 most important workflow studies are immunoglobulin-free light chain assay, immunofixation of serum and urine for kappa and lambda immunoglobulins and a technetium pyrophosphate scan. In a patient with a monoclonal protein and a clinically suspicious ECHO, the finding of a monoclonal protein should be considered a high index of suspicion for AL amyloidosis. Abnormalities of the immunoglobulin-free light chain assay are not only helpful in pointing to the correct diagnosis but the light chains are also part of the staging system and predict outcomes in amyloidosis AL. Serialized measurements of the light chain are used to monitor the impact of therapy and the response depth is a function of the percentage reduction of the involved immunoglobulin light chain. Although endomyocardial biopsy will be the gold standard of diagnosis these invasive biopsies are not required to establish the diagnosis. As patients with a monoclonal gammopathy will require a bone marrow biopsy to exclude multiple myeloma a Congo red stain can be conducted on the bone marrow biopsy and will be positive in 50% of patients. The subcutaneous fat aspirate an outpatient procedure conducted under local whereby milligrams of fat are removed from the abdominal wall will demonstrate amyloid deposits in 70% of patients.[19] We have also increased the utilization of lip biopsy which is easily accessible in can be conducted in patients on anticoagulant therapy with a 70% positivity rate for amyloid.

The presence of a positive pyrophosphate scan (**Fig. 4**) is highly sensitive for the diagnosis of TTR amyloidosis.[20] In the absence of a monoclonal protein a scan that is graded 2 or 3 in uptake is considered diagnostic of ATTR amyloidosis without biopsy.[21] However, if a monoclonal protein is present and a technetium pyrophosphate scan is positive, tissue biopsy is required to establish a diagnosis. Approximately 25% of patients with TTR cardiac amyloidosis have a detectable abnormality of immunoglobulins. The presence of both makes it difficult to distinguish ATTR from AL amyloidosis and the distinction is important given the differences in therapies for the 2 forms of amyloidosis. All patients with suspect ATTR amyloidosis based on a pyrophosphate scan should have the TTR gene sequenced. Once considered rare, mutations in the ATTR gene are seen in 3.5% of African Americans (V142I) and

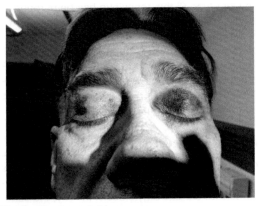

Fig. 2. Classic amyloid purpura.

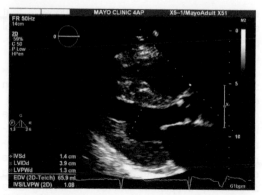

Fig. 3. 2D echo demonstrating marked thickening of the left ventricular septum and free wall.

this inherited form of amyloid cardiomyopathy is almost certainly under diagnosis because the median age at recognition is more than 70 years and the etiology of the heart failure can be misattributed to other more common forms of heart disease. The allele has been found in 10% of African Americans older than age 65 with severe congestive heart failure.[22] Recent artificial intelligence algorithms have been developed that can analyze the echocardiogram and the EKG for wild-type TTR cardiac amyloidosis providing a positive predictive value of 3% to 4%. This automated strategy would increase the detection of cardiac amyloidosis.[23]

Classification of Type

When a pathologist reports out a tissue positive biopsy demonstrating Congo red uptake with green birefringence the task remains incomplete. All positive amyloid biopsies require classification of type

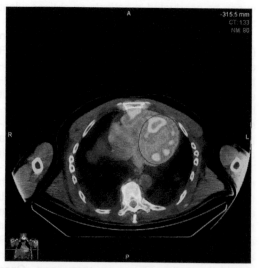

Fig. 4. Technetium pyrophosphate scan showing 3+ uptake in the myocardium with a SPECT image demonstrating the radionucleotide localizes to the ventricle.

because the similarities between AL and ATTR do not allow the discrimination of the 2 types based on clinical features alone. Historically immunohistochemistry was used to classify the various types of amyloid. This technique has fallen out of favor for several reasons. There are more than 20 proteins reported to form amyloid fibrils. These include apolipoproteins, fibrinogen, lysozyme, and insulin among others. This would require a very large panel of antisera and multiple tissue sections for classification which is beyond the scope of most routine immunohistochemistry laboratories. Commercial antisera used in immunohistochemistry are generally directed to the constant portion of the immunoglobulin light chain when trying to diagnose AL amyloidosis. Amyloid deposits raise 2 major barriers. Most light chain amyloid deposits represent only fragments of the intact immunoglobulin light chain with the constant portion deleted and are not present in the amyloid deposit and therefore will not be recognized by commercial antisera. Secondly amyloid fibrils are characterized by the misfolding of the protein which often hides the epitope from antibody recognition. In prospective studies immunohistochemistry will fail to definitively diagnose the amyloid protein subunit in upwards of 20% of specimens.[24] Mass spectrometry can be performed on the tissue while still on the glass slide and does not require paraffin blocks or frozen tissue samples. A sample stained with Congo red can be directly excised from the glass slide placed into a cuvette and the individual peptides can be separated by molecular weight in a mass spectrometer and sequenced. Peptides are compared with a library of sequenced proteins. Samples will demonstrate positive control seen in all amyloid deposits such as serum amyloid P protein.[25] The failure rate with this technique is less than 5% and is usually because the amyloid deposits are present in trace amounts. This has become the new gold standard for the identification of the amyloid type.[26] this technique has been reported in the diagnosis of 21 different established forms of amyloidosis. Amino acid substitutions in cases of hereditary amyloidosis were diagnosed with 100% specificity. The median age of A TTR amyloidosis was 74.4 years. AL amyloidosis represented 59% of patients and ATTR amyloidosis represented 28% of patients[27]

Prognosis

Over the past 2 decades, multiple parameters have been identified that predict outcomes in patients with cardiac amyloidosis. Initially, the echocardiogram was used and the ejection fraction,

Table 2
Staging systems cardiac amyloidosis

AL	Points	Stage	Median Survival, mo.
	0	I	>120
	1	II	69
	2	III	16
	3	IV	6
ATTR	0	I	69.2
	1	II	46.7
	2	III	24.1

AL 1 point each for dFLC greater than 180 mg/L; NTproBNP greater than 1800 pg./mL; HS TroponinT ≥40 ng/L.[61] ATTR 1 point each for NTproBNP greater than 300 ng/L; eGFR less than 45 mL/min.[62]

deceleration time, wall thickness, granular sparkling appearance, and atrial failure had all been associated with survival.[28] Global longitudinal strain is particularly useful in the diagnosis of amyloid based on the presence of apical sparing but has been prognostic as well and should be regularly measured in these patients.[29] The use of echocardiography to predict outcomes, however, has been crit a size due to interobserver variability and the fact that echocardiographic parameters do not retain their significance in multivariable models. Cardiac magnetic resonance imaging has also provided predictors of survival, particularly by measurements of extracellular volume. Extracellular volume measurements have a greater diagnostic sensitivity compared with late gadolinium enhancement and native T1. Extracellular volume provides high diagnostic and prognostic utility for the assessment of cardiac amyloidosis.[30] Several staging systems have been proposed in light chain amyloidosis. All of them have validity and some are better at predicting early mortality the others have long-term survival. The most common in use today is the Mayo 2018 staging system which measures the N terminal fragment of brain natriuretic peptide, high sensitivity troponin T, and the difference between the involved and uninvolved immunoglobulin-free light chain levels. For ATTR cardiac amyloidosis, the most common staging system use combines the BNP with eGFR. These systems are listed in **Table 2**.

Supportive Management of Amyloidosis

The mainstay of therapy is the reduction of preload with the use of loop diuretics. Because of superior absorption torsemide is preferred to furosemide in our practice. For patients that have refractory edema, metolazone can be quite useful but aggressive use can lead to profound hypokalemia and hypotension leading to syncope. Patients with significant amyloid cardiomyopathy require higher intravascular fluid volumes and higher filling pressures to fill the noncompliant ventricle.

Most patients have significant tachycardia required to maintain cardiac output. Most patients' beta-blockade to reduce the cardiac rate will result in the exacerbation of symptoms. Even in patients that have significant supraventricular tachyarrhythmias digoxin is to be preferred to metoprolol or carvedilol. Contrary to earlier reports digoxin use for rate control in atrial fibrillation is safe. No deaths were attributed to digoxin use or toxicity.[31] Afterload reduction plays little role in patients with diastolic heart failure and the use of angiotensin-converting enzymes inhibitors or angiotensin receptor blocker inhibitors will result in hypotension with no improvement in cardiac output.

Atrial arrhythmias occur commonly, among 25 patients with cardiac amyloidosis that underwent cardioversion for atrial arrhythmias, sinus rhythm was restored in 96% of patients but 36% of patients experience procedural complications an 80% had a recurrence of atrial a rhythm is at 1 year. This suggests that cardioversion in cardiac amyloidosis is not efficient for achieving long-term rate control.[32] The placement of a pacemaker can be useful in patients that have significant bradycardia but the value of implantable cardiac defibrillators remains controversial.[33] Multiple case series have been published with mixed results and no clear demonstrable survival prolongation. Many patients die with electrical mechanical dissociation, and it is unclear whether the defibrillator impulse can capture in an amyloid-involved ventricle. Among 472 patients with cardiac amyloidosis with implantable cardiac defibrillators, the 1-year mortality was 27% more than double patients receiving an ICD for nonamyloid heart disease. The most powerful predictor of death was syncope.[34] In a report of 15 patients undergoing autologous stem cell transplantation with cardiac defibrillators, 5 had detectable arrhythmias and 2 had defibrillator discharges.[35] Transplant related mortality was 6.7% Intraventricular assist devices have also been used but most patients with amyloidosis have very small left ventricular chambers due to the massive infiltration of the ventricular wall and major technical difficulties exist in the safe placement of an assist device in amyloid laden myocardium.[36] One case report in a patient with AL lambda amyloidosis underwent left ventricular assist device implantation and 90 days after hospital discharge had not had complications or hospital readmission. Implanting the inflow cannula into the left atrium via a conduit may reduce the risks of complications.[37]

Orthostatic hypotension is common in patients with amyloidosis and may reflect autonomic failure or moderate to severe cardiac involvement with aggressive diuretic therapy. Standard therapies for orthostatic hypotension include fludrocortisone and midodrine. Recently droxidopa a norepinephrine precursor was reported to be self and well-tolerated with improvement in presyncope symptoms in 80% of patients.[38]

Specific Treatment Directed Against the Amyloidosis

Amyloid transthyretin (ATTR)

Currently available therapies for the management of ATTR amyloidosis fall into 2 categories gene silencing and tetramer stabilizers. Transthyretin is a protein found in all mammals. It is responsible for the transportation of thyroxine and retinol-binding protein. In the native state, it circulates as a tetramer with a central pocket that binds to thyroxine much in the same way as four globin chains form a tetramer and bind to oxygen in the central pocket. When there is a mutation in transthyretin the tetrameric form of the protein becomes unstable and will dissociate under physiologic conditions. The monomers which are not present in normal adults will miss fold into amyloid Proto fibrils and subsequently fully formed amyloid fibrils capable of depositing in heart peripheral and autonomic nerves and the vitreous chamber of the eye. The 1st stabilizer diflunisal is a nonsteroidal agent that prevents the tetramer from dissociating. It was shown in a double-blind placebo-controlled trial to reduce the neurologic impairment in patients with mutant TTR amyloid polyneuropathy.

Tafamidis is a stabilizer that was tested both in wild-type and mutant TTR amyloid cardiomyopathy. Eligibility required a minimum NT proBNP of 600 pg. per mL. This trial that had a composite endpoint of all-cause survival and cardiac hospitalization showed significant benefit for the treated arm leading to its approval. This is an oral medication administered once daily with a very favorable toxicity profile.[39] AG-10 is an investigational stabilizing agent that is currently in clinical trial.[40] AG10 is also an ATTR stabilizer. In a randomized double-blind placebo controlled study of orally administered Ag 10 in healthy adults, the drug was well-tolerated with no safety signals. The drug half-life is 25 hours. More than 90% stabilization of TTR was observed at a steady state at the highest dose. Stabilization resulted in an increase in TTR levels. It would be predicted to be potentially beneficial for both mutant and wild-type ATTR.[41]

Gene silencing medications are either small interfering RNAs or antisense oligonucleotides. Both have tested their value in mutant TTR peripheral neuropathy and have demonstrated improvement in neurologic impairment and quality of life when compared with a 15 to 18-month placebo arm in phase 3 trials. Both agents patisiran [42,43] and inotersen are undergoing testing in amyloid cardiomyopathy of both mutant and wild-type. In the analysis of a randomized double-blind placebo-controlled trial of patisiran, the drug improved absolute global longitudinal strain compared with placebo at 18 months with the greatest differential increase observed in the basal region. The agent seems to prevent the deterioration of global longitudinal strain by attenuating disease progression in the basal region.[44] Vutrisiran which can silence the TTR gene is administered subcutaneously once every 3 months has completed accrual in a placebo-controlled trial in patients with amyloid cardiomyopathy (Helios B).

In vitro studies have demonstrated that doxycycline also can act as a stabilizer of the transthyretin tetramer. Retrospective case-control studies have suggested that the use of doxycycline improves outcome in patients with cardiac amyloidosis but the evidence is weak and no prospective studies demonstrating benefit have been published to date.[45]

There is active research into the use of monoclonal antibodies in the treatment of ATTR cardiac amyloidosis. A selective anti-ATTR antibody has been developed having been cloned following the comprehensive analysis of B-cells derived from healthy elderly subjects. This antibody binds selectively to disease-associated ATTR aggregates both wild-type and mutant ATTR but does not bind to physiologic transthyretin. This antibody binds and activates macrophages which will remove ATTR deposits from patient-derived myocardium by macrophages. The activity of ATTR removal has led to the development of an ongoing phase 1 clinical trial in patients with ATTR cardiomyopathy.[46] CRISPR-Cas9–based in vivo gene editing has been used in the management of variant TTR amyloidosis. Six patients were treated with a lipid nanoparticle encapsulated messenger RNA for Cas9 protein. At the higher dose level reduction in serum, TTR protein concentration was 87% adverse events were mild. This targeted knock out of TTR may translate into slowing of disease progression or potential improvement in neuropathy.[47]

Amyloid light-chain

As the source of the amyloid fibril subunit in light chain amyloidosis is a clonal population of plasma cells in the bone marrow all therapies to date are directed to the eradication of the plasma cell clone thereby disrupting light chain synthesis. Response to therapy in light chain amyloidosis is assessed by the difference between the involved and uninvolved immunoglobulin-free light chain (dFLC). The use of the immunoglobulin-free light chain ratio can be misleading and is discouraged.[48] The best-reported responses occur in those patients who achieve a complete response as measured by the normalization of the difference between involved and uninvolved free light chain with immunofixation negativity of the serum and urine. Further refinement of the response criteria has demonstrated even better outcomes when the dFLC falls less than 10 mg per liter. At this level of response, increased organ response and an extended survival has been demonstrated in 2 independent cohorts.[49]

The Backbone of therapy for light chain amyloidosis is the use of weekly subcutaneous bortezomib. In an observational study of 915 patients, the median overall survival with bortezomib was 72 months. Cardiac responses were 61% in those that achieve stringent dFLC response.[50] A prospective randomized trial adding daratumumab in anti-CD 38 monoclonal antibody to 3 chemotherapy agents bortezomib cyclophosphamide and dexamethasone showed a 3-fold increase in the hematologic complete response rate and a doubling of the cardiac response rate as defined by 30% reduction in the NT proBNP level.[51] The method of grading response of the heart in AL amyloidosis is defined as a 30% to 59% reduction in NT proBNP (partial response, PR); a greater than or equal to 60% reduction in NT proBNP (very good partial response, VGPR); and a complete response defined as an NT proBNP less than 450 µg per milliliter. Cardiac progression or relapse is [52] finding a 30% increase in the NT proBNP. Currently, a widely accepted chemotherapy approach would be the use of daratumumab combined with bortezomib cyclophosphamide dexamethasone for 6 months followed by monthly daratumumab for a total of 24 months of therapy. Survival outcome has not been reported.

For more than 25 years autologous stem cell transplantation has been used to achieve hematologic an organ response is in the management of light chain amyloidosis.[53] Myeloablative chemotherapy must be undertaken with extreme caution in patients with cardiac amyloidosis. Patients who undergo autologous stem cell transplantation have a period of severe neutropenia ranging from 6 to 10 days. During this period, the development of bacteremia and sepsis is common. When patients with cardiac amyloidosis develop sepsis-induced hypotension their cardiac reserve is insufficient to compensate for the fall in vascular resistance. Patients can develop hypotension, lactic acidosis, and ultimately death. In early studies of autologous stem cell transplantation patients with cardiac amyloidosis had mortality rates in excess of 20%.[54] Current selection criteria require new York Heart Association class 2 or better, a systolic blood pressure more than 90 and a high sensitivity troponin level generally less than 75 ng per liter. With current techniques mortality associated with stem cell transplantation is approximately 3%. Reported response rates for renal, cardiac, and liver were 54%, 62%, and 56%, respectively. Organ response was strongly associated with prolonged survival.[55]

Currently, there are no validated techniques for removing amyloid fibrils in tissue. Two monoclonal antibodies are about to be tested in patients who are therapy I with Mayo stage IV cardiac amyloidosis. In both trials the monoclonal antibody developed to remove the amyloid deposits will be combined with bortezomib cyclophosphamide dexamethasone and compared with placebo bortezomib cyclophosphamide dexamethasone. The antibodies CAEL-101[56] and birtamimab [57] are currently activated and accruing patients. Both antibodies have demonstrated in vitro activity by leading to macrophage activation following binding to the amyloid deposits and subsequent proteolysis. It is hypothesized that by combining antiamyloid antibodies with antiplasma cell chemotherapy deeper response a longer survival will be achieved.

Organ Transplantation

Before the development of highly effective antiplasma cell chemotherapy, the outcomes of cardiac transplantation for AL amyloidosis were poor often due to the recurrence of amyloid both in the transplanted heart as well as the gastrointestinal tract and kidney. With the introduction of highly effective chemotherapy, outcomes have improved substantially. A recent report of 46 patients was reported of whom 7 were bridged to cardiac transplantation with a ventricular assist device. The 1-year survival for the entire cohort was 91%, 83% with AL amyloidosis, and 94% with TTR amyloidosis. In the group with AL amyloidosis all received chemotherapy before heart transplant, 5 of 8 patients subsequently received autologous stem cell transplant an average of 1 year after the cardiac allograft.[58] A 2nd series of 31 patients, 13 light chain amyloid 18, ATTR reported no significant difference in mortality between amyloid cardiomyopathy and heart transplantation for other indications. Extracardiac amyloidosis was not considered a contraindication to transplantation. Posttransplant chemotherapy included both bortezomib-based chemotherapy as well as autologous stem cell transplantation. Sixteen patients underwent heart transplantation for AL amyloidosis with stem cell transplantation performed in 9 patients at a median of 13.5 months following heart transplantation. One-year survival was 87.5%- and 5-year survival was 76.6%. The strategy of stem cell transplant 1 year after heart transplant was feasible, safe, and resulted in excellent outcomes.[59] Survival at 8 years was more than 80%.[60] Patients with wild-type TTR amyloidosis can be transplanted, the anticipated time to recurrence is quite long. The primary limitation is the advanced age of most patients with symptomatic cardiac failure and wild-type TTR amyloidosis.

SUMMARY

The major gap in the management of patients with amyloidosis revolves around early diagnosis. All patients with thickened ventricular walls without a history of hypertension and those with HFpEF should include immunoglobulin-free light chain measurements and technetium pyrophosphate scanning as part of the initial evaluation. The former should raise the suspicion of light chain amyloidosis and lead to subcutaneous fat aspiration and bone marrow for Congo red staining. Endomyocardial biopsy is generally not required to establish the diagnosis. Patients with strong uptake in the myocardium on pyrophosphate scanning that lack a monoclonal protein can be considered as having TTR amyloidosis. Genetic testing should be performed to ensure that the amyloidosis is not a mutation. Early diagnosis is important because all forms of amyloidosis have FDA-approved therapies that have been shown to improve outcomes.

CLINICS CARE POINTS

- If the echocardiogram shows wall thickening consistent with hypertension amyloidosis should be considered.
- The most important blood test when amyloidosis is being considered is the immunoglobulin-free light chain assay.
- Prognosis is determined by troponin or (NT-pro) BNP.
- The most valuable imaging study is the PYP scan which is sensitive but not specific as both AL and TTTR amyloidosis can be positive.

FUNDING

NCI SPORE MM SPORE 5P50 CA186781-04CA90628-21 Pal Calabresi K12 Career Development Award.

REFERENCES

1. McCausland KL, White MK, Guthrie SD, et al. Light Chain (AL) Amyloidosis: The Journey to Diagnosis. Patient 2018;11(2):207–16.
2. van den Berg MP, Mulder BA, Klaassen SHC, et al. Heart failure with preserved ejection fraction, atrial fibrillation, and the role of senile amyloidosis. Eur Heart J 2019;40(16):1287–93.
3. Vitarelli A, Lai S, Petrucci MT, et al. Biventricular assessment of light-chain amyloidosis using 3D speckle tracking echocardiography: Differentiation from other forms of myocardial hypertrophy. Int J Cardiol 2018;271:371–7.
4. Alexander KM, Orav J, Singh A, et al. Geographic Disparities in Reported US Amyloidosis Mortality From 1979 to 2015: Potential Underdetection of Cardiac Amyloidosis. JAMA Cardiol 2018;3(9):865–70.
5. Mohammed SF, Mirzoyev SA, Edwards WD, et al. Left ventricular amyloid deposition in patients with heart failure and preserved ejection fraction. JACC Heart Fail 2014;2(2):113–22.
6. Maurizi N, Rella V, Fumagalli C, et al. Prevalence of cardiac amyloidosis among adult patients referred to tertiary centres with an initial diagnosis of hypertrophic cardiomyopathy. Int J Cardiol 2020;300:191–5.
7. Wisniowski B, McLeod D, Adams R, et al. The epidemiology of amyloidosis in Australia. Amyloid 2019; 26(sup1):132–3.
8. Kyle RA, Larson DR, Kurtin PJ, et al. Incidence of AL Amyloidosis in Olmsted County, Minnesota, 1990 through 2015. Mayo Clin Proc 2019;94(3):465–71.
9. Rezk T, Lachmann HJ, Fontana M, et al. Cardiorenal AL amyloidosis: risk stratification and outcomes based upon cardiac and renal biomarkers. Br J Haematol 2019;186(3):460–70.
10. Zegri-Reiriz I, de Haro-Del Moral FJ, Dominguez F, et al. Prevalence of Cardiac Amyloidosis in Patients with Carpal Tunnel Syndrome. J Cardiovasc Transl Res 2019;12(6):507–13.
11. Sueyoshi T, Ueda M, Jono H, et al. Wild-type transthyretin-derived amyloidosis in various ligaments and tendons. Hum Pathol 2011;42(9):1259–64.
12. Galat A, Guellich A, Bodez D, et al. Aortic stenosis and transthyretin cardiac amyloidosis: the chicken or the egg? Eur Heart J 2016;37(47):3525–31.
13. Ripoll-Vera T, Álvarez Rubio J, Iglesias M, et al. Association between aortic stenosis and hereditary transthyretin amyloidosis. Rev Esp Cardiol (Engl Ed 2021;74(2):185–7.

14. Kim D, Lee GY, Choi JO, et al. Associations of Electrocardiographic Parameters with Left Ventricular Longitudinal Strain and Prognosis in Cardiac Light Chain Amyloidosis. Sci 2019;9(1).

15. Tung-Chen Y, Arnau MA. Amyloid cardiomyopathy: a hidden heart failure cause that is often misdiagnosed. Acta Clin Belg 2018;73(6):460–1.

16. Martinez-Naharro A, Kotecha T, Norrington K, et al. Native T1 and Extracellular Volume in Transthyretin Amyloidosis. JACC Cardiovasc Imaging 2019; 12(5):810–9.

17. Kim SH, Kim YS, Kim SJ. Diagnostic performance of PET for detection of cardiac amyloidosis: A systematic review and meta-analysis. J Cardiol 2020;76(6): 618–25.

18. Cuddy SAM, Bravo PE, Falk RH, et al. Improved Quantification of Cardiac Amyloid Burden in Systemic Light Chain Amyloidosis: Redefining Early Disease? JACC Cardiovasc Imaging 2020;13(6): 1325–36.

19. De Larrea CF Verga L, Morbini P, Klersy C, et al. A practical approach to the diagnosis of systemic amyloidoses. Blood 2015;125(14):2239–44.

20. Castano A, Haq M, Narotsky DL, et al. Multicenter Study of Planar Technetium 99m Pyrophosphate Cardiac Imaging: Predicting Survival for Patients With ATTR Cardiac Amyloidosis. JAMA Cardiol 2016;1(8):880–9.

21. Gertz M, Adams D, Ando Y, et al. Avoiding misdiagnosis: expert consensus recommendations for the suspicion and diagnosis of transthyretin amyloidosis for the general practitioner. BMC Fam Pract 2020; 21(1):198.

22. Buxbaum JN, Ruberg FL. Transthyretin V122I (pV142I) cardiac amyloidosis: an age-dependent autosomal dominant cardiomyopathy too common to be overlooked as a cause of significant heart disease in elderly African Americans. Genet Med 2017; 19(7):733–42.

23. Goto S, Mahara K, Beussink-Nelson L, et al. Artificial intelligence-enabled fully automated detection of cardiac amyloidosis using electrocardiograms and echocardiograms. Nat Commun 2021;12(1):2726.

24. Schonland SO, Hegenbart U, Bochtler T, et al. Immunohistochemistry in the classification of systemic forms of amyloidosis: A systematic investigation of 117 patients. Blood 2012;119(2):488–93.

25. Vrana JA, Theis JD, Dasari S, et al. Clinical diagnosis and typing of systemic amyloidosis in subcutaneous fat aspirates by mass spectrometry-based proteomics. Haematologica 2014;99(7):1239–47.

26. Rezk T, Gilbertson JA, Mangione PP, et al. The complementary role of histology and proteomics for diagnosis and typing of systemic amyloidosis. J Pathol Clin Res 2019;5(3):145–53.

27. Dasari S, Theis JD, Vrana JA, et al. Amyloid Typing by Mass Spectrometry in Clinical Practice: a Comprehensive Review of 16,175 Samples. Mayo Clin Proc 2020;95(9):1852–64.

28. Pradel S, Magne J, Jaccard A, et al. Left ventricular assessment in patients with systemic light chain amyloidosis: a 3-dimensional speckle tracking transthoracic echocardiographic study. Int J Cardiovasc Imaging 2019;35(5):845–54.

29. Barros-Gomes S, Williams B, Nhola LF, et al. Prognosis of Light Chain Amyloidosis With Preserved LVEF: Added Value of 2D Speckle-Tracking Echocardiography to the Current Prognostic Staging System. JACC Cardiovasc Imaging 2017;10(4): 398–407.

30. Pan JA, Kerwin MJ, Salerno M. Native T1 Mapping, Extracellular Volume Mapping, and Late Gadolinium Enhancement in Cardiac Amyloidosis: A Meta-Analysis. JACC Cardiovasc Imaging 2020;13(6):1299–310.

31. Donnelly JP, Sperry BW, Gabrovsek A, et al. Digoxin Use in Cardiac Amyloidosis. Am J Cardiol 2020;133: 134–8.

32. Loungani RS, Rehorn MR, Geurink KR, et al. Outcomes following cardioversion for patients with cardiac amyloidosis and atrial fibrillation or atrial flutter. Am Heart J 2020;222:26–9.

33. Hamon D, Algalarrondo V, Gandjbakhch E, et al. Outcome and incidence of appropriate implantable cardioverter-defibrillator therapy in patients with cardiac amyloidosis. Int J Cardiol 2016;222:562–8.

34. Higgins AY, Annapureddy AR, Wang Y, et al. Survival Following Implantable Cardioverter-Defibrillator Implantation in Patients With Amyloid Cardiomyopathy. J Am Heart Assoc 2020;9(18):e016038.

35. Phull P, Sanchorawala V, Brauneis D, et al. High-dose melphalan and autologous peripheral blood stem cell transplantation in patients with AL amyloidosis and cardiac defibrillators. Bone Marrow Transplant 2019;54(8):1304–9.

36. Swiecicki PL, Edwards BS, Kushwaha SS, et al. Left ventricular device implantation for advanced cardiac amyloidosis. J Heart Lung Transpl 2013;32(5):563–8.

37. Lim CP, Lim YP, Lim CH, et al. Ventricular Assist Device Support in End-Stage Heart Failure From Cardiac Amyloidosis. Ann Acad Med Singap 2019; 48(12):435–8.

38. McDonell KE, Preheim BA, Diedrich A, et al. Initiation of droxidopa during hospital admission for management of refractory neurogenic orthostatic hypotension in severely ill patients. J Clin Hypertens (Greenwich) 2019;21(9):1308–14.

39. Rigopoulos AG, Ali M, Abate E, et al. Advances in the diagnosis and treatment of transthyretin amyloidosis with cardiac involvement. Heart Fail Rev 2019; 24(4):521–33.

40. Judge DP, Heitner SB, Falk RH, et al. Transthyretin Stabilization by AG10 in Symptomatic Transthyretin Amyloid Cardiomyopathy. J Am Coll Cardiol 2019; 74(3):285–95.

41. Fox JC, Hellawell JL, Rao S, et al. First-in-Human Study of AG10, a Novel, Oral, Specific, Selective, and Potent Transthyretin Stabilizer for the Treatment of Transthyretin Amyloidosis: A Phase 1 Safety, Tolerability, Pharmacokinetic, and Pharmacodynamic Study in Healthy Adult Volunteers. Clin Pharmacol Drug Dev 2020;9(1):115–29.

42. Solomon SD, Adams D, Kristen A, et al. Effects of Patisiran, an RNA Interference Therapeutic, on Cardiac Parameters in Patients With Hereditary Transthyretin-Mediated Amyloidosis. Circulation 2019;139(4):431–43.

43. Gertz MA, Scheinberg M, Waddington-Cruz M, et al. Inotersen for the treatment of adults with polyneuropathy caused by hereditary transthyretin-mediated amyloidosis. Expert Rev Clin Pharmacol 2019;12(8):701–11.

44. Minamisawa M, Claggett B, Adams D, et al. Association of Patisiran, an RNA Interference Therapeutic, With Regional Left Ventricular Myocardial Strain in Hereditary Transthyretin Amyloidosis: The APOLLO Study. JAMA Cardiol 2019;4(5):466–72.

45. Karlstedt E, Jimenez-Zepeda V, Howlett JG, et al. Clinical Experience With the Use of Doxycycline and Ursodeoxycholic Acid for the Treatment of Transthyretin Cardiac Amyloidosis. J Card Fail 2019;25(3):147–53.

46. Michalon A, Hagenbuch A, Huy C, et al. A human antibody selective for transthyretin amyloid removes cardiac amyloid through phagocytic immune cells. Nat Commun 2021;12(1):3142.

47. Gillmore JD, Gane E, Taubel J, et al. CRISPR-Cas9 In Vivo Gene Editing for Transthyretin Amyloidosis. N Engl J Med 2021;385(6):493–502.

48. Zhao L, Tian Z, Fang Q. The prognostic value of baseline serum free light chain in cardiac amyloidosis. Zhonghua Nei Ke Za Zhi 2016;55(3):186–90.

49. Godara A, Toskic D, Albanese J, et al. Involved free light chains <10 mg/L with treatment predict better outcomes in systemic light-chain amyloidosis. Am J Hematol 2021;96(1). E20-e3.

50. Manwani R, Cohen O, Sharpley F, et al. A prospective observational study of 915 patients with systemic AL amyloidosis treated with upfront bortezomib. Blood 2019;134(25):2271–80.

51. Palladini G, Kastritis E, Maurer MS, et al. Daratumumab plus CyBorD for patients with newly diagnosed AL amyloidosis: safety run-in results of ANDROMEDA. Blood 2020;136(1):71–80.

52. Eckhert E, Witteles R, Kaufman G, et al. Grading cardiac response in AL amyloidosis: implications for relapse and survival. Br J Haematol 2019;186(1):144–6.

53. Sidiqi MH, Aljama MA, Buadi FK, et al. Stem Cell Transplantation for Light Chain Amyloidosis: Decreased Early Mortality Over Time. J Clin Oncol 2018;36(13):1323–9.

54. Al Saleh AS, Sidiqi MH, Muchtar E, et al. Outcomes of Patients with Light Chain Amyloidosis Who Had Autologous Stem Cell Transplantation with 3 or More Organs Involved. Biol Blood Marrow Transplant 2019;25(8):1520–5.

55. Szalat R, Sarosiek S, Havasi A, et al. Organ responses after highdose melphalan and stemcell transplantation in AL amyloidosis. Leukemia 2021;35(3):916–9.

56. Varga C, Lentzsch S, Comenzo RL. Beyond NEOD001 for systemic light-chain amyloidosis. Blood 2018;132(18):1992–3.

57. Gertz MA, Landau H, Comenzo RL, et al. First-in-human phase I/II study of NEOD001 in patients with light chain amyloidosis and persistent organ dysfunction. J Clin Oncol 2016;34(10):1097–103.

58. Chen Q, Moriguchi J, Levine R, et al. Outcomes of Heart Transplantation in Cardiac Amyloidosis Patients: A Single Center Experience. Transpl Proc 2021;53(1):329–34.

59. Trachtenberg BH, Kamble RT, Rice L, et al. Delayed autologous stem cell transplantation following cardiac transplantation experience in patients with cardiac amyloidosis. Am J Transplant 2019;19(10):2900–9.

60. Barrett CD, Alexander KM, Zhao H, et al. Outcomes in Patients With Cardiac Amyloidosis Undergoing Heart Transplantation. JACC Heart Fail 2020;8(6):461–8.

61. Kumar S, Dispenzieri A, Lacy MQ, et al. Revised prognostic staging system for light chain amyloidosis incorporating cardiac biomarkers and serum free light chain measurements. J Clin Oncol 2012;30(9):989–95.

62. Gillmore JD, Damy T, Fontana M, et al. A new staging system for cardiac transthyretin amyloidosis. Eur Heart J 2018;39(30):2799–806.

Clinical Practice Guidelines in Cardio-Oncology

Darryl P. Leong, MBBS, MPH, MBiostat, PhD[a],*, Daniel J. Lenihan, MD[b]

KEYWORDS

- Cardio-oncology • Guidelines • Cardiotoxicity • Heart failure • Left ventricular dysfunction
- Cancer therapy–related cardiac dysfunction

KEY POINTS

- The International Cardio-Oncology Society (IC-OS) has recently developed criteria for identifying cancer therapy–related cardiac dysfunction (CTRCD) based on left ventricular ejection fraction, echocardiographic global longitudinal strain, and blood biomarkers.
- The major cancer therapeutics that can cause CTRCD or heart failure are: anthracyclines, trastuzumab, pertuzumab, immune checkpoint inhibitors, certain tyrosine kinase inhibitors, cyclophosphamide, and radiotherapy (where the heart is within the therapeutic field).
- Baseline evaluation of cardiac function before the administration of potentially cardiotoxic cancer therapy is recommended. Echocardiography is the preferred imaging modality because of its safety, availability, and (especially for three-dimensional imaging) reproducibility. Surveillance strategies during cancer therapy vary according to the cancer therapy being administered with modest evidence to inform the optimal strategy.
- Angiotensin-converting enzyme inhibitors (ACE-I), angiotensin receptor blockers (ARB), and β-blockers are not recommended as primary prevention in unselected patients with preserved systolic left ventricular function receiving potentially cardiotoxic cancer therapies but should be considered in specific individuals.
- Dexrazoxane should be considered for the prevention of CTRCD in individuals with advanced breast cancer and other cancers in whom cumulative doses of doxorubicin ≥300 mg/m^2 (or equivalent) are planned.

INTRODUCTION

Because of the rapid growth of cardio-oncology (CO) and the need to provide health care professionals with clinical practice guidance, there have been a variety of "white papers" and consensus statements released during the last 5 years from the European Society of Medical Oncology (ESMO),[1] the European Society of Cardiology (ESC),[2] the American Society of Clinical Oncology (ASCO),[3] the American Society of Echocardiography (ASE), and the European Association of Cardiovascular Imaging (EACVI).[4] There are also other documents that have attempted to provide clarity for complex topics, such as all major cardiovascular (CV) toxicity that is related to cancer therapy, as recently organized by the International Cardio-Oncology (IC-OS).[5] Given that CO is a new discipline, data to inform these recommendations are evolving, and so, many important details may vary in the absence of conclusive supportive evidence. To provide some clarity and perspective, the objectives of this review article are to (1) summarize the published CO guidelines as they pertain to heart failure (HF) and left ventricular (LV) function, (2) compare and contrast the guidelines and position statements promoted by the different professional societies, and (3) discuss

[a] The Population Health Research Institute and Department of Medicine, McMaster University and Hamilton Health Sciences, C2-238 David Braley Building, Hamilton General Hospital, 237 Barton St. East, Hamilton, ON L8L 2X2b, Canada; [b] International Cardio-Oncology Society, 465 Laverne Avenue, Tampa, FL 33606, USA
* Corresponding author.
E-mail address: Darryl.Leong@phri.ca

Heart Failure Clin 18 (2022) 489–501
https://doi.org/10.1016/j.hfc.2022.02.002
1551-7136/22/© 2022 Elsevier Inc. All rights reserved.

heartfailure.theclinics.com

the evidence underpinning key published recommendations.

DISCUSSION
Definitions and Classification of Heart Failure

The classification of the severity of HF and LV dysfunction as indicators of cancer therapy cardiotoxicity are widely disparate (**Table 1**). The American Heart Association and American College of Cardiology describe HF as a spectrum from (cardiotoxic) risk factor exposure (stage A) to asymptomatic cardiac dysfunction (stage B) to symptomatic HF (stage C) to refractory HF (stage D).[6] This classification has some overlap with the commonly used New York Heart Association (NYHA) HF classification scheme of I (asymptomatic), II (mild symptoms, slight limitation during ordinary activity), III (marked limitation because of symptoms with less than ordinary activity), or IV (symptoms at rest). The ESC endorses the use of the NYHA HF classification scheme for the purposes of describing the severity of HF symptoms.[7] In addition, the ESC categorizes HF based on LV ejection fraction (LVEF) into HF with reduced (≤40%), mildly reduced (41%–49%), and preserved (≥50%) LVEF. The National Cancer Institute of the US National Institutes of Health, in its Common Terminology Criteria for Adverse Events (CTCAE version 5.0), classifies HF as asymptomatic with biomarker abnormalities (grade 1), symptomatic with moderate exertion (grade 2), new symptoms or symptoms with minimal exertion (grade 3), life-threatening HF requiring intervention (grade 4), and fatal (grade 5). The American Heart Association/American College of Cardiology, NYHA, and CTCAE classification schemes share enough similarity to allow for potential harmonization of data from different sources. However, these classification schemes were either not created with cardiotoxicity in mind (and so, do not address some relevant nuances in CO, such as the high burden of patients with subclinical LV dysfunction identified on surveillance) or were not developed with the understanding of cardiotoxicity that we now have. Recently, the IC-OS provided a consensus for these definitions by incorporating all the known cardiotoxicity classification systems for HF that have been used for the past 10 to 15 years in CO.[5]

In addition to symptomatic HF as an adverse CV event during cancer therapy and clinical trials, the CTCAE, which is primarily a tool to describe these adverse events in a codified manner, also describes LV systolic dysfunction as either a symptomatic fall in LVEF responsive to intervention (grade 3) or HF because of a fall in LVEF that is not responsive to intervention (grade 4), with no grade assigned to asymptomatic declines in LVEF. The ASE and the EACVI define cancer therapeutics–related cardiac dysfunction (CTRCD) as an absolute decrease in LVEF of greater than 10% to a value less than 53%.[4] According to this definition, a fall in LVEF from 55% to 45% would not be considered CTCRD, although such a decline might be considered of high clinical importance. In addition, the ASE and EACVI recommend confirmation of CTCRD 2 to 3 weeks after the first abnormal study (although the feasibility of this recommendation in resource-constrained environments is not considered, nor is the possibility that LVEF can normalize rapidly following the discontinuation of some cardiotoxic cancer therapies or if another causal stressor is removed). This group then classifies CTRCD as reversible (if to within 5% of baseline LVEF), partially reversible (improved by ≥10% from the nadir but remaining >5% below baseline), or irreversible (improved by <10% from the nadir and remaining >5% below baseline). Although this classification scheme may be applied to CTRCD that affects predominantly systolic LV function, it does not include thresholds for abnormalities in LV strain, nor does it enable the classification of cancer therapeutics–related HF with preserved LVEF. The ESMO guidelines suggest that in asymptomatic individuals, the finding of global longitudinal strain (GLS) that has reduced by greater than or equal to 12% in relative magnitude or by greater than or equal to 5% in absolute magnitude should prompt consideration of changes in cardiac disease management.

In the recent IC-OS consensus statement on the definitions of cardiotoxicities,[5] the previous definitions for CTRCD are synthesized and revised definitions of CTRCD are proposed. CTRCD is divided into asymptomatic (including [1] a relative decline in GLS of >15% and/or a new increase in cardiac biomarkers in individuals with LVEF ≥50%; [2] a reduction in LVEF to 40%–49% [accompanied by a relative decline in GLS of >15% and/or a new increase in cardiac biomarkers if the reduction in LVEF is <10%]; or [3] a fall in LVEF to <40%) versus symptomatic (characterized by HF symptoms with supportive LVEF and diagnostic biomarkers).

None of the guidelines explicitly incorporate diastolic LV or right ventricular parameters into their definitions of CTRCD. In a systematic review of studies evaluating changes in diastolic parameters associated with anthracycline-based chemotherapy, Mincu, and colleagues[8] reported that these regimens were associated with decreases in E′ and the E/A ratio. In a small series of women treated with trastuzumab, Mazzutti, and colleagues[9] found that

Table 1
Definitions for cancer treatment–related cardiac dysfunction

Cardiac Review and Evaluation Committee, Definition of Chemotherapy-induced Cardiotoxicity[36]

Any one of the following:
1. Reduction of LVEF, either global or specific in the interventricular septum
2. Symptoms of congestive HF
3. Signs associated with HF, such as S3 gallop, tachycardia, or both
4. Reduction in LVEF from baseline ≥5% to <55% in the presence of signs or symptoms of HF, or a reduction in LVEF ≥10% to <55% without signs or symptoms of HF

NYHA classification	Class I No symptoms	Class II Mild symptoms and slight limitation during ordinary activity	Class III Marked limitation because of symptoms, even with less than ordinary activity	Class IV Symptoms at rest
ACCF/AHA stages of HF	Stage A At high risk for HF but without structural disease or symptoms of HF	Stage B Structural heart disease but without signs or symptoms of HF	Stage C Structural heart disease with prior or current symptoms of HF	Stage D Refractory HF requiring specialized interventions
CTCAE version 5.0 Ejection Fraction Decreased[a]		Grade 2 Resting ejection fraction 50%–40%; 10%–19% drop from baseline	Grade 3 Resting ejection fraction 39%–20%; ≥20% drop from baseline	Grade 4 Resting ejection fraction <20%
CTCAE version 5.0 LV Systolic Dysfunction[a]			Grade 3 Symptomatic because of drop in ejection fraction responsive to intervention	Grade 4 Refractory or poorly controlled HF caused by drop in ejection fraction; intervention, such as ventricular-assist device, intravenous vasopressor support, or heart transplant indicated
CTCAE version 5 Heart Failure[a]	Grade 1 Asymptomatic with laboratory (eg, BNP) or cardiac imaging abnormalities	Grade 2 Symptoms with moderate activity or exertion	Grade 3 Symptoms at rest or with minimal activity or exertion; hospitalization; new onset of symptoms	Grade 4 Life-threatening consequences; urgent intervention indicated (eg, continuous IV therapy or mechanical hemodynamic support)

Guideline	Therapy	Subclinical / Mild	Moderate	Severe
2014 Echo Guidelines for Subclinical LV Dysfunction[37]		Subclinical LV dysfunction: >15% relative drop in GLS from baseline; should be confirmed by repeat testing within 2–3 wk	CRTCD: Drop in LVEF of >10% points to a level <53%; should be confirmed by repeat testing within 2–3 wk	
2016 ESC Position Statement		Mild (asymptomatic) LVEF <50% or LVEF reduction >10% from baseline, should be repeated within 3–4 wk	Moderate (symptomatic from HF) LVEF <50%	
2017 ASCO Guideline		Cardiotoxicity not specifically defined		
2020 ESMO Guideline	All cancer therapy	Mild (asymptomatic) LVEF >15% from baseline if LVEF >50%	Moderate Symptomatic HF regardless of LVEF	Severe LVEF <40%
	Anthracycline or trastuzumab related		Moderate LVEF ≥10% from baseline, or any drop of LVEF to <50% but ≥40%	

Abbreviations: ACCF, American College of Cardiology Foundation; AHA, American Heart Association; BNP, brain natriuretic peptide; CTCAE, common terminology criteria for adverse events; CRTCD, Cancer-therapeutics Related Cardiac Dysfunction; GLS, global longitudinal strain; LVEF, left ventricular ejection fraction; NYHA, New York Heart Association.

[a] Oncology trial investigators can choose to classify a given event under "ejection fraction decreased," "LV systolic dysfunction," or "heart failure" with associated grades if they decide the adverse effect is related to the intervention. This contributes to difficulty in comparing results of trials and effects of cancer therapies. Grade 1 to grade 4 = mild to severe; grade 5 = death. No grade 5 for "ejection fraction decreased."

Modified from Herrmann J, Lenihan D, Armenian S, Barac A, Blaes A, Cardinale D, Carver J, Dent S, Ky B, Lyon AR, López-Fernández T, Fradley MG, Ganatra S, Curigliano G, Mitchell JD, Minotti G, Lang NN, Liu JE, Neilan TG, Nohria A, O'Quinn R, Pusic I, Porter C, Reynolds KL, Ruddy KJ, Thavendiranathan P, Valent P. Defining cardiovascular toxicities of cancer therapies: an International Cardio-Oncology Society (IC-OS) consensus statement. Eur Heart J. 2022 Jan 31;43(4):280-299.

right ventricular GLS and fractional area change decrease with therapy independently of changes in LV function. In another study of patients with breast cancer treated with anthracycline and undergoing serial cardiac MRI, right ventricular ejection fraction decreased during 9 months' observation and right ventricular extracellular volume increased.[10] With increasing evidence of the potential importance of these measures of LV and right ventricular function, future definitions incorporating these parameters may be helpful clinically to discern early evidence of cardiotoxicity or for potentially validating research findings.

Cancer Therapies that Can Cause Left Ventricular Systolic Dysfunction

The ASCO guidelines recognize that anthracyclines, trastuzumab, and radiotherapy can cause cardiac dysfunction (**Fig. 1**). This document also acknowledges that for anthracyclines and radiotherapy, the degree of risk is closely correlated with the dose to which the heart is exposed. Doses of doxorubicin greater than or equal to 250 mg/m^2, epirubicin greater than or equal to 600 mg/m^2, or radiotherapy greater than or equal to 30 Gy (where the heart is within the treatment field) are considered high risk. The ESMO guideline additionally identifies cyclophosphamide, ifosfamide, and several tyrosine kinase inhibitors of different classes as potential causes of HF. It also distinguishes pertuzumab as an uncommon cause of HF as compared with trastuzumab, which is considered a common cause of HF or LV dysfunction. However, recent evidence from randomized, controlled trials indicates that pertuzumab leads to a two-fold increase in the risk of HF (relative risk, 1.97;

95% confidence interval [CI], 1.05–3.70; $I^2 = 0\%$).[11] In addition, given the novelty and increasing use of several cancer therapies, new associations with HF are reported on an ongoing basis. For instance, cabozantinib and gilteritinib are not linked with HF in the ESMO guideline; however, associations of a plausibly causal nature have been reported.[12,13] The ESC position paper lists similar cancer therapies as potential causes of LV dysfunction to the ESMO document but, in addition, it cites an incidence of LV dysfunction of 2.3% to 13% with docetaxel. However, these estimates are from a trial where docetaxel was administered with doxorubicin and cyclophosphamide, and a trial where the only HF cases were in participants who also received trastuzumab. Therefore, the reported corresponding incidence rates of HF of 1.6% and 1.0% may be more attributable to concomitant therapies than to docetaxel and it is likely that the incidence of LV dysfunction attributed to docetaxel is lower than 2.3% to 13%.[14]

The ASE/EACVI guideline dichotomizes cardiotoxicity mechanisms into type I (dose-dependent with myocyte necrosis) and type II (not dose-dependent; less myocyte necrosis). This dichotomy was primarily used to contrast myocardial damage from anthracycline with myocardial injury from trastuzumab.[15] However, it does not adequately describe immune checkpoint inhibitor myocarditis as a potential cause of HF and its relevance to myocardial injury from other potentially cardiotoxic therapies is unclear. It is likely that the pathologic findings and natural history of CTRCD caused by different drug classes are nuanced and the broader relevance of the ASE/EACVI dichotomy is therefore limited in the current

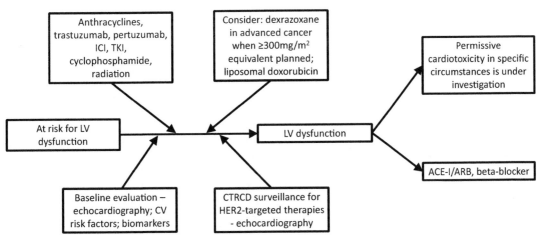

Fig. 1. Summary of guidelines for the identification, prevention, surveillance, and management of CTRCD. ACE-I, angiotensin-converting enzyme inhibitor; ARB, angiotensin receptor blocker; ICI, immune checkpoint inhibitor; TKI, tyrosine kinase inhibitor.

landscape of potentially cardiotoxic cancer therapies.

Cardiovascular Risk Factors

The ASCO and ESMO broadly recommend the evaluation of modifiable CV risk factors (see **Fig. 1**), but no specific guidance is given with respect to their management beyond recommending that abnormalities be treated. The ESC provides recommendations specifically related to hypertension in the context of vascular endothelial growth factor inhibitor use, where they recommend treatment in accordance with other general clinical practice guidelines. No specific guidance is included in any professional societal guideline with respect to cholesterol targets, diabetes management, smoking cessation alternatives, ideal body weight, or anthropometrics. This may relate to a paucity of data on the relationship between these risk factors and clinical outcomes in populations with active cancer.

The appropriateness of extrapolating CV risk factor treatment targets and strategies from the general population to individuals with cancer, especially advanced cancer, is unproven. For example, the benefits of aggressive lowering of low-density lipoprotein cholesterol in the general population may not be realized in those with advanced cancers because of the competing risk of cancer death. Blood glucose levels may vary widely in patients with malignancies or who have undergone hemopoietic stem cell transplantation who are treated with corticosteroids. Blood glucose levels may be elevated during corticosteroid therapy but may normalize when off corticosteroids or because of anorexia related to the cancer or its treatment. Although targeting weight in those in the general population with a body mass index greater than 30 kg/m^2 is recommended, the benefit of this recommendation among those with active cancer is unclear because weight loss may also occur with cachexia, which is an ominous prognostic sign. Therefore, further data are required to inform more specific recommendations on CV risk factor control in patients with active cancers.

Baseline Evaluation of Cardiac Function

All guidelines recommend the evaluation of cardiac function before the initiation of potentially cardiotoxic cancer therapy (**Table 2**). In general, emphasis is placed on using the same imaging modality that would be used during follow-up (to maximize test reproducibility and to minimize the sequelae of measurement error) and on avoiding unnecessary radiation. For these reasons, echocardiography is the preferred approach over multigated acquisition (MUGA). Three-dimensional echocardiography has a high level of interobserver and intraobserver reliability and test-retest reliability.[16] In expert centers, GLS may also be highly reproducible in patients with cancer.[17] However, the reproducibility of strain measurements in less experienced centers is less clear. Cardiac MRI may be considered for the baseline and serial evaluation of cardiac function before and during potentially cardiotoxic cancer therapies but is likely less accessible than echocardiography in the contemporary imaging environment.[18,19]

Beyond advocating the evaluation of baseline LV function, only the ESMO guideline provides specific recommendations if the baseline LVEF is impaired. It suggests that individuals with a baseline LVEF less than 50% should only receive anthracycline with caution and alternatives to anthracycline should be considered if possible.

Baseline Measurement of Blood Biomarkers

According to the ESC, ESMO, and ASE/EACVI troponin measurement is considered before initiating cancer therapies with potential cardiotoxicity (although notably, the ASCO does not recommend the measurement of troponin in asymptomatic individuals). Although troponin measurement in this context is the most studied blood biomarker, most data are from a single Italian center. In the study from this institution, 703 patients with various cancers receiving diverse chemotherapy regimens had troponin I measured early after chemotherapy initiation and again at 1 month.[20] The composite outcome of cardiac death, HF, life-threatening arrhythmia, or asymptomatic fall in LVEF of greater than or equal to 25% occurred in 1% of the 495 patients whose troponin I remained negative; 37% of the 125 whose initial troponin I was positive but whose late troponin I was negative; and 84% of those with a persistently elevated troponin I. In a more recent multicenter study that included 78 patients with HER2-positive breast cancer treated with anthracycline-containing chemotherapy and trastuzumab, a panel of cardiac biomarkers was measured at baseline, following anthracycline completion, and after 3 months of trastuzumab.[21] An increase in troponin I seemed to be the strongest biomarker predictor of cardiotoxicity. Given the modest data from heterogeneous populations receiving varied chemotherapy regimens, all guideline documents indicate that more data are needed before a stronger recommendation to measure troponin at baseline (or during therapy) is made.

Table 2
Recommendations for the baseline evaluation of patients in preparation for potentially cardiotoxic cancer therapies

Baseline	ESC	ASCO[3]	ESMO
Conventional cardiovascular risk factors	May be performed by oncologists; cardiology referral recommended for high-risk individuals	Recommended (including lipid panel and diabetes screening)	Recommended (including lipid panel and cardiac biomarkers)
LVEF	Recommended	Recommended	Recommended
Diastolic LV function	Not stated	Not stated	Recommended
Troponin	May be considered	No definitive recommendation	May be considered
BNP or NT-proBNP	May be considered	Not routinely supported	May be considered

Abbreviations: BNP, brain natriuretic peptide; NT-proBNP, amino-terminal pro-brain natriuretic peptide.

The enthusiasm for the routine baseline measurement of brain natriuretic peptide (BNP)/amino-terminal pro-brain natriuretic peptide (NT-proBNP) among professional societies was lower than for troponin, because of less available data.

Primary Prevention of Cardiotoxicity

The primary prevention of cardiotoxicity refers to the implementation of strategies to prevent CTRCD in patients with normal baseline cardiac function. In a systematic review, in five randomized, controlled trials, dexrazoxane reduced the risk of HF with relative risk of 0.21 (95% CI, 0.13–0.33; $I^2 = 0\%$). At present, the European Medicines Agency and the US Food and Drug Administration recommend that dexrazoxane be used in adults with advanced or metastatic breast cancer (reflecting the trials of dexrazoxane to date) who have received a cumulative dose of doxorubicin greater than or equal to 300 mg/m^2 (or epirubicin $\geq$540 mg/m^2).[22,23] They explicitly recommend against its use in children and adolescents because of an increased risk of acute myeloid leukemia and myelodysplastic syndrome.[22,23]

According to the ESMO guidelines, liposomal doxorubicin was thought not to have sufficient supportive evidence to justify its recommendation. This recommendation, without elaboration, seems to contrast with the cited evidence: a systematic review of anthracyclines found that in four randomized trials comparing liposomal with standard doxorubicin, the relative risk of HF with the liposomal formulation was 0.18 (95% CI, 0.08–0.38; $I^2 = 0\%$) and the relative risk of cardiotoxicity was 0.31 (95% CI, 0.20–0.48; $I^2 = 48.5\%$).[24] The trials included in this systematic review seemed to be of generally high quality (**Table 3**). Therefore, there would seem to be a

reasonable rationale for the consideration of liposomal doxorubicin. This was the position of the ASCO and ESC guidelines, in which liposomal doxorubicin and dexrazoxane were included as potential strategies that could be considered for the primary prevention of cardiotoxicity under select circumstances. However, the optimal use of these approaches remains to be fully defined.

There have been several trials evaluating the role of angiotensin-converting enzyme inhibitors (ACE-I), angiotensin receptor blockers (ARB), β-blockers, and statins for the primary prevention of LV systolic dysfunction in patients treated with potentially cardiotoxic cancer therapies. The ASCO highlights the limitations of these trials, including small sample sizes and lack of long-term follow-up or clinical markers of efficacy. It therefore does not recommend the routine use of these medications for the primary prevention of CTRCD in the absence of another indication for their use. Similarly, the ASE, EACVI, and ESC do not provide any recommendations for the use of these agents given the limited supportive data available, especially among patients with low baseline risk of cardiotoxicity. The ESMO indicates that further research is needed to identify populations of patients who may benefit from primary cardiotoxicity prevention with ACE-I/ARB or β-blockers.

Mineralocorticoid receptor antagonists and SGLT2-inhibitors are effective treatments for HF across a wide spectrum of LVEF values. It is therefore intuitive to hypothesize that these drug classes may prevent the development of CTRCD. Small randomized, controlled trials of eplerenone and spironolactone have come to divergent conclusions with regards to the ability of these mineralocorticoid receptor antagonists to prevent CTRCD, with the trial of spironolactone suggesting a beneficial

Table 3
Randomized trials comparing liposomal doxorubicin with standard doxorubicin

Study	Population	Treatments	Outcomes	Blinding
Batist et al,[38] 2001 (n = 297)	Metastatic breast cancer	Liposomal doxorubicin 60 mg/m² vs doxorubicin 60 mg/m² every 3 wk until disease progression or dose-limiting toxicity (cyclophosphamide given to all participants)	Primary: decrease in LVEF ≥20% from baseline to ≥50% or ≥10% to <50%; or clinical heart failure Primary efficacy outcome: objective tumor response	Outcomes evaluated blinded to allocation
Harris et al,[39] 2002 (n = 244)	Metastatic breast cancer	Liposomal doxorubicin 75 mg/m² vs doxorubicin 75 mg/m² every 3 wk until disease progression or dose-limiting toxicity	Primary: tumor response rate Primary safety outcome: decrease in LVEF ≥20% from baseline to ≥50% or ≥10% to <50%; or clinical heart failure	Outcomes evaluated blinded to allocation
O'Brien et al,[40] 2004 (n = 504)	Metastatic breast cancer	Pegylated liposomal doxorubicin 50 mg/m² every 4 wk vs doxorubicin 60 mg/m² every 3 wk	Noninferiority for progression-free survival; safety outcome: decrease in LVEF ≥20% from baseline to ≥ LLN or ≥10% to < LLN %; or clinical heart failure	Open-label
Rifkin et al,[41] 2006 (n = 192)	Multiple myeloma	Pegylated liposomal doxorubicin 40 mg/m² on Day 1 of each of 4 cycles vs doxorubicin 9 mg/m²/d on Days 1–4 of each of 4 cycles	Primary: objective response	Outcomes evaluated blinded to allocation

effect, whereas the trial of eplerenone showed no difference as compared with placebo.[25,26] Evidence to support the role of SGLT2-inhibitors for this indication is scant, although theoretically attractive.[27] Thus, there are insufficient data at present to recommend the routine use of mineralocorticoid receptor antagonists and SGLT2-inhibitors for the primary prevention of CTRCD.

CARDIOTOXICITY SURVEILLANCE

The professional societies have provided recommendations on the role of surveillance for cardiotoxicity (**Table 4**). However, because of the limited evidence available to inform these recommendations, they are generally limited in granularity. The ESMO indicates that LVEF and diastolic LV function should be assessed before the initiation of cancer therapy that is associated with LV dysfunction or HF. The ESC document has provided more detailed recommendations on which patient groups should have LV function assessed and at what time points. Recommendations vary according to cancer therapy. In anthracycline recipients, it recommends assessment of cardiac function before and after chemotherapy. In those receiving HER2-targeted therapies, there was no definitive recommendation; however, it acknowledged that 3-monthly assessment of cardiac function is typical (see **Fig. 1**). The origin of this practice is traced to landmark trastuzumab clinical trials that led to their registration. In these trials, measurement of LVEF was required approximately every 3 months during trastuzumab, a practice that was then translated to the drug product monograph. However, it is important to recognize that the clinical trial protocols were designed to ensure participant safety; the real-world effectiveness, feasibility, or cost-effectiveness of this intensity of LVEF surveillance were not evaluated in these trials and it is unknown whether less intensive monitoring would confer acceptable clinical safety. In the BCIRG-006 trial, 1050 patients were randomized to receive doxorubicin, cyclophosphamide, and docetaxel; 1068 to receive doxorubicin, cyclophosphamide, followed by docetaxel and trastuzumab; and 1075 to receive docetaxel, carboplatin, and trastuzumab.[28] Participants' LVEF was measured seven times during the trial. Per protocol, asymptomatic decreases in LVEF were addressed by withholding trastuzumab for an LVEF greater than or equal to 10% less than baseline and 1% to 5% less than the lower limit of normal and for any LVEF greater than or equal to 6% less than the lower limit of normal. In this trial, cardiotoxicity, defined as a relative greater than 10% reduction in LVEF from baseline, occurred in 11%, 19%, and 9% of these three respective groups. HF was reported in 0.7%, 2.0%, and 0.4% of the treatment groups, respectively, and no cardiac deaths occurred during the trial. It is not known if the incidence of HF would be higher in the absence of such rigorous monitoring of LV function.

LVEF and GLS thresholds that are consistent with the presence of cardiotoxicity have been proposed. The ASE and the EACVI consensus is that decreased LVEF is associated with an increased risk of future adverse cardiac events; and that change in GLS (relative change >15%) is likely to be helpful in the detection of early, subclinical LV dysfunction; but that there is insufficient evidence to indicate that abnormalities in diastolic LV function predict future abnormalities in systolic LV function.[4]

The ASE and the EACVI also provide guidance on the role of MUGA in monitoring for LV systolic dysfunction among anthracycline-treated patients[4] (see **Table 4**). These recommendations were based on retrospective data from 1983, in which 29 patients prescribed doxorubicin were monitored using MUGA over a mean of 6 months. In the 12 patients who received a cumulative dose greater than 350 mg/m^2, LV ejection fell from 48% ± 4% to 43% ± 8% ($P < .05$).[29] This was followed by another retrospective analysis of data from 282 patients (46 of whom developed clinical HF) from the same institution.[30] Among those whose LVEF remained within 10% of baseline, HF was not observed. Given the relative paucity of data on MUGA, the exposure to radiation and the lack of information on right ventricular, valvular, or diastolic LV function, echocardiography is preferred over MUGA for cardiotoxicity surveillance.[3]

The ASE and the EACVI also concluded that elevated troponin levels may be a sensitive indicator of cardiotoxicity. However, they highlight barriers to the widespread implementation of troponin surveillance, including uncertainty over the optimal time (relative to therapy administration) to measure troponin and uncertainty over the optimal troponin threshold for the identification of cardiotoxicity. Also cited are several studies of modest size in which BNP or NT-proBNP was measured. Based on this evidence, no guidance was provided on the role of BNP or NT-proBNP in surveillance for cardiotoxicity.

The Management of Cardiotoxicity

The role of ongoing cancer therapy

The ASCO explicitly states that no recommendations can be made regarding the continuation or discontinuation of cancer therapy if cardiotoxicity occurs. Rather, the ESC and ASCO indicate that

Table 4
Recommendations for the surveillance of CTRCD during therapy

Tool	ESC[2]	ASCO	ASE/EACVI[4]	ESMO
Echocardiography	Recommended periodically during therapy in patients receiving potentially cardiotoxic cancer therapy	Recommended in those with symptoms or signs of cardiac dysfunction and in asymptomatic individuals at increased risk of cardiotoxicity	Generally recommended without specific recommendations on frequency	Recommended in preference to MUGA
MUGA	Echocardiography preferred over MUGA for CTRCD surveillance	Recommended if echocardiography and CMR unavailable	In those receiving anthracycline with LVEF >50% at baseline, remeasure LVEF at cumulative doxorubicin equivalent dose 250–300 mg/m², at 450 mg/m² then before each dose >450 mg/m². If LVEF <50% at baseline, measure LVEF before each subsequent dose	Echocardiography preferable
Troponin	Increase identifies patients treated with high-dose chemotherapy who may benefit from ACE-I	Recommended in those with symptoms or signs of cardiac dysfunction	Although troponin elevation during cancer therapy may be sensitive for the detection of cardiotoxicity, no specific recommendations provided	Periodic measurement is considered
BNP/NT-proBNP	Routine role unclear	Recommended in those with symptoms or signs of cardiac dysfunction	Not generally recommended for the early identification of CTRCD	Periodic measurement is considered

Abbreviation: CMR, cardiac magnetic resonance.

the role and timing of withholding or discontinuing cancer therapy need to be individualized, weighing the patient's risks and potential benefits.

Permissive cardiotoxicity and HER2-targeted therapy

Current recommendations, including those of the UK National Cancer Research Institute, which are endorsed by the ESC, indicate that LVEF decreases to less than 45% or by greater than 10% to 45% to 49% following HER2-targeted therapy should be managed by therapy interruption.[31] Given that HER2-targeted therapies tend not to cause cardiomyocyte necrosis and that related CTRCD is often reversible, there has been interest in whether a strategy of permissive cardiotoxicity (in which mild, minimally symptomatic LV dysfunction is accepted to allow ongoing HER2 therapy) is feasible. There have been two small, prospective single-arm trials addressing this question.[32,33] In both trials, ongoing HER2-targeted therapy for LVEF greater than 40%, accompanied by the administration of an ACE-I/ARB and/or β-blocker, was evaluated. The findings from the trials were remarkably consistent, with 10% of participants in both studies needing to discontinue HER2-targeted therapy because of HF or LVEF less than 40%. Therefore, although this strategy of permissive cardiotoxicity may be feasible, ongoing research is needed to evaluate whether the benefit of this approach outweighs the risk of HF.

The ESMO recommends that if anthracycline is considered essential in individuals with baseline LVEF less than 50%, LVEF should be measured at least before every second treatment cycle and there should be consideration for the use of dexrazoxane as a cardioprotective agent.

Selection and duration of heart failure therapies

In a single-center, open-label, randomized, controlled trial, among 114 patients who exhibited an elevated troponin I level soon after initiation of high-dose chemotherapy, enalapril preserved LVEF as compared with control.[34] In this trial, enalapril was continued for 12 months after chemotherapy. In patients exhibiting CTRCD, ACE-I/ARB and β-blockers are generally recommended. However, the optimal duration of these agents is unclear; in particular, if markers of cardiac function normalize, the safety of discontinuing ACE-I/ARB and β-blockers is unknown. In a pilot randomized, controlled trial, the withdrawal of HF in therapy in individuals with dilated cardiomyopathy whose LVEF had recovered led to worse LV function than those in whom such therapy was continued.[35] It is not known whether this evidence should be

extrapolated to patients with CTRCD. Because of the heterogeneity in CTRCD, it is possible that these drugs could be safely discontinued following some cardiotoxic therapies, whereas in other cardiotoxicities (eg, anthracycline-related), the associated myonecrosis confers sufficiently high risk of relapse that HF medication should be continued indefinitely.

SUMMARY

Although the existing white papers and consensus statements have broad similarities in cancer therapy cardiotoxicity definitions, primary prevention, and surveillance recommendations, there are important knowledge gaps that are highlighted in these consensus statements. Further research is needed to inform future recommendations on specific aspects of CTRCD surveillance and especially the role of blood biomarkers and management strategies for those who develop overt cardiotoxicity.

CLINICS CARE POINTS

- Patients who plan to receive potentially cardiotoxic cancer therapies, including anthracyclines, trastuzumab, pertuzumab, immune checkpoint inhibitors, tyrosine kinase inhibitors, cyclophosphamide, ifosfamide, and radiotherapy (where the heart is within the therapeutic field) should have their cardiac function evaluated before initiating therapy. Surveillance cardiac imaging is considered, depending on the specific cancer treatment administered and on imaging availability.

- Asymptomatic CTRCD is characterized by: (1) a relative decline in global longitudinal strain of greater than 15% and/or a new increase in cardiac biomarkers in individuals with LVEF greater than or equal to 50%, (2) a reduction in LVEF to 40% to 49% (accompanied by a relative decline in global longitudinal strain of >15% and/or a new increase in cardiac biomarkers if the reduction in LVEF is <10%), or (3) a fall in LVEF to less than 40%.

- Angiotensin-converting enzyme inhibitors, angiotensin receptor blockers, and β-blockers are not recommended as routine in patients with preserved systolic left ventricular function receiving potentially cardiotoxic cancer therapies, but is considered in select individuals.

- Dexrazoxane should be considered for the prevention of CTRCD in individuals with advanced breast cancer in whom cumulative doses of doxorubicin greater than or equal to 300 mg/m² (or equivalent) are planned.

DISCLOSURE

DPL and DJL have no disclosures related to this paper. DPL has received unrelated research support from Novartis and consulting fees from Abbvie, Ferring Pharmaceuticals, Janssen, Myovant Sciences, Novartis, Pfizer, Sanofi, Paladin and Tolmar. DJL has received research funding from Myocardial Solutions and consulting fees from Intellia, OncXerna, SecuraBio, Astra Zeneca, Clementia, Eidos, Myocardial Solutions.

REFERENCES

1. Curigliano G, Lenihan D, Fradley M, et al. Management of cardiac disease in cancer patients throughout oncological treatment: ESMO consensus recommendations. Ann Oncol 2020; 31(2):171–90.

2. Zamorano JL, Lancellotti P, Rodriguez Munoz D, et al. 2016 ESC Position Paper on cancer treatments and cardiovascular toxicity developed under the auspices of the ESC Committee for practice guidelines: the task force for cancer treatments and cardiovascular toxicity of the European Society of Cardiology (ESC). Eur Heart J 2016;37(36):2768–801.

3. Armenian SH, Lacchetti C, Barac A, et al. Prevention and monitoring of cardiac dysfunction in survivors of adult cancers: American Society of Clinical Oncology Clinical Practice Guideline. J Clin Oncol 2017;35(8):893–911.

4. Plana JC, Galderisi M, Barac A, et al. Expert consensus for multimodality imaging evaluation of adult patients during and after cancer therapy: a report from the American Society of Echocardiography and the European Association of Cardiovascular Imaging. Eur Heart J Cardiovasc Imaging 2014; 15(10):1063–93.

5. Herrmann J, Lenihan D, Armenian S, et al. Defining cardiovascular toxicities of cancer therapies: an International Cardio-Oncology Society (IC-OS) consensus statement. Eur Heart J 2021. https://doi.org/10.1093/eurheartj/ehab674.

6. Yancy CW, Jessup M, Bozkurt B, et al. 2013 ACCF/AHA guideline for the management of heart failure: a report of the American College of Cardiology Foundation/American Heart Association task force on practice guidelines. Circulation 2013;128(16): e240–327.

7. McDonagh TA, Metra M, Adamo M, et al. 2021 ESC Guidelines for the diagnosis and treatment of acute and chronic heart failure. Eur Heart J 2021;42(36): 3599–726.

8. Mincu RI, Lampe LF, Mahabadi AA, et al. Left ventricular diastolic function following anthracycline-based chemotherapy in patients with breast cancer without previous cardiac disease: a meta-analysis.

J Clin Med 2021;10(17). https://doi.org/10.3390/jcm10173890.

9. Mazzutti G, Pivatto Junior F, Costa GOM, et al. Right ventricular function during trastuzumab therapy for breast cancer. Int J Cardiovasc Imaging 2021. https://doi.org/10.1007/s10554-021-02470-2.

10. de Souza TF, Silva TQ, Antunes-Correa L, et al. Cardiac magnetic resonance assessment of right ventricular remodeling after anthracycline therapy. Sci Rep 2021;11(1):17132.

11. Alhussein M, Mokbel A, Cosman T, et al. Pertuzumab cardiotoxicity in patients with HER2-positive cancer: a systematic review and meta-analysis. CJC Open 2021;3(11):1372–82.

12. Alhussein M, Hotte SJ, Leong DP. Reversible cabozantinib-induced cardiomyopathy. Can J Cardiol 2019;35(4):544.e1–2.

13. Kim L, Fowler B, Campbell CM, et al. Acute cardiotoxicity after initiation of the novel tyrosine kinase inhibitor gilteritinib for acute myeloid leukemia. Cardiooncology 2021;7(1):36.

14. Martin M, Pienkowski T, Mackey J, et al. Adjuvant docetaxel for node-positive breast cancer. N Engl J Med 2005;352(22):2302–13.

15. Ewer MS, Lippman SM. Type II chemotherapy-related cardiac dysfunction: time to recognize a new entity. J Clin Oncol 2005;23(13):2900–2.

16. Thavendiranathan P, Grant AD, Negishi T, et al. Reproducibility of echocardiographic techniques for sequential assessment of left ventricular ejection fraction and volumes: application to patients undergoing cancer chemotherapy. J Am Coll Cardiol 2013;61(1):77–84.

17. Lambert J, Lamacie M, Thampinathan B, et al. Variability in echocardiography and MRI for detection of cancer therapy cardiotoxicity. Heart 2020;106(11): 817–23.

18. Giusca S, Korosoglou G, Montenbruck M, et al. Multiparametric early detection and prediction of cardiotoxicity using myocardial strain, T1 and T2 mapping, and biochemical markers: a longitudinal cardiac resonance imaging study during 2 years of follow-up. circulation cardiovascular imaging 2021; 14(6):e012459.

19. O'Quinn R, Ferrari VA, Daly R, et al. Cardiac magnetic resonance in cardio-oncology: advantages, importance of expediency, and considerations to navigate pre-authorization. JACC CardioOncol 2021;3(2):191–200.

20. Cardinale D, Sandri MT, Colombo A, et al. Prognostic value of troponin I in cardiac risk stratification of cancer patients undergoing high-dose chemotherapy. Circulation 2004;109(22):2749–54.

21. Ky B, Putt M, Sawaya H, et al. Early increases in multiple biomarkers predict subsequent cardiotoxicity in patients with breast cancer treated with doxorubicin, taxanes, and trastuzumab. J Am Coll Cardiol 2014; 63(8):809–16.

22. European Medicines Agency. Dexrazoxane. Available at: https://www.ema.europa.eu/en/medicines/human/referrals/dexrazoxane. Accessed December 19, 2021.

23. U.S. Food and Drug Administration. Highlights of prescribing information. Available at: https://www.accessdata.fda.gov/drugsatfda_docs/label/2014/020212s017lbl.pdf. Accessed December 19, 2021.

24. Smith LA, Cornelius VR, Plummer CJ, et al. Cardiotoxicity of anthracycline agents for the treatment of cancer: systematic review and meta-analysis of randomised controlled trials. BMC Cancer 2010;10:337.

25. Akpek M, Ozdogru I, Sahin O, et al. Protective effects of spironolactone against anthracycline-induced cardiomyopathy. Eur J Heart Fail 2015;17(1):81–9.

26. Davis MK, Villa D, Tsang TSM, et al. Effect of eplerenone on diastolic function in women receiving anthracycline-based chemotherapy for breast cancer. JACC CardioOncol 2019;1(2):295–8.

27. Lau KTK, Ng L, Wong JWH, et al. Repurposing sodium-glucose co-transporter 2 inhibitors (SGLT2i) for cancer treatment: a review. Rev Endocr Metab Disord 2021;22(4):1121–36.

28. Slamon D, Eiermann W, Robert N, et al. Adjuvant trastuzumab in HER2-positive breast cancer. N Engl J Med 2011;365(14):1273–83.

29. Choi BW, Berger HJ, Schwartz PE, et al. Serial radionuclide assessment of doxorubicin cardiotoxicity in cancer patients with abnormal baseline resting left ventricular performance. Am Heart J 1983;106(4 Pt 1):638–43.

30. Schwartz RG, McKenzie WB, Alexander J, et al. Congestive heart failure and left ventricular dysfunction complicating doxorubicin therapy. Seven-year experience using serial radionuclide angiocardiography. Am J Med 1987;82(6):1109–18.

31. Jones AL, Barlow M, Barrett-Lee PJ, et al. Management of cardiac health in trastuzumab-treated patients with breast cancer: updated United Kingdom National Cancer Research Institute recommendations for monitoring. Br J Cancer 2009;100(5):684–92.

32. Lynce F, Barac A, Geng X, et al. Prospective evaluation of the cardiac safety of HER2-targeted therapies in patients with HER2-positive breast cancer and compromised heart function: the SAFE-HEaRt study. Breast Cancer Res Treat 2019. https://doi.org/10.1007/s10549-019-05191-2.

33. Leong DP, Cosman TL, Alhussein MM, et al. A phase I trial evaluating the safety of continuing trastuzumab despite mild cardiotoxicity. JACC CardioOncology 2019;1(1):1–9.

34. Cardinale D, Colombo A, Sandri MT, et al. Prevention of high-dose chemotherapy-induced cardiotoxicity in high-risk patients by angiotensin-converting enzyme inhibition. Randomized controlled trial. Circulation 2006;114(23):2474–81.

35. Halliday BP, Wassall R, Lota AS, et al. Withdrawal of pharmacological treatment for heart failure in patients with recovered dilated cardiomyopathy (TRED-HF): an open-label, pilot, randomised trial. Lancet 2018. https://doi.org/10.1016/S0140-6736(18)32484-X.

36. Seidman A, Hudis C, Pierri MK, et al. Cardiac dysfunction in the trastuzumab clinical trials experience. J Clin Oncol 2002;20(5):1215–21.

37. Plana JC, Galderisi M, Barac A, et al. Expert consensus for multimodality imaging evaluation of adult patients during and after cancer therapy: a report from the American Society of Echocardiography and the European Association of Cardiovascular Imaging. J Am Soc Echocardiogr 2014;27(9):911–39.

38. Batist G, Ramakrishnan G, Rao CS, et al. Reduced cardiotoxicity and preserved antitumor efficacy of liposome-encapsulated doxorubicin and cyclophosphamide compared with conventional doxorubicin and cyclophosphamide in a randomized, multicenter trial of metastatic breast cancer. J Clin Oncol 2001;19(5):1444–54.

39. Harris L, Batist G, Belt R, et al. Liposome-encapsulated doxorubicin compared with conventional doxorubicin in a randomized multicenter trial as first-line therapy of metastatic breast carcinoma. Cancer 2002;94(1):25–36.

40. O'Brien ME, Wigler N, Inbar M, et al. Reduced cardiotoxicity and comparable efficacy in a phase III trial of pegylated liposomal doxorubicin HCl (CAELYX/Doxil) versus conventional doxorubicin for first-line treatment of metastatic breast cancer. Ann Oncol 2004;15(3):440–9.

41. Rifkin RM, Gregory SA, Mohrbacher A, et al. Pegylated liposomal doxorubicin, vincristine, and dexamethasone provide significant reduction in toxicity compared with doxorubicin, vincristine, and dexamethasone in patients with newly diagnosed multiple myeloma: a phase III multicenter randomized trial. Cancer 2006;106(4):848–58.

Training and Career Development in Cardio-Oncology Translational and Implementation Science

Sherry-Ann Brown, MD, PhD[a],*, Eric H. Yang, MD[b], Mary Branch, MD, MS[c], Craig Beavers, PharmD[d], Anne Blaes, MD, MS[e], Michael G. Fradley, MD[f], Richard K. Cheng, MD, MSc[g]

KEYWORDS

• Cardio-oncology • Trainees • Education • Cardiology • Oncology

KEY POINTS

- The necessity of training in cardio-oncology increases as the number of cancer survivors with cardiovascular complications increases.
- Many variables need to be considered when establishing a cardio-oncology program.
- With the increase of social media, there are multiple new formats and avenues for training and career development.

INTRODUCTION

The cancer population continues to increase with approximately 1.9 million new cases projected for 2021[1] and more than 20 million cancer survivors projected to be alive in the United States by the next decade.[2] In response, the multidisciplinary field of cardio-oncology has emerged rapidly in order to provide clinical care and research initiatives to address the cardiovascular care of this unique and vulnerable population. This field within cardiology is unique due to the necessity of harmonizing care between 2 major fields within Medicine, in addition to the dynamic demands of addressing the numerous and heterogeneous treatment strategies of the different kinds of cancer. Finally, a current and ongoing challenge is trying to understand, detect, and treat the cardiotoxicities that may accompany both historical agents and the deluge of novel therapeutics that are being developed at an unprecedented pace.

With the successful establishment of cardio-oncology as a major subspecialty within the fields of cardiology and oncology, a fundamental objective is to define an effective strategy of training and providing education to scientists and health care professionals (eg, physicians, nurse practitioners,

[a] Cardio-Oncology Program, Division of Cardiovascular Medicine, Medical College of Wisconsin, 8701 West Watertown Plank Road, Milwaukee, WI 53226, USA; [b] UCLA Cardio-Oncology Program, Division of Cardiology, Department of Medicine, University of California at Los Angeles, UCLA Cardiovascular Center, 100 Medical Plaza, Suite 630, Los Angeles, CA 90095, USA; [c] Section of Cardiovascular Medicine, Wake Forest University, 1834 Wake Forest Road, Winston-Salem, NC 27109, USA; [d] University of Kentucky College of Pharmacy, 40506, 789 South Limestone, Lexington, KY 40508, USA; [e] Division of Hematology/Oncology, University of Minnesota, 3 Morrill Hall, 100 Church Street Southeast, Minneapolis, MN 55455, USA; [f] Division of Cardiology, Department of Medicine, Cardio-Oncology Center of Excellence, Perelman School of Medicine at the University of Pennsylvania, 3400 Civic Center Boulevard, Philadelphia, PA 19104, USA; [g] Cardio-oncology Program, Division of Cardiology, University of Washington, 1959 Northeast Pacific Street, Seattle, WA 98195, USA
* Corresponding author.
E-mail addresses: drbrowncares@gmail.com; shbrown@mcw.edu
Twitter: @drbrowncares (S.-A.B.); @datsunian (E.H.Y.); @DocBanks84 (M.B.); @beaverspharmd (C.B.); @BlaesAnne (A.B.); @Richardkcheng2 (R.K.C.)

Heart Failure Clin 18 (2022) 503–514
https://doi.org/10.1016/j.hfc.2022.02.014
1551-7136/22/© 2022 Elsevier Inc. All rights reserved.

pharmacists, and others) who wish to pursue research endeavors in and achieve clinical competence in the field, respectively. Such efforts, if successful, will allow for cardio-oncology to develop a sustainable model of education and research that will lead to growth of the field on a wide scale. Such desired objectives would include (1) structured, standardized training curricula for research and clinical trainees in cardiology and hematology/oncology programs; (2) establishment of private and public sector–funded research programs that can provide not only a platform for scientific discovery and advancement but also cyclical funding for both training and research programs; and (3) the development of competent, knowledgeable health care workers who are able to provide high-quality clinical care to the cardio-oncology population within a variety of health care systems, with the ability to continue lifelong self-learning with the dynamic nature of the field. All of this occurs best in the context of established comprehensive cardio-oncology programs or centers of excellence.

In this report, the authors provide an overview of optimal infrastructure for training and career development in cardio-oncology translational and implementation science (**Fig. 1**). They lay the foundation for building cardio-oncology programs with emphasis on collaborations among clinicians and scientists. The authors also highlight the role of the multidisciplinary cardiovascular team for both research and patient care. Opportunities for cardio-oncology training in general cardiology fellowship, hematology/oncology fellowship, dedicated cardio-oncology clinical fellowship with research, and cardio-oncology research fellowship are described, with proposed training for the multidisciplinary cardiovascular team (**Fig. 2**).

INFRASTRUCTURE FOR TRAINING
Cardio-Oncology Program

Although the cardio-oncology literature has several reviews on strategies to establish a cardio-oncology program,[3–9] each institution has its unique challenges based on varying degrees of institutional, faculty, financial, and logistical support. In addition to this, cardio-oncology is unique in that it is a field that depends on another subspecialty of Medicine—for multidisciplinary collaboration and the referral of its unique cancer patient population. Advocates who are invested in starting and/or building a cardio-oncology program at their own institution need to begin identifying gaps in support and champions both within cardiology and oncology divisions to promote this multidisciplinary collaboration. Identifying cardiovascular needs within an institution's oncology population and generating services lines for clinical referrals based on these needs may be an initial effective strategy for program building and the subsequent integration of didactics and training of house-staff into their curriculum to help garner support in the realms of clinical care and research. Depending on programmatic funding, whether it is based on clinical revenue and/or research funding, such financial sources of support also need to be identified and prioritized in order to develop the building blocks necessary for an effective training program.

In order for an effective training program to exist, whether its focus is on clinical care, research, or both, it can be argued that a robust cardio-oncology program needs to be a prerequisite in order to expose the trainee to the diverse spectrum of malignancies and related cardiotoxicities. Analogously, it would be presumed that in order for an effective training program in structural

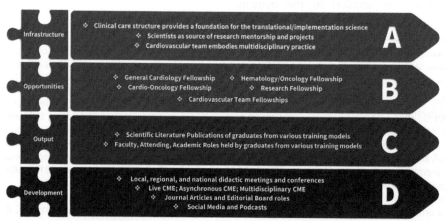

Fig. 1. Components of training and career development in cardio-oncology translational and implementation science.

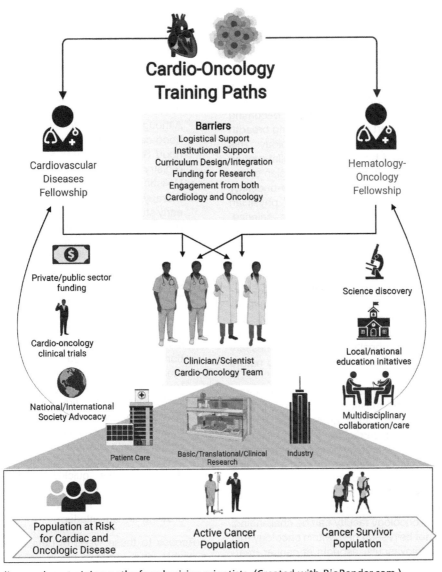

Fig. 2. Cardio-oncology training paths for physician scientists. (Created with BioRender.com.)

cardiovascular interventions and imaging to be successful, there would need to be preexisting high-volume cardiac catheterization laboratory with cardiothoracic surgery, advanced imaging capacity, and a heart team approach to these cases. Already, many health care centers with cardiology fellowships have begun these efforts; a survey conducted in 2017 revealed that approximately 51% of those who responded (n = 81) were part of institutions spread across the United States that provided dedicated cardio-oncology services, and almost a half of those responders were providing cardio-oncology–related didactics. At the time of the survey, programs had dedicated training opportunities specific to cardio-oncology, ranging from clinical observerships to training programs ranging from less than 6 months to at least a year.[10] In addition, in the same format as the American College of Cardiology (ACC) Core Cardiovascular Training Symposium (COCATS) training (the standardized training documents to achieve competency in Cardiovascular training), the ACC Cardio-Oncology Section Council also devised a proposed curriculum that would allow for training at 3 levels of competency, depending on the extent of immersion that a trainee would strive to aim for during their general fellowship training.[11] However, it is also acknowledged that cancer-related clinical services can be highly variable and heterogeneous in health care systems across the country, and it is possible that not all programs will have the same degree of exposure to all cancer states and drug classes that can cause cardiotoxicity.

Cardio-Oncology Research

Care of patients in cardio-oncology programs is driven by expert recommendations and scientific statements.[12–18] More guidelines are becoming available, in large part due to the growing breadth of research conducted in cardio-oncology. This research is pursued by scientists in collaboration with clinicians and oftentimes by physician scientists. A fundamental objective of cardio-oncology training is therefore the production of physician scientists, whether focused on basic science, translational, clinical, or population health research. The International Cardio-Oncology Society (ICOS) and Canadian Cardiac Oncology Network (CCON) training statement highlighted the importance of translational research in understanding cardiotoxicity, as a thorough understanding of the underlying biological pathways can inform screening and treatment.[19] Similarly, clinical and population health research is necessary in an iterative manner, given the dynamic nature of cancer treatment.

In programs with established cardio-oncology faculty, the major question is finding a project that aligns with the career goals of the trainee. For those in general cardiology training or a clinically based cardio-oncology program, a dedicated clinical or population health study with preexisting data may be more manageable than a more time-intensive basic science or translational study. Identification of mentorship at sites without dedicated cardio-oncology faculty can be challenging. There may not be researchers within oncology that focus on cardiovascular aspects of cancer treatment. Likewise, not all centers will have cardiologists with a particular interest in the cancer population, and this can be overcome by identifying an established mentor in cardiology or oncology and focusing on cardio-oncology–specific questions within their existing research infrastructure; this may ultimately be advantageous by creating a niche for the trainee in that working group.

Within the limited training time horizon of either 1 or 2 years for most cardio-oncology training programs, there needs to be a finite defined period for research, as the balance between producing a well-rounded clinician and importance for research has to be considered. Hence, early identification of a mentor is crucial.

Although the field is rapidly advancing, there remain many areas in need of further study and gaps in knowledge.

Some of these examples include the following:

- Better understanding of mechanistic pathways of cardiotoxicity from targeted therapies including the different classes of tyrosine kinase inhibitors.
- Improved understanding of long-term cardiovascular risk in adult cancer survivors. Although long-term follow-up exists in childhood cancer survivors via the St. Jude Childhood Survivor Study,[20] a similar longitudinal registry remains lacking in adults.
- Holistic and long-term impact of immunotherapy on cardiovascular health. Although early studies identified risk for immune-checkpoint–associated myocarditis[21] and more recent work has noted increased risk for atherosclerosis,[22] the effects of immune checkpoint inhibitors on the cardiovascular system remain incompletely understood.
- The concept of cardio-immuno-oncology, including immune checkpoint inhibitors, chimeric antigen receptor T cells, and bispecific T-cell engagers.[23] Long-term implications of the increasing use of cancer therapies modulating the immune system, leading to sustained negative changes to the cardiovascular system related to cytokine release, systemic inflammation, and other bidirectional mechanisms. This is a rapidly changing field in which data regarding cardiotoxicities and drug development for immunotherapy evolve quickly. Thus, a robust training and research environment for cardio-oncology is needed to address this growing armamentarium.

Access to these types of data is not typically available and requires close collaboration between cardiology and oncology teams at the individual institution and on a multiinstitutional level. The advent of cardio-oncology as an established subspecialty and creation of networks with key stakeholders from the different disciplines will create opportunities. These networks can also facilitate collaborative funding opportunities, such as demonstrated by the recent awarding of the American Heart Association's (AHA) Strategically Focused Research Networks (SFRN). More than $11 million was awarded during the current round of SFRN funding, with a focus of disparities in cardio-oncology, meeting an urgent and important need.

Cardiovascular Team

It has been well documented that the multidisciplinary team, including, but not limited to, nurse practitioners, physician assistants, pharmacists, nurses, and social workers, in cardio-oncology improve patient care through optimizing outcomes, preventing complications, and reducing cost of care.[24] Often, the clinical challenges toward advancing patient care require various and complementary expertise of the cardiovascular team. By nature, implementation research also requires a transdisciplinary team.[25] Thus, it is critical to develop members of the team to be engaged in cardio-oncology implementation research and science. Given this critical point, the need to promote and advance training for the whole team is required. In addition, many funding mechanisms require a diverse team in order to successfully achieve funding. Although the full scope of each professions education and training pathway could not be discussed due to the space limitations of the paper, there are common elements that exist for the ability to integrate both cardio-oncology and implementation research training into each profession's respective degree programs as well as in any postgraduate training opportunities, such as fellowships and/or residencies. Furthermore, the development of informal programs is needed to train team-based investigators. There are many questions germane to team science that have not been addressed in the literature including the effects of various research structures and funding mechanisms.[26] However, the structure, focus, opportunities, and challenges to this paradigm would not differ drastically from what has been described earlier regarding the physician pathway.[11]

OPPORTUNITIES FOR TRAINING
Cardio-Oncology Training in General Cardiology Fellowship

As new cancer therapeutics arise and cancer survivorship is improving, there is a strong need for attentive cardiac care. Risk factors for many cancers coincide with cardiovascular disease, and cardiotoxic (ie, adverse effects of cancer therapy on the heart) cancer therapeutics further perpetuate the risk of heart disease in these patients.[17,27–29] The ICOS and the ACC have each produced articles describing variations on a proposed conceptual framework with comprehensive training goals and standards for this subspecialty.[11,19] In addition, a roadmap for incorporating cardio-oncology training during general cardiology fellowship was recently published by a group of worldwide experts.[30]

Training in cardio-oncology should include a multimodality and multidisciplinary approach to address the needs of this high-risk population.

The required curriculum must include extensive educational and clinical experience with cardiovascular risk assessment before cancer therapy, management of cardiotoxicities associated with cancer treatment, ongoing cardiovascular issues in cancer patients with cancer undergoing therapy or cancer survivors, and long-term effects after immunotherapy.[31] To screen patients with cancer for cardiotoxicity during treatment, clinicians in this field require expertise in assessing electrocardiogram (ECG) (eg, for QTc prolongation in the setting of certain cancer therapies), incorporating pertinent cardiac-specific biomarkers into practice (eg, troponin in the setting of immune checkpoint inhibitors with risk of myocarditis), and having advanced knowledge of echocardiography (including strain imaging), cardiac MRI, and coronary computed tomography (CT).[16,19,31–35] Considering the diversity of adverse cardiac effects in response to cancer therapies, it is essential to have educational sessions with other advanced subspecialists in fields such as electrophysiology and advanced heart failure. Trainees should be exposed to cancer therapy clinical trials and be familiar with modern medical oncologic treatments.

During the clinical years, a trainee can request to work in the continuity clinic of the onsite cardio-oncologist as well as subscribe to the Journals of the American College of Cardiology (JACC): CardioOncology. To further keep up with the field and network in cardio-oncology, social media can be an engaging platform. Ultimately, the goal is to prevent, protect, and monitor patients with cancer in order to facilitate the use of life-saving cancer therapeutics. A clinician building a knowledge base in cardio-oncology will need to work with a multidisciplinary team and be involved with comprehensive care, often in structured meetings (eg, tumor board). This team typically includes hematologist-oncologists, pharmacists, and nurse navigators. Through this interdisciplinary approach, general cardiology fellows can develop a substantial cardio-oncology knowledge base. Training facilities should have at least 100 unique patients with cancer yearly.

Many general cardiology fellowships allow for up to 12 to 18 months of research during fellowship; this is sometimes strengthened by a National Institutes of Health (NIH) T32 training grant. Planning a research year dedicated to cardio-oncology research is a great opportunity to focus on cardio-oncology topics and work on individual novel research projects. For fellows without a formal research year, research can be otherwise incorporated concurrent with clinical training. On completion of research projects, trainees can present at national cardio-oncology, cardiology, and hematology/oncology meetings. These societies and meetings include ICOS, the ACC's Advancing the Cardiovascular Care of the Oncology Patient, and the national scientific sessions of the AHA, ACC, and the American Society for Clinical Oncology (ASCO).

Cardio-Oncology Training in Hematology/Oncology Fellowship

Within a hematology/oncology fellowship training, competency is required for cancer prevention, diagnosis, care, health promotion, and the treatment of patients across genders and ages throughout the stages of a hematologic and malignant illness. Hematology and oncology fellows learn about the use of chemotherapeutic drugs and biological agents including the mechanisms of action, pharmacokinetics, and associated toxicities. These toxicities encompass both acute and chronic toxicities, such as cardiotoxicities of all types across the spectrum of heart failure, ischemic heart disease, myocarditis/pericarditis, pericardial effusions, and arrhythmias. As described by the Institute of Medicine's Crossing the Quality Chasm: A New Health System for the 21st Century, "Quality patient care is safe, effective, timely, efficient, patient-centered, equitable, and designed to improve population health, while reducing per capita costs" and remains an essential component of the hematology/oncology curriculum.[36,37] Although Accreditation Council for Graduate Medical Education (ACGME) requirements outline specific recommendations around addressing toxicities from cancer therapies including cardiotoxicities, there remains opportunity to expand specific cardio-oncology education within the hematology/oncology training programs.[11,19]

Embedding rotations to a cardio-oncology clinic and detailing discussions within a cardio-oncology grand rounds may be useful in addressing close collaborations between cardiology and oncology. Similarly, attending cardio oncology meetings such as the ICOS and ACC cardio-oncology meetings may be useful in expanding the oncologist's knowledge around the pathophysiology of cardiac-specific complications, the prevention of cardiac toxicities, and the long-term health of cancer survivors. In hematology/oncology fellowships as well for clinicians in practice currently, there is a growing emphasis on training in cancer survivorship.

With more than 16 million cancer survivors now in the United States,[38] there is increasing recognition of the need to train hematology/oncology fellows (in both adult and pediatric programs) in the long-term manifestations of health consequences after cancer treatment, the most common of which are second malignancies and cardiovascular disease.[39–41] In many situations, cancer survivors are more likely to die of cardiovascular disease itself as compared with recurrent cancer.[42] Embedded within many fellowship curricula, there are opportunities to rotate within survivorship or long-term follow-up clinics for pediatric, adult, and bone marrow transplant survivors. Ensuring this curriculum in each program as opposed to select ones is essential in expanding the growth and knowledge of the cardio-oncology field. Ongoing continuing medical education (CME) events such as Cancer Center Survivorship Research Forums (ccsrf.umn.edu), the American Society of Clinical Oncology's survivorship compendium, and George Washington University's E-learning series on cancer survivorship are also valuable resources in embedding cardio-oncology curricula within hematology and oncology training.

Dedicated Cardio-Oncology Clinical Fellowship with Research

With the increasing complexity of cancer therapeutics and their potential cardiovascular side effects, there is increasing emphasis on dedicated fellowship training in cardio-oncology. Multiple cardio-oncology fellowship programs currently exist throughout the world including those affiliated with the University of Pennsylvania, Washington University in St. Louis, Vanderbilt University, and the Royal Brompton Hospital in London.[43] Because cardio-oncology is not yet an ACGME-accredited fellowship, various training models currently exist.[11,19,30] Although most programs are designed to prepare board-certified/board-eligible cardiologists to manage these conditions, some programs enroll trainees who have completed internal medicine training without further subspecialization and others matriculate individuals with a medical oncology background. Most programs try to integrate both clinical and research training; however, this is not necessarily universal. The training structure needs to be tailored to the different background and skill sets of the learner. For example, a cardiology-trained cardio-oncology fellow may also want to augment their cardiovascular procedural skills, whereas a trainee without cardiology background will need to spend a significant amount of time learning the basics of cardiovascular disease management.

When working to develop a cardio-oncology fellowship, the authors suggest 3 areas of focus over at least 1 year of training: clinical care, didactics, and research/scholarly endeavors.[11,31] A periodic evaluation of the program's educational quality and compliance with the program's requirements will be formally implemented through the faculty and the fellow. Faculty will complete standard evaluation documents for the fellow. The ultimate success of the training will be gauged by the fellow's ability to obtain a cardio-oncology faculty position and/or develop and lead cardio-oncology programs once their training is complete.

Clinical care

A mentored experience is provided for the cardiovascular assessment of oncology patients with attention to the specific cardiotoxicities of chemotherapeutics, targeted therapies, immuno- and cell-based therapies, and radiation therapy as well as the appropriate application and interpretation of cardiac diagnostic tests (eg, ECG, imaging, and biomarkers). Specific topics that the cardio-oncology fellow will be expected to master include precancer treatment cardiovascular risk assessment, management of cancer-treatment associated cardiotoxicities, cardiac implantable device management in radiation oncology, and cardiovascular disease management in the cancer survivor.[11,19,31,44] The fellow will be required to have no less than 100 unique patient encounters over the course of the year, as outlined in the ICOS and the CCON training document.[19]

The fellow will be expected to regularly participate in the established outpatient cardio-oncology clinics. In addition, he/she will be encouraged to attend outpatient oncology clinics as well as other advanced cardiology practices such as heart failure or preventative cardiology. The fellow should also participate in inpatient/acute consultative cardio-oncology services. Moreover, they are encouraged to round with different oncology inpatient services (solid tumors, liquid tumors, stem cell transplant/cellular therapies) based on individual preferences for more advanced/detailed cancer instruction. It is encouraged (but not required) that the fellow identify a particular area of focus within cardio-oncology. Over the duration of this fellowship, the trainee may tailor the experience to fit their individual needs with exposure to multimodality cardiovascular imaging (echo, nuclear cardiology, CT/MRI), advanced heart failure, preventative cardiology, or electrophysiology.

Didactic education

The cardio-oncology fellow should also receive regular didactic lectures on topics inherent to cardio-oncology including a thorough understanding of cancer therapeutics and their potential cardiotoxicities.[11,31,44] They will be encouraged to attend national and international cardio-oncology educational meetings including the ACC-sponsored "Advancing the Cardiovascular Care of the Cancer Patient" or the Global Cardio-Oncology Summit. Finally, the cardio-oncology fellow should also create their own didactic lectures for the general cardiovascular fellows and internal medicine residents, as this is a great method to improve knowledge and engagement. The fellow is expected to adequately complete all 7 ACGME core competencies within this fellowship. Fellows should be expected to complete the ICOS board examination at the completion of their training.

Scholarly research

Fellows will also be expected to participate in scholarly research activities that align with their clinical interests, resulting in an abstract presentation and/or article publication, as the success of the field is contingent on enhancing our knowledge of cardiotoxicities through science.[11,31,44]

Cardio-Oncology Research Fellowship

Given the lack of formal accreditation for cardio-oncology programs, variation exists on an individual program level that may cater to the strengths of a particular program.[11] Research training may co-exist within the patient care framework in a clinically oriented program or be a more dedicated research-focused training in hybrid programs. One of the challenges within cardiology is the increasing duration of training across many of the subspecialties. In order to justify the incremental time spent beyond the years of training in internal medicine, general cardiology, and clinical cardio-oncology, the research aspects should serve as a foundation for next steps when transitioning into a faculty position. Ideally, it should lead to external funding opportunities from industry or from NIH/National Cancer Institute (NCI). A recent ACC training statement suggests a research project for trainees in cardio-oncology.[11] Level II trainees are expected to participate in a research project, whereas level III trainees are expected to complete at least 1 research project, leading to publication during their training.[11] In a recent survey of 16 graduated fellows from 6 institutions who completed training commensurate with level II to III cardio-oncology–specific competency between 2014 and 2020, fellows averaged 5 to 6 months of research during their 3 to 4 years of training.[45]

A distinct benefit of training in cardio-oncology is the opportunity to collaborate with expansive teams with experts from both cardiology and oncology. This overlap and synergy provide access to multiple potential sources of mentors and funding. As an example, at the authors' institution the cardiology fellow working on epidemiologic breast cancer research receives guidance from a cardio-oncologist, breast oncologist, and cancer epidemiologist, ensuring a high-quality product. Although the mentor is a cardiologist/cardio-oncologist, funding for the data source is from NIH/NCI, and statistical support is provided by the oncology research team.

Training the Multidisciplinary Cardiovascular Team

The need to train the cardiovascular team in the general and specialized concepts of cardio-oncology and implementation research is critical to advancing the care of this complex population.[46] At the time of this writing there is no formalized training programs within any of the current pathways of any professions that systematically encompasses structured training and evaluation of nonphysician members of the cardiovascular team. In the present state, cardiovascular or oncology education and training is occurring in silos and either occurs through didactic means or on the job training. There exist opportunities to work collaboratively between the various cardiovascular team members professional and the cardiovascular/oncology societies to promote and develop the competencies, training programs, and certifications required to assure a competent, effective, and knowledgeable team. Ideally, the foundation education and training would encompass and mirror the same elements found for the physician teams but there will be slight modifications that would be tailored to each profession's expertise and scope.[11] There would need to be some urgency to the development of these programs, given the rapid expansion and ever evolving cardio-oncology field. In addition, there would need to be programs to train clinicians who are already in practice and transitioning into cardio-oncology as well as development of future cardio-oncology team members; this could be accomplished through a combination of fellowships, residencies, certification programs, and other educational programs. Finally, it is critical these programs be interdisciplinary with a research component to create a symphony within the team.

CAREER DEVELOPMENT
Journal Articles and Editorial Boards

Several journals are dedicated solely to cardio-oncology or have cardio-oncology sections, such as JACC: CardioOncology (by the *ACC*), CardioOncology (hosted on BMC by Springer Nature), Frontiers in Cardiovascular Medicine (Cardio-Oncology Section), Current Oncology Reports, and Current Treatment Options in Oncology. Serving as a reviewer for these journals can provide opportunities to access the most cutting-edge scientific research well before the research becomes public; this helps reviewers stay current on research and begin examining their own work through critical lens. Indeed, peer review enables improvement as a writer and, ultimately, as a published author. Peer review requires critical thinking skills that can inform subsequent academic work and assist in further developing scientific inquiry methods in one's academic career. Reviewing teaches how to be critical of one's own research. Identifying the strengths and weaknesses of others' research increases the likelihood of incorporating the strengths and avoiding the same weaknesses. As a result, serving as a cardio-oncology journal article reviewer can provide substantial benefits, expand field of vision, and generate new ideas for future research. Participating on the journals' editorial board additionally facilitates gaining an understanding of the editorial process, which will enhance one's own article submissions. Being on editorial boards also offers pathways to contribute to journal and specialty development. Serving as a reviewer then as an editorial board member can help advance lifelong learning in cardio-oncology translational and implementation science.

Didactic Meetings and Conferences

Formal and structured continuing education (CE) is also of importance for training in cardio-oncology translational and implementation science; this is relevant for all members of the multidisciplinary cardiology team, including clinicians, nurses, advanced practice providers, pharmacists, trainees, and others.[1] Among clinicians and trainees, specialties represented should include, at a minimum, cardiology (particularly cardio-oncology), medical oncology, hematology, surgical oncology, and radiation oncology. CE should be pursued by those who have completed formal training in cardio-oncology and also by those who may just be starting out in the field. CE can take many forms, especially leveraging innovative platforms and methods of learning in the Digital Era. Given the current accessibility of the global learning community, several options for collaborative CE should be considered.

These options include attendance online or in-person at local, regional, national, and international didactic courses, meetings, and conferences, as well as participation in synchronous and asynchronous CME offerings, in addition to engaging with social media posts (eg, educational polls, quizzes, tutorials, live chats) and podcasts, along with being abreast of the latest relevant articles that are published or in press, or under consideration if encountered in the role of journal reviewer or editorial board member. The primary national meetings relevant to cardio-oncology translational and implementation science training and research are the annual scientific sessions of the AHA and ACC, the ACC Cardio-oncology course titled Advancing the Cardiovascular Care of the Oncology Patient, and the annual scientific sessions of the ASCO.

Also available are various summits, conferences, and symposia hosted by various academic organizations in the United States (eg, Memorial Sloan Kettering Cancer Center, Mayo Clinic, Scripps, Rush University, Duke, Washington University, Ohio State University, and the FDA). International options are also available and include the Global Cardio-Oncology Summit, Cardiology Oncology Innovation Network (COIN) Summit, Cardio Oncology Society of Southern Africa, Israel Society Cardio Oncology, Cardio-oncology International Virtual Symposium, International Colloquium on Cardio-Oncology, and National Institute on Aging/American Geriatrics Society Conference on Cancer and Cardiovascular Disease. Several institutions (eg, University of Tennessee Health Sciences Center, Moffitt Cancer Center, Duke University, and Vanderbilt University) also provide public access to their cardio-oncology grand round series. These local, regional, national, and international meetings frequently offer accredited CE and many maintain these offerings online for review long after completion of the live meetings. Innovative platforms for education are being used, with the most common being customized mobile health applications.

Role of Social Media

Social media has the potential to revolutionize CME.[47] Social media–based learning is asynchronous, allowing for access to educational content at any time or location and at one's own pace, transforming learning into something that is portable, real-time, and collaborative.[47] The microblogging site Twitter is an innovative platform for delivering continuing medical education to the health care

community, leveraging the advantages and practicalities of an untethered and collaborative learning environment.[47] Twitter enables the expansion of educational opportunities in cardio-oncology, especially during the COVID-19 pandemic.

Activities related to networking and education in the cardio-oncology social media community (commonly referred to on the microblogging platform Twitter as #CardioOnc) frequently occur around the time of major national scientific sessions for major professional societies in Cardiology and Oncology, such as the ACC, AHA, European Society of Cardiology, and ASCO.[48] Most of the participants in the social chatter surrounding these conferences are actively tweeting pearls and insights from the sessions or reactions to the scientific data. Such efforts by those in attendance and those remotely "listening" to conference chatter on social media help to increase engagement and conference-related education among cardiologists, oncologists, and hematologists worldwide, even if they are unable to attend in person; this increases access to continuing educational materials that would otherwise be restricted to in-person attendees. In particular, tweeting specifically from and about cardio-oncology sessions, posters, and gatherings at these conferences or at dedicated cardio-oncology conferences educates others currently practicing or in training to meet the growing needs of cancer survivors, which remains an important need.[49]

Numerous meetings and scientific sessions have been canceled as a result of the COVID-19 pandemic. Twitter has therefore been leveraged to spread the word about educational webinars and published material in the pandemic; this will continue in the Digital Era even beyond the pandemic. #CardioTwitter is an excellent platform for reporting live from various medical conferences around the world, allowing for immediate knowledge transfer, idea exchange, and lively discussion. Perhaps this was most evident during the COVID19 pandemic, when numerous conferences went virtual.[50] Online journal clubs, chats, tutorials, and podcasts are additional emerging methods for increasing health care professionals' engagement with educational efforts on SoMe.[51]

Journal club

The purpose of Twitter-based journal clubs is to connect clinicians, educators, and researchers in order to discuss recent research and facilitate its dissemination.[52] Twitter-based journal clubs that meet virtually and provide a forum for participants from a variety of disciplines and across the globe are becoming increasingly prevalent.[51] Twitter journal clubs are frequently journal-sponsored and can affect journal metrics.[47] Journal clubs may be moderated by a journal social media editor and feature at least one study investigator or special guest.[47]

Twitter chat

Twitter chats are discussions that take place on Twitter at a predetermined time and date about a specific subject. Each Twitter chat is identified by a hashtag, which enables everyone on Twitter to attend or participate. To add a comment or respond to a question, Twitter users can include the chat hashtag in their tweets. Notably, a Twitter Chat campaign focused on education and advocacy in cardio-oncology accumulated ~ 1.2 million impressions (views by Twitter users) in 24 hours.[53] High engagement was noted, with tweets demonstrating (1) knowledge impartation (K), (2) advocacy awareness (A), (3) interdisciplinary collaboration (I), and (4) learning impact (L), termed "KAIL."[53]

Tweetorials

SoMe are a brief series of multimedia tweets that contain clinical bullet point educational content on a particular subject.[54] Tweetorials are essentially condensed lectures composed entirely of linked tweets.[55] Often, tweetorials are interactive, with polls to solicit participation, step-by-step disclosure of diagnostic clues, and opportunities for questions and feedback.[54] Some educators have compiled multimedia slides into GIFs (Graphics Interchange Format) or Twitter Moments in order to deliver teaching points.[54] Many SoMe users use Threader.app to consolidate their tweetorials into a single continuous webpage posted on Twitter for easy reading.

Podcasts

Podcasts are digital audio recordings typically in the form of a series of discussions, typically with new installments delivered automatically to subscribers. Podcasts have now become frequently accessed for succinct descriptions of classic and up-to-date cardio-oncology material, and are often posted on Twitter.

SUMMARY

Heart health is becoming particularly crucial for cancer survivors, as improved survival rates have resulted in an increased frequency of survivors suffering from cardiovascular disease. As a result, the interdisciplinary field of cardio-oncology has expanded rapidly in recent years to meet the cardiovascular care needs of this distinct population through clinical care and research initiatives.

Herein, the authors have reviewed an advantageous infrastructure and system of training for career development in cardio-oncology translational and implementation science, with emphases on collaborations among scientists and the role of the multidisciplinary cardiovascular team in both research and patient care and the impact of social media in the Digital Era. Such an approach will be key to incorporate health services research training in cardio-oncology guided by appropriate implementation science frameworks. This important approach will therefore continue to be applied and assessed in the setting of established and ongoing translational and implementation science practice and training models.

DISCLOSURE

This publication was supported by the National Center for Advancing Translational Sciences, National Institutes of Health, through Grant Numbers UL1TR001436 and KL2TR001438. Its contents are solely the responsibility of the authors and do not necessarily represent the official views of the NIH. The authors have no other relevant disclosures.

REFERENCES

1. Siegel RL, Miller KD, Fuchs HE, et al. Cancer statistics, 2021. CA Cancer J Clin 2021;71(1):7–33.
2. Miller KD, Nogueira L, Mariotto AB, et al. Cancer treatment and survivorship statistics, 2019. CA Cancer J Clin 2019;69(5):363–85.
3. Snipelisky D, Park JY, Lerman A, et al. How to develop a cardio-oncology clinic. Heart Fail Clin 2017;13(2):347–59.
4. Brown SA, Patel S, Rayan D, et al. A virtual-hybrid approach to launching a cardio-oncology clinic during a pandemic. Cardiooncology 2021;7(1):2.
5. Herrmann J, Loprinzi C, Ruddy K. Building a cardio-onco-hematology program. Curr Oncol Rep 2018; 20(10):81.
6. Fradley MG, Brown AC, Shields B, et al. Developing a comprehensive cardio-oncology program at a cancer institute: the moffitt cancer center experience. Oncol Rev 2017;11(2):340.
7. Sadler D, Chaulagain C, Alvarado B, et al. Practical and cost-effective model to build and sustain a cardio-oncology program. Cardiooncology 2020;6: 9.
8. Okwuosa TM, Akhter N, Williams KA, et al. Building a cardio-oncology program in a small- to medium-sized, nonprimary cancer center, academic hospital in the USA: challenges and pitfalls. Future Cardiol 2015;11(4):413–20.

9. Sundlöf DW, Patel BD, Schadler KC, et al. Development of a cardio-oncology program in a community hospital. JACC CardioOncol 2019;1(2):310–3.

10. Hayek SS, Ganatra S, Lenneman C, et al. Preparing the cardiovascular workforce to care for oncology patients: JACC review topic of the week. J Am Coll Cardiol 2019;73(17):2226–35.

11. Alvarez-Cardona JA, Ray J, Carver J, et al. Cardio-oncology education and training: JACC Council perspectives. J Am Coll Cardiol 2020;76(19):2267–81.

12. Fradley MG, Beckie TM, Brown SA, et al. Recognition, prevention, and management of arrhythmias and autonomic disorders in cardio-oncology: a scientific statement from the american heart association. Circulation 2021;144(3):e41–55.

13. Gilchrist SC, Barac A, Ades PA, et al. Cardio-oncology rehabilitation to manage cardiovascular outcomes in cancer patients and survivors: a scientific statement from the american heart association. Circulation 2019;139(21):e997–1012.

14. Campia U, Moslehi JJ, Amiri-Kordestani L, et al. Cardio-oncology: vascular and metabolic perspectives: a scientific statement from the American heart association. Circulation 2019;139(13):e579–602.

15. Asnani A, Moslehi JJ, Adhikari BB, et al. Preclinical models of cancer therapy-associated cardiovascular toxicity: a scientific statement from the American heart association. Circ Res 2021;129(1):e21–34.

16. Plana JC, Galderisi M, Barac A, et al. Expert consensus for multimodality imaging evaluation of adult patients during and after cancer therapy: a report from the American Society of Echocardiography and the European Association of Cardiovascular Imaging. Eur Heart J Cardiovasc Imaging 2014;15(10):1063–93.

17. Armenian SH, Lacchetti C, Barac A, et al. Prevention and monitoring of cardiac dysfunction in survivors of adult cancers: american society of clinical oncology clinical practice guideline. J Clin Oncol 2017;35(8):893–911.

18. Iliescu CA, Grines CL, Herrmann J, et al. SCAI Expert consensus statement: evaluation, management, and special considerations of cardio-oncology patients in the cardiac catheterization laboratory (endorsed by the cardiological society of india, and sociedad Latino Americana de Cardiología intervencionista). Catheter Cardiovasc Interv 2016;87(5):E202–23.

19. Lenihan DJ, Hartlage G, DeCara J, et al. Cardio-oncology training: a proposal from the international cardioncology society and canadian cardiac oncology network for a new multidisciplinary specialty. J Card Fail 2016;22(6):465–71.

20. The Childhood Cancer Survivor Study. Available at: https://ccss.stjude.org/. Accessed January 1, 2021.

21. Mahmood SS, Fradley MG, Cohen JV, et al. Myocarditis in patients treated with immune checkpoint inhibitors. J Am Coll Cardiol 2018;71(16):1755–64.

22. Drobni ZD, Alvi RM, Taron J, et al. Association between immune checkpoint inhibitors with cardiovascular events and atherosclerotic plaque. Circulation 2020;142(24):2299–311.

23. Zaha VG, Meijers WC, Moslehi J. Cardio-immuno-oncology. Circulation 2020;141(2):87–9.

24. Lancellotti P, Suter TM, López-Fernández T, et al. Cardio-oncology services: rationale, organization, and implementation: a report from the ESC cardio-oncology council. Eur Heart J 2018;40(22):1756–63.

25. Bauer MS, Damschroder L, Hagedorn H, et al. An introduction to implementation science for the nonspecialist. BMC Psychol 2015;3:32.

26. Aarons GA, Reeder K, Miller CJ, et al. Identifying strategies to promote team science in dissemination and implementation research. J Clin Translational Sci 2020;4(3):180–7.

27. Bradshaw PT, Stevens J, Khankari N, et al. Cardiovascular disease mortality among breast cancer survivors. Epidemiology 2016;27(1):6–13.

28. Moslehi JJ. Cardiovascular toxic effects of targeted cancer therapies. N Engl J Med 2016;375(15):1457–67.

29. Iacopo F, Branch M, Cardinale D, et al. Preventive cardio-oncology: cardiovascular disease prevention in cancer patients and survivors. Curr Treat Options Cardiovasc Med 2021;23(1):1–23.

30. Tuzovic M, Brown S-A, Yang EH, et al. Implementation of cardio-oncology training for cardiology fellows. Washington DC: American College of Cardiology Foundation; 2020.

31. Fradley MG. Cardio-oncology fellowship training and education. Curr Treat Options Cardiovasc Med 2019;21(6):27.

32. Cardinale D, Sandri MT. Role of biomarkers in chemotherapy-induced cardiotoxicity. Prog Cardiovasc Dis 2010;53(2):121–9.

33. Pistillucci G, Ciorra AA, Sciacca V, et al. [Troponin I and B-type Natriuretic Peptide (BNP) as biomarkers for the prediction of cardiotoxicity in patients with breast cancer treated with adjuvant anthracyclines and trastuzumab]. Clin Ter 2015;166(1):e67–71.

34. Thavendiranathan P, Poulin F, Lim KD, et al. Use of myocardial strain imaging by echocardiography for the early detection of cardiotoxicity in patients during and after cancer chemotherapy: a systematic review. J Am Coll Cardiol 2014;63(25 Pt A):2751–68.

35. Stoodley PW, Richards DA, Meikle SR, et al. The potential role of echocardiographic strain imaging for evaluating cardiotoxicity due to cancer therapy. Heart Lung Circ 2011;20(1):3–9.

36. America IoMUCoQoHCi. Crossing the Quality Chasm: A New Health System for the 21st Century. 2001.

37. Berwick DM, Nolan TW, Whittington J. The triple aim: care, health, and cost. Health Aff (Millwood) 2008; 27(3):759–69.

38. Bluethmann SM, Mariotto AB, Rowland JH. Anticipating the "Silver Tsunami": prevalence trajectories and comorbidity burden among older cancer survivors in the United States. Cancer Epidemiol Biomarkers Prev 2016;25(7):1029–36.

39. Suh E, Stratton KL, Leisenring WM, et al. Late mortality and chronic health conditions in long-term survivors of early-adolescent and young adult cancers: a retrospective cohort analysis from the Childhood Cancer Survivor Study. Lancet Oncol 2020;21(3): 421–35.

40. Chao C, Bhatia S, Xu L, et al. Chronic comorbidities among survivors of adolescent and young adult cancer. J Clin Oncol 2020;38(27):3161–74.

41. Guida JL, Ahles TA, Belsky D, et al. Measuring aging and identifying aging phenotypes in cancer survivors. J Natl Cancer Inst 2019;111(12):1245–54.

42. Blaes AH, Shenoy C. Is it time to include cancer in cardiovascular risk prediction tools? Lancet 2019; 394(10203):986–8.

43. Brown S-A. Cardio-Oncology Fellowships. Available at: https://www.cardioonctrain.com/fellowships. Accessed January 1, 2021.

44. Johnson MN, Steingart R, Carver J. How to develop a cardio-oncology fellowship. Heart Fail Clin 2017; 13(2):361–6.

45. Tuzovic M, Brown SA, Yang EH, et al. Implementation of cardio-oncology training for cardiology fellows. JACC CardioOncol 2020;2(5):795–9.

46. Brown SA, Sandhu N. Proposing and meeting the need for interdisciplinary cardio-oncology subspecialty training. J Card Fail 2016;22(11):934–5.

47. Thamman R, Gulati M, Narang A, et al. Twitter-based learning for continuing medical education? Eur Heart J 2020;41(46):4376–9.

48. Jackson S, Tanoue M, Shahandeh N, et al. Reaching across the digital aisle: a comparison of cardio-oncology-related tweets at cardiology and oncology conferences from 2014-2018. J Am Coll Cardiol CardioOnc. 2021 Sep, 3 (3) 457-460. https://www.jacc.org/doi/10.1016/j.jaccao.2021.08.003.

49. Brown SA, Daly RP, Duma N, et al. Leveraging social media for cardio-oncology. Curr Treat Options Oncol 2020;21(10):83.

50. Masri A, Remme CA, Jneid H. #Cardiotwitter: the global cardiology fellowship. J Am Heart Assoc 2021;10(14):e020719.

51. Parwani P, Choi AD, Lopez-Mattei J, et al. Understanding social media: opportunities for cardiovascular medicine. J Am Coll Cardiol 2019;73(9): 1089–93.

52. Wray CM, Auerbach AD, Arora VM. The adoption of an online journal club to improve research dissemination and social media engagement among hospitalists. J Hosp Med 2018;13(11):764–9.

53. Conley CC, Goyal NG, Brown SA. #CardioOncology: twitter chat as a mechanism for increasing awareness of heart health for cancer patients. Cardiooncology 2020;6:19.

54. Parwani P, Choi AD, Swamy P, et al. Social media: the new paradigm for cardiovascular case reports. JACC Case Rep 2019;1(3):452–6.

55. Cifu AS, Vandross AL, Prasad V. Case reports in the age of twitter. Am J Med 2019;132(10):e725–6.

Spectrum of National Institutes of Health-Funded Research in Cardio-Oncology

A Basic, Clinical, and Observational Science Perspective

Bishow B. Adhikari, PhD[a,*], Scarlet Shi, PhD[b], Eileen P. Dimond, BSN, MSN[c], Nonniekaye Shelburne, CRNP, MS, AOCN[d], Patrice Desvigne-Nickens, MD[e], Lori M. Minasian, MD[f]

KEYWORDS

- Cardiotoxicity • Cardiovascular toxicity • Cardiovascular complications • Cancer therapy
- Cancer treatment • Chemotherapy • Cardiac toxicity • Radiation injury

KEY POINTS

- Although survival from cancer is improving dramatically with newer and improved therapies, the incidence and impact of cancer treatment-related cardiotoxicity also has grown. In response, the National Institutes of Health (NIH) is supporting a broad range of basic/translational, clinical/interventional, and observational studies in cardio-oncology. The National Cancer Institute (NCI) and the National Heart, Lung, and Blood Institute (NHLBI) jointly held workshops to identify gaps and future research opportunities and released funding opportunity announcements to advance the science in this area.
- With the improvements in cancer treatments and survival, research opportunities exist to better predict, mitigate, and manage the acute, chronic, and late-onset cardiovascular effects of cancer therapy and improve the quality of life for cancer survivors.
- A review of recently funded cardio-oncology research during the past decade shows that NIH research support on cardiotoxicity has been increasing. Most studies have focused on anthracyclines or anthracycline-containing treatment regimens (eg, with trastuzumab and/or radiotherapy). Future research could also address the potential cardiovascular complications of emerging therapeutics and treatment regimens.
- Understanding, predicting, and managing cancer treatment-induced cardiovascular adverse events could be addressed by a collaborative and multi-disciplinary research approach to synergize research advances across cardiovascular and oncology science.

[a] Division of Cardiovascular Sciences, National Heart, Lung, and Blood Institute, NIH6705 Rockledge Drive, Room 313-J, MSC 7956, Bethesda, MD 20892-7956, USA; [b] Division of Cardiovascular Sciences, NHLBI, NIH, 6705 Rockledge Drive, Room 313-H, MSC 7956, Bethesda, MD 20817, USA; [c] Division of Cancer Prevention, NCI, NIH, 9609 Medical Center Drive Room 5E332, Bethesda, MD 20892, USA; [d] Division of Cancer Control and Population Sciences, NCI, NIH, 9609 Medical Center Drive Room 4E110, Bethesda, MD 20892, USA; [e] Division of Cardiovascular Sciences, NHLBI, NIH, 6705 One Rockledge Drive, Room 312-B2, Bethesda, MD 20892-7940, USA; [f] Division of Cancer Prevention, NCI, NIH, 9609 Medical Center Dr. Room 5E342, Bethesda, MD 20892, USA
* Corresponding author.
E-mail address: adhikarb@mail.nih.gov

Heart Failure Clin 18 (2022) 515–528
https://doi.org/10.1016/j.hfc.2022.01.001

INTRODUCTION

Cardiovascular complications from cancer therapy remain a significant and growing health challenge. Nowhere is this more apparent than in the rising population of cancer survivors who are at an increased risk of cardiovascular complications. In the US today, there are ~17 million pediatric and adult cancer survivors, a nearly 1.2-fold increase from ~14 million in 2012 and projected to increase to ~22 million by 2030.[1–3] This positive trend of survival is welcome news for patients with cancer and clearly demonstrates the dramatic improvements in the efficacy of many anticancer treatments in recent years.[4] However, improved survival is associated with a parallel rise in the incidence of cancer treatment-related cardiovascular toxicity and increased morbidity and mortality in survivors.[5–8] Longer survival duration together with age-related comorbidities and newer therapies with unknown cardiotoxicity potential in pediatric and adult patients with cancer may result in further increases in cardiotoxicity risk in survivors. Anticancer therapies continue to improve and expand rapidly from the traditional cytotoxic chemotherapies and radiation to targeted immunomodulatory agents and newer immuno-based therapies, such as immune checkpoint inhibitors (ICI) and chimeric antigen receptor T-cell (CAR-T) immunotherapies.[9–11] Increasingly, these therapies are used in multiple combined treatment regimens across numerous cancer types at the time of diagnosis, progression, and relapse. As new cancer therapies continue to emerge and expand rapidly, as treatment regimens become more complex and as cancer survival continues to improve, we can expect cancer treatment-induced cardiotoxicity to remain a highly significant health challenge.

Cardiotoxicity generally refers to all forms of cardiovascular complications. Although cardiotoxicity has been an established consequence of anthracyclines such as doxorubicin, the explosion of approved anticancer agents has led to a rethinking of the full spectrum of cardiovascular adverse effects that can result from targeting new pathways, stimulating the immune system, and revising radiation strategies. Cardiovascular sequelae may manifest as acute, chronic, or late-onset adverse events. Acute cardiotoxicity that occurs during or immediately after therapy may lead to dose modifications, dose delays, and even cessation of cancer therapy. Patients on chronic cancer therapy, with or without co-existing cardiovascular disease or comorbidities, may develop chronic or cumulative cardiovascular complications. Late-onset cardiotoxicity that occurs years or decades after

cancer treatments may lead to increased morbidity and early mortality due to what is thought to mimic an accelerated treatment-induced cardiovascular disease progression.[12–14] While the methods of diagnosis and monitoring may be similar, the management strategies and implementation of cardioprotective interventions for acute, chronic, and late-onset cardiotoxicity require distinctly different approaches, implying that cardiovascular complications can be progressive and may involve a highly nonuniform or complex pathogenic process.

Risk assessment tools, which aid the prevention and management of cardiotoxicity risk, are currently lacking for many cancer treatments. The risk of cardiovascular toxicity depends greatly on the treatment regimen. In addition, other factors such as cardiovascular health status, age, genetics, social determinants of health, and environmental stress may further add to an individual's risk of cardiovascular complications. Unfortunately, how these risk factors combine to determine the timing of onset, clinical and subclinical presentations, and clinical outcomes are not fully understood for most anticancer treatment regimens. As a result, it has been challenging to critically assess the individual risk profile of cardiotoxicity and develop effective management strategies for prevention, treatment, and monitoring. These challenges are hindering improvements in clinical outcomes and quality of life in cancer survivors. Furthermore, clinical guidelines for managing the risk of cardiotoxicity from specific cancer treatment regimens have focused primarily on managing the cardiovascular adverse effects from Adriamycin and radiation.[15–20] To date, limited evidence exists to support clinical guidelines for other cancer treatment regimens. Enhanced research collaborations between cardiologists and oncologists could generate the evidence needed to support more comprehensive guidelines.

The development of new diagnostic and cardioprotective approaches requires advances in the mechanistic understanding of cardiovascular injury. Despite undergoing extensive safety testing during development, nearly all anticancer therapeutic agents have the potential to cause cardiovascular complications.[21,22] The known adverse cellular and tissue impacts of cancer therapies include dysfunction of the cardiac myocytes and other cells of the cardiovascular system, such as vascular endothelial cells, cardiac macrophages, cardiac fibroblasts, and myofibroblasts; injury to the vasculature; cardiac valvular dysfunction; hemodynamic flow alterations; thrombotic events; and radiation-mediated tissue damage.[9,23]

However, the molecular mechanisms of the injury remain unclear. This uncertainty is illustrated by the case for anthracyclines, one of the earliest and most common classes of anticancer therapeutic agents. Reported molecular mechanisms of anthracycline (eg, doxorubicin) cardiotoxicity include topoisomerase 2β (Top2b) mediated DNA damage; mitochondrial dysfunction; alterations of calcium, cell survival, and metabolic signaling pathways; excessive reactive oxygen species (ROS); dysregulation of neuregulin-1 and endothelin-1 signaling; and ultimately, autophagy and apoptosis.[24] While such research advances have contributed to new diagnostics and cardioprotective approaches, anthracycline cardiotoxicity remains an active research area and new research findings continue to reveal additional mechanisms by which these therapeutic agents cause cardiovascular complications. For other more recent pharmacologic, biologic, targeted therapeutic agents, radiation therapy, or combination treatment regimens, much less is known about the cellular and molecular mechanisms that lead to cardiovascular injury.

The goals of research advances in cancer treatment-induced cardiotoxicity are to optimize cancer treatment efficacy while minimizing cardiotoxicity risk. This broad research field spans risk assessment, prevention, diagnosis, monitoring, treatment, and management. As cancer treatments continue to improve and expand, early assessment of whether the treatments pose cardiotoxicity sequelae might support more effective integration of preventive and cardioprotective approaches. Recently, several pathogenic mechanisms have been recognized as common elements in cancer and cardiac disorders; thus, studies of cardiovascular effects of anticancer agents have the potential to inform basic and translational mechanisms in cardiovascular disease.[25] Although NIH-supported research continues to support significant scientific advances, major research gaps remain in areas such as the mechanistic understanding of cardiovascular injury, preclinical risk evaluations, preclinical disease models, chronic and late-onset mechanisms, and development and assessment of preventive and cardioprotective approaches.

NATIONAL INSTITUTES OF HEALTH WORKSHOPS AND FUNDING OPPORTUNITY ANNOUNCEMENTS

To address the growing research challenges and gaps in cancer treatment-related cardiotoxicity, the NCI and NHLBI cosponsored a workshop entitled "Cancer Treatment-Related Cardiotoxicity: Understanding the Current State of Knowledge and Future Research Priorities" in March 2013.[26] The goals of the workshop were to identify knowledge gaps and research barriers and to help determine how best to prioritize research opportunities, allocate resources, and establish needed infrastructure. While recognizing the broad scope of multiple cardiotoxicity disorders, this initial workshop focused primarily on hypertension and heart failure and included all cancer treatment modalities in use at that time. Over 40 scientific knowledge gaps and research opportunities were identified by the workshop.[26] In addition, several resources and infrastructure for the research community were identified. The workshop helped increase collaborations among the cardiovascular and cancer research investigators who are involved in cardiotoxicity research.

An early concern regarding cardiotoxicity that became evident during the discussions at the workshop was the nonuniform and poorly defined cardiotoxicity terms used to record the various cardiovascular complications across different clinical studies at the time. To address this issue, 2 working groups were established following the workshop that was facilitated by the NCI: one for adverse event reporting and another for data collection in randomized clinical trials. These working groups have continued to refine, standardize, and harmonize cardiotoxicity terms in clinical data across the different adverse events reporting and clinical trial studies and this effort has enhanced the sharing and utility of the collected data.[27] Additionally, the recognition of this issue by the cardio-oncology research community subsequently led to the revision of the clinical care guidelines for pediatric and adult cancer survivors which were published by the American Society of Cardio-Oncology in 2017[15,27] and by the European Society of Medical Oncology in 2020.[28]

A follow-on workshop entitled "Changing Hearts and Minds: Improving Outcomes in Cancer Treatment-Related Cardiotoxicity" was held in June 2018 to evaluate progress, reassess research gaps, identify emerging areas of research opportunities, and update the scientific priorities since the 2013 workshop.[29] This workshop included all forms of cardiotoxicity as defined by cardiac and/or vascular specific common terminology criteria for adverse events. Significant research challenges remained despite the substantial progress since the first workshop, such as an expanded cardiotoxicity portfolio of NIH research awards, establishment of interdisciplinary working groups within cardiology and oncology, initiation of several prevention and management trials, and development of cardio-oncology specific clinical guidelines. These challenges were, in part, due to the proliferation of new and improved cancer treatments and continued improvement in survival duration. Over 20 additional research gaps and emerging research opportunities were identified by the second workshop.[29] Together with the research gaps identified by the earlier workshop, the updated knowledge gaps and research priorities provide a comprehensive and detailed roadmap of research opportunities in the field and serve as a useful resource of information for researchers who are interested in pursuing cardio-oncology research.

In November 2015, NCI and NHLBI released the first set of 2 Funding Opportunity Announcements (FOAs) aimed at addressing the broad research gaps in cancer treatment-related cardiotoxicity (**Table 1**). The reason for having 2 FOAs was to allow both exploratory (ie, R21, PA16–036) as well as standard (ie, R01, PA16–035) research project grant proposals. The goal of the solicitations was to encourage collaborative applications from cardiology and oncology researchers to focus on the identification and characterization of patients at risk of developing cancer treatment-related cardiotoxicity and developing mitigation/prevention strategies to minimize cardiovascular dysfunction while optimizing cancer outcomes. Innovative methods designed to evaluate cardiac risk before treatment and integrate evidence-based cancer treatment regimens with screening, diagnostic, and/or management strategies were encouraged. These FOAs were subsequently renewed twice, first in November 2017 (PA18–003 and PA18–013) and again in December 2018 (PA19–111 and PA19–112), and covered 11 grant application receipt cycles over a period of nearly 5 years (see **Table 1**).

SPECTRUM OF NATIONAL INSTITUTES OF HEALTH -SUPPORTED RESEARCH PROJECTS

To date, NCI and NHLBI have supported 33 research project grants through the above FOAs amounting to nearly $26M[a] in research support (*data accessed on August 4, 2021*). Four of the funded exploratory R21 research awards led to subsequent funding of the larger R01 research awards. The research awards have supported the careers of 5 early-stage investigators and 2 new investigators. In addition, the FOAs have resulted in the funding of several clinical trials.

Most of the awarded research projects have begun recently and thus the research work is ongoing. The topics of research supported by these R21 and R01 awards are included below under the research categories.

Beyond the FOAs, NIH has been supporting cancer treatment-related cardiotoxicity research through the investigator-initiated research projects. To get an idea of the approximate extent of research support and potential research gaps and trends, a keyword search was conducted on the database of NIH-funded research projects over a 10-year period, from the fiscal year 2011 to 2020.[30] The search was limited to the title, abstract and specific aims sections of the awarded grant applications. Only new or competing renewal projects were counted to avoid duplicate counting of multi-year awarded projects. The output of the search was verified to ensure that the resulted list of grant awards contained the keywords used for the search in those sections. The list was then adjudicated by the authors to ensure that at least one or more aims of the projects were focused on cancer treatment-related cardiotoxicity. Duplicates, intramural projects, or inadvertent grants were removed, and the grants were separated into 3 broad categories: basic and translational, clinical trials and interventions, and observational. For most of the awards, the categorization was unanimous, for a few where there was disagreement, discussion among the reviewers facilitated consensus. It should be noted that the keyword search strategy may miss or overestimate the actual number of research projects that focus on cancer treatment-related cardiotoxicity. Additionally, the categorization is subjective. The list of the funded research projects identified here thus is a representative spectrum of NIH support on this topic rather than a comprehensive portfolio analysis.

Over the 10-year period, the search yielded a set of 102 awarded research projects amounting to a cumulative total of approximately $94M in NIH grant research support (**Fig. 1**). The NIH uses three-character activity codes to indicate the type of award mechanism (https://grants.nih.gov/grants/funding/ac_search_results.htm). The research projects in the list fell into 4 activity types: research project grants (activity codes: R01, R21, R56, R03, R15), training/career grants (activity codes: F32, K01, K08, K23, K24, K99, L30), small-business innovation research (SBIR) and technology transfer (STTR) grants (activity codes:

---

[a]All dollar values reported in this paper are in 2021 dollars, converted using the Biomedical Research and Development Price Index (BRDPI): https://officeofbudget.od.nih.gov/gbipriceindexes.html Accessed, August 27, 2021

Table 1
Workshops and funding opportunity announcements

NIH Workshops

Title	Date	Reference
Cancer Treatment-Related Cardiotoxicity: Understanding the Current State of Knowledge and Developing Future Research Priorities	3/20–21/2013	https://epi.grants.cancer.gov/events/cardiotoxicity/ Publication with the summary of future research opportunities[26]:
Changing Hearts and Minds: Improving Outcomes in Cancer Treatment-Related Cardiotoxicity	6/25–26/2018	https://epi.grants.cancer.gov/events/cardiotoxicity/improving-outcomes.html Publication with summary of future research opportunities:[29]

Funding Opportunity Announcements

Title	Number	Date	Website address
Improving Outcomes in Cancer Treatment-Related Cardiotoxicity (R01 & R21)	R01: PA16–035 R21: PA16–036	11/17/2015–1/24/2018	https://grants.nih.gov/grants/guide/pa-files/PA-16-035.html https://grants.nih.gov/grants/guide/pa-files/PA-16-036.html
Improving Outcomes in Cancer Treatment-Related Cardiotoxicity (R01 & R21, Clinical Trial Optional)	R01: PA-18–003 R21: PA-18–013	11/2/2017–12/17/2018	https://grants.nih.gov/grants/guide/pa-files/PA-18-003.html https://grants.nih.gov/grants/guide/pa-files/PA-18-013.html
Improving Outcomes in Cancer Treatment-Related Cardiotoxicity (R01 & R21, Clinical Trial Optional)	R01: PA-19–112 R21: PA-19–111	12/17/2018–1/8/2022	https://grants.nih.gov/grants/guide/pa-files/PA-19-112.html https://grants.nih.gov/grants/guide/pa-files/PA-19-111.html

R41, R43, U42, R44), and an "other" type to indicate exploratory resource-related grants (activity code: P20). The types of research projects and their respective funding are shown in **Fig. 1**A. It shows that, in terms of the number of projects, the largest percentage was research project grants (70%), followed by training (16%), small business SBIR/STTR (14%), and other (1%). The respective funding supports were 90% for the research project grants, 4% for training, 5% for small business SBIR/STTR, and 0.3% for the other grant award. The NHLBI and NCI each supported the largest numbers of research projects numbering 59 and 33, respectively, followed by the National Institute of General Medical Sciences (NIGMS), the National Institute of Biomedical Imaging and Bioengineering (NIBIB), the National

Institute of Allergy and Infectious Diseases (NIAID), and the National Institute of Environmental Health Sciences (NIEHS) supporting 5, 3, 1, and 1 awards, respectively (see **Fig. 1**B). Most of the projects were categorized as basic and translational (N = 63, 62%), followed by observational (N = 30, 29%), and clinical trials and interventions (N = 9, 9%) (see **Fig. 1**C).

The number of funded projects and the funding amounts for each year over the 10-year period are shown in **Fig. 1**D. The numbers inside the bars in **Fig. 1**D indicate the total number of awards in that year. Interestingly, although only a few awards were made every year between 2011 and 2013, the number of awards in 2014 increased dramatically to 14 awards, coinciding with a 1-year period following the first workshop held in

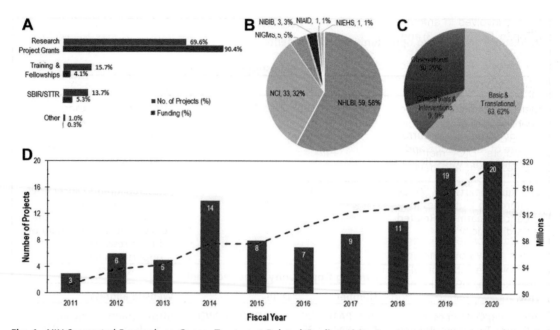

Fig. 1. *NIH-Supported Research on Cancer Treatment-Related Cardiotoxicity.* Representative spectrum of awarded research projects over a 10-year period (fiscal year 2011–2020) obtained by a keyword search of the title, abstract, and specific aims sections of the awarded grants from the NIH database of funded projects.[30] Total number of projects and funding were 102 and $94M, respectively. (*A*). In terms of the proportion of the types of research projects and respective funding, most of the projects and funding were for research project grants (70%, 90%), followed by training (16%, 4%), small business (SBIR/STTR) (14%, 5%), and other (1%, 0.3%, eg, resource) grants. (*B*). Number of projects and their corresponding Institute assignments. NHLBI and NCI supported the largest numbers of research projects, 59 and 32, respectively, followed by, NIGMS, NIBIB, NIAID, and NIEHS supporting 5, 3, 1, and 1, respectively. (*C*). Funded projects were categorized, based on the research aims, into basic and translational, clinical trials and interventions, and observational. As indicated, the majority were basic and translational (N = 63, 62%), followed by observational (N = 30, 29%) and clinical trials and interventions (N = 9, 9%). (*D*). The number of projects (*bar chart*, left y-axis) and approximate support amounts (*dotted line*, right vertical axis) for each year over the 10-year period. The numbers within the bars indicate the total number of awarded projects in that year. The number of projects began modestly between the years 2011 to 2013, jumped in year 14, then decreased again, and remained at 11 or below in years 2015 to 2018. The number of projects has recently risen significantly as seen in years 2019 and 2020. The corresponding funding support shows a gradual rise over the 10-year period, likely due to the multi-year funding periods (eg, 2–4 years) of the research projects.

2013. The number of awards dropped to 11 or less thereafter in years 2015 to 2018, but rose again significantly in years 2019 and 2020 (see **Fig. 1**D). Research funding shows a gradual increase in all years, likely due to the multi-year research funding period which typically ranges from 2 to 4 years for each research project (see **Fig. 1**D). The recent increase in the number of funded research awards and corresponding funding amounts reflect the potential positive impact of the second workshop augmented by the grants funded by the recent FOAs. The data indicate that research interest in cancer treatment-related cardiotoxicity in recent years has increased.

Basic and translational studies

In the basic and translational category, there were 37 grants with activity codes R01 and R21, which

are the activity codes for primary research-oriented projects. The aims of these research projects ranged from mechanistic studies and research model development to biomarkers of risk, development of clinical imaging methods for early subclinical cardiovascular injury, and novel cardioprotective therapeutic strategies. The focus of these basic research studies included understanding of cardiovascular injury mechanisms primarily related to anthracyclines (eg, doxorubicin) and a few related to radiation injury or adverse effects of other agents such as trastuzumab and tyrosine kinase inhibitors. Additional basic studies included the influence of sex differences, cancer cachexia, late-onset mechanisms, clonal hematopoiesis, and innate immune mechanisms. Several studies explored mitochondrial dysfunction and mechanistic understanding of metabolic or hypoxia-related cellular and molecular signaling pathways involved in anthracycline cardiotoxicity (eg, Top2b, CCR5, BAG3) and potential cardioprotective or therapeutic strategies to mitigate such cardiotoxicity. A few projects focused on the development of new *in vitro* human induced pluripotent stem cell-derived cardiomyocyte (iPSC-CM) models and animal models (eg, swine models for clinical imaging, cross-species validation, and so forth). Biomarker-related research included genetic factors, DNA methylation, biomarkers for risk assessment, and development of iPSC-CM-based *in vitro* methods for risk screening. Clinical imaging methods included improvements of imaging probes and imaging methods such as PET, SPECT-CT, and cardiac MRI for early injury evaluation. Cardioprotective and therapeutic studies included a few novel therapeutic agents such as small-molecule inhibitor of the serine–threonine protein kinase, p90RSK, new chemical analogs of doxorubicin, neuregulin-1 directed therapy to improve the potency of doxorubicin and alleviate its cardiotoxicity, a novel small peptide therapeutic to reduce radiation injury, liposome-encapsuled doxorubicin for ultrasound activated treatment and exercise.

In addition to the research project grants, there were 12 small business SBIR/STTR research projects in the basic and translational categories. The focus of these projects included the development of cardiac imaging probes for early detection of doxorubicin-induced cardiotoxicity, a cardiac MRI image-analysis tool to assess subclinical cardiac injury, a method to develop mature human iPSC-CMs for preclinical safety screening, a real-time microfluidic biosensor-based assay to monitor chemotherapy levels in blood, and several new therapeutic agents to reduce cardiotoxicity.

Clinical trials and interventional studies

There were a total of eight R01 and R21 research projects in the clinical trials and interventional studies category as shown in **Table 2**. The projects included the following:

- An evaluation of cardiac-sparing whole lung intensity-modulated radiation therapy (IMRT) aimed at reducing cardiovascular injury of radiotherapy treatment of lung metastases in young adults;
- Two randomized trials testing the effectiveness of statins in preserving left ventricular function following anthracycline treatment—one for triple-negative breast cancer and the other for non-Hodgkin's lymphoma;
- A trial evaluating whether early timing of and reduced-dose dexrazoxane is effective in

reducing doxorubicin-induced cardiotoxicity in patients with HER2-negative breast cancer;
- A pilot study to determine if a cardioprotective strategy guided by the biomarker, NT-proBNP, in patients with high-risk breast cancer or patients with lymphoma treated with doxorubicin is feasible, well-tolerated, and superior to usual care;
- Three trials on carvedilol:
  o A randomized, placebo-controlled trial to evaluate the cardioprotective effect of carvedilol on high-dose anthracycline treated childhood cancer survivors;
  o A randomized, placebo-controlled pilot trial to assess whether a risk-guided prior treatment with carvedilol is safe, feasible, well-tolerated, and effective in reducing cardiotoxicity in patients with high-risk breast cancer;
  o A trial to determine optimal preventive treatment strategy with carvedilol to reduce cardiomyopathy in patients with breast cancer undergoing trastuzumab therapy.

The IMRT radiotherapy and one of the earlier statin studies have concluded while the remaining 6 studies are ongoing (see **Table 2**). NCI sponsors several clinical trials networks to evaluate novel anticancer agents, compare standard versus experimental cancer treatment regimens, address cancer treatment toxicity via symptom mitigation research, and evaluate the effectiveness of cancer care delivery. In these networks, it is possible to integrate cardiotoxicity assessments as well as develop trials to answer cardiotoxicity questions[31]

Observational studies

There were a total of 19 R21 and R01 research project grants in the observational category. The majority were focused on the evaluation and validation of early cardiovascular risk assessment or detection of subclinical cardiovascular injury using ongoing patient trial data or data from cohorts of survivors following cancer therapies to inform and improve clinical outcomes in survivors. These include cardiac magnetic resonance (CMR) imaging, CMR-based algorithms, echocardiography or echocardiography-derived parameters, serum biomarkers, or combined imaging and serum biomarkers, maximum Vo_2 as a measure of cardiac reserve, CMR-derived aortic stiffness as a measure of early subclinical injury to the vasculature, and automated electronic health record (EHR)-based or genetics-based risk management tools. Several of the studies were ancillary studies that used clinical data from recent or ongoing clinical

Table 2
Clinical trials and interventions

Title, NCT#	Intervention	Goals	Study Population	Enrollment	Dates
Cardiac Sparing Whole Lung Intensity-Modulated Radiation Therapy (IMRT) in Children and Young Adults with Lung Metastases, NCT01586104	Whole lung intensity-modulated radiation therapy (WL-IMRT)	Demonstrate feasibility, dosimetric advantages, and short-term efficacy of WL-IMRT over the standard of care whole lung irradiation.	Children and young adults with lung metastases from Wilms tumor, rhabdomyosarcoma, and Ewing Sarcoma.	20 participants	2/2011–9/2015
Preventing Anthracycline Cardiovascular Toxicity with Statins (PREVENT), NCT01988571	Atorvastatin (a generic statin)	Double-blind, randomized, placebo-controlled trial to determine if atorvastatin administration attenuates deterioration in left ventricular ejection fraction (LVEF) in women receiving adjuvant anthracycline-based chemotherapy for breast cancer.	Women receiving anthracycline-based chemotherapy for triple-negative breast cancer.	279 participants	2/2014–9/2020
Prevention of Heart Failure induced by Doxorubicin with Early Administration of Dexrazoxane (PHOENIX1), NCT03930680	Dexrazoxane	Determine whether reduced dose and early administration of dexrazoxane prevent doxorubicin-induced cardiotoxicity.	Patients with nonmetastatic, HER2-negative, breast cancer HER2-negative, stage I–III female patients with breast cancer.	25 participants	6/2021–6/2023
Reducing the risk of anthracycline-related heart failure after childhood cancer (PREVENT-HF), NCT02717507	Carvedilol (beta-blocker)	Randomized, placebo-controlled trial of low-dose carvedilol (beta-blocker) to determine the impact of a 2-year course of carvedilol on left ventricular function.	Asymptomatic childhood cancer survivors with prior exposure to high-dose anthracyclines ($\geq$300 mg/m^2).	182 participants	4/2016–7/2022

Study	Drug/Strategy	Description	Population	Participants	Dates
Statins to prevent Cardiotoxicity from Anthracyclines (STOP-CA), NCT02943590	Atorvastatin (a generic statin)	Randomized placebo-controlled trial to determine whether statins preserve LVEF 12 months after the initiation of chemotherapy.	Patients with non-Hodgkin's Lymphoma undergoing anthracycline-based chemotherapy.	270 participants	1/2017–10/2023
Strategies in Cardiotoxicity Risk Reduction with Breast Cancer Therapy, NCT04023110	Risk-guided Carvedilol (beta-blocker)	A randomized, placebo-controlled pilot study to determine if a risk-guided treatment strategy that initiates carvedilol in high-risk patients before cancer therapy will be feasible, safe, well-tolerated, and result in decreases in cardiotoxicity measures, compared with placebo.	Patients from Penn Cardiotoxicity of Cancer Therapy (Penn CCT) study population, a longitudinal cohort study of 630 patients with breast cancer.	110 participants	8/2019–12/2023
The Feasibility of a Biomarker-Guided Strategy in Anthracycline Cardiotoxicity, NCT04737265	Biomarker (NT-proBNP) guided therapy strategy	Pilot study to determine if a biomarker-guided strategy (NT-proBNP) to identify and treat patients with high CV risk is feasible, well-tolerated, and superior to usual care in patients with breast cancer or lymphoma treated with doxorubicin.	Patients from Penn Cardiotoxicity of Cancer Therapy (Penn CCT) study population, a longitudinal cohort study of 630 patients with breast cancer.	100 participants	3/2021–3/2025
Trastuzumab Cardiomyopathy Therapeutic Intervention with Carvedilol (TACTIC) Trial, NCT03879629	Carvedilol (beta-blocker)	Determine the best management strategy (ie, pre-emptive or preventive) for the initiation and duration of beta-blocker carvedilol treatment to reduce cardiotoxicity in patients with breast cancer undergoing treatment with trastuzumab.	Patients with adult breast cancer undergoing trastuzumab therapy.	450 participants	8/2019–9/2025

trials such as the AH-HA,[32] the RadComp,[33] the PREVENT trial (see **Table 2**), or prior cohort studies such as the Women's Health Initiative (WHI) Life and Longevity After Cancer (LILAC).[34] The remaining few research projects were focused on identifying radiotherapies with reduced cardiotoxicity risk (ie, photon vs proton), assessing long-term impact of dexrazoxane cardioprotective strategy, studies of sex differences, and racial differences in venous thromboembolism risk. The observational category also included 2 small business SBIR/STTR grants and both were focused on the development of a clinical tool to analyze cardiac MRI images for detection of subclinical cardiac injury and to provide clinical assessments as a service to clinicians.

RESEARCH TRAINING AND FELLOWSHIPS

Support for research training of the next generation of scientists is an important component of the NIH mission. Nearly 16% of the awarded grants were related to research training which included a loan repayment, 2 fellowships, and 13 mentored career development awards over the 10-year period. The awards supported the research training of 15 early career scientists and accounted for about 4% of the total funding. Most of these awards were supported by the NHLBI, 2 by the NCI, and one by the NIBIB. In terms of the categories, one was a clinical trial/interventional study, six were observational studies, and 9 were basic/translational research projects. The topics of the supported research are included under the categories above. Existing training-related funding opportunities were used to apply for these awards and the recipients included both basic researchers and physician-scientists whose stated long-term career goals were cardio-oncology research. The number of awards per year was low for the years 2011 to 2016, varying between zero and one, except for the year 2014 which had three awards. The number of awards per year increased to 2 in the years 2017 to 2019 and 4 in the year 2020. Five of the earlier awardees have been successful in receiving subsequent investigator-initiated R01 research project grants. The data show a growing interest in cardio-oncology research by early career scientists. Their success in obtaining the training and subsequent research grants demonstrates that cardio-oncology is emerging as an important investigative field at the intersection of cardiovascular disease, cancer biology, and therapeutics, with excellent opportunities to make impactful research advances in all 3 research areas.[35]

SUMMARY AND FUTURE DIRECTIONS

As cancer survival outlook continues to improve with expanded and improved treatments, it is reasonable to expect that the significance and potential risk of cardiovascular complications for survivors will remain high in the near future. The goal of cancer treatment-related cardiotoxicity research is to mitigate the cardiovascular dysfunction of cancer therapy without compromising its therapeutic efficacy and thereby improve patient outcomes. As most cancer treatments carry the potential risk of cardiovascular complications and complete elimination of such risk may not be feasible, it may be helpful to consider a cardiotoxicity risk management strategy that optimizes the balance of cardiovascular risk with cancer therapy benefit (**Fig. 2**). Such strategy would require, for every cancer treatment regimen, an assessment of cardiovascular risk factors, including the existing history of cardiovascular disease risk and potential comorbidities, evaluation of the treatment's potential impact on cardiovascular health, and implementation of appropriate cardioprotective interventions. Significantly, the different cardiotoxicity stages (ie, acute, chronic, and late-onset) may require different mitigation approaches. It is also important to recognize that cardiovascular health, cancer disease, and cancer therapy are not independent entities, but are interconnected and changes in any one of these entities may impact the other 2 (see **Fig. 2**). Cancer therapies continue to evolve rapidly from pharmacotherapies and molecularly targeted agents to immunotherapies, expanding treatment options greatly, but also bringing potentially unknown cardiotoxicity risks. Recognizing the opportunities to address critical research gaps in this field with increasing importance, NIH has supported and continues to support a broad portfolio of FOA-solicited and investigator-initiated research projects on cardiotoxicity.

It is important to recognize that the burdens of cancers, cardiovascular diseases and cancer treatment-related cardiotoxicity remain highly disproportionate among minority and under-resourced populations.[36,37] For example, Black and under-represented minority populations have higher risk and higher prevalence of cancers and cardiovascular diseases compared to their non-Hispanic White counterparts.[38–40] Similarly, although the data remains limited, the incidence of cancer-treatment related cardiotoxicity following anthracycline or trastuzumab treatments is higher in Black patients compared to White patients.[41–43] Disproportionately higher risk for poor cancer prognosis coupled with a higher burden of cardiovascular disease before cancer treatment

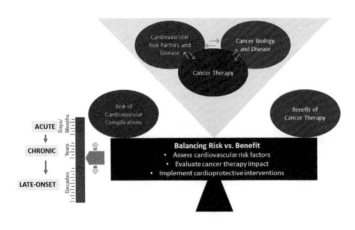

Fig. 2. *Research Strategy: Optimize the Balance of Cardiotoxicity with Cancer-Therapy Benefit.* The goal of cancer treatment-related cardiotoxicity research is to reduce cardiovascular complications of cancer therapy without compromising efficacy and thereby improve patient outcomes. As all cancer therapies carry a potential risk of cardiovascular complications and complete elimination of such risk may not be achievable, a cardiotoxicity management strategy that optimizes the risk-benefit balance, as depicted, may offer the best practical approach. For every cancer therapy, this would require the assessment of cardiovascular risk factors (including existing disease and comorbidities), evaluation of potential cardiotoxicity impact of cancer therapy, and implementation of appropriate cardioprotective interventions. Cardiotoxicity stage, that is, acute, chronic, or late-onset, is an important consideration in this approach as it may impact the risk-benefit balance. It is also important to recognize that cardiovascular health, cancer disease, and cancer therapy are interconnected and changes in any one may impact the other 2. (*Adapted from* Minasian L, Dimond E, Davis M, et al. The Evolving Design of NIH-Funded Cardio-Oncology Studies to Address Cancer Treatment-Related Cardiovascular Toxicity. JACC CardioOncol. 2019;1(1):105–113).

likely contribute to the disparities in post-treatment cardiotoxicity outcomes. Some of the key recognized barriers to health equity are related to structural racism and include under representation in research, mistrust, socioeconomic and cultural factors, and lack of access to specialty care.[37] Consistent with the NIH's commitment to address broader health inequities and significant recent efforts aimed towards a vision of inclusive excellence[44], future research in cancer treatment-related cardiotoxicity needs to recognize and prioritize potential health inequities early and address the barriers effectively.

The participants of the 2 NIH workshops identified a comprehensive list of potential gap area topics,[26,29] and the recent FOAs and investigator-initiated research projects are beginning to address many of these identified research gaps. However, many research challenges remain and research questions related to new cancer treatments and potential impact of comorbidities associated with longer survival duration remain unaddressed. Research discoveries and advances in cardiotoxicity are highly amenable to translation into human applications and disease management across populations; such opportunities remain underexplored.[45,46] As research in this field is informative and conducive to both cardiovascular and cancer research advances, the cross-talk between cardiovascular diseases and cancer biology is of particular interest.

NIH-supported research projects over the previous 10 years indicate that most of the research projects were focused on anthracycline or anthracycline-combined therapies and cancers that require these therapies such as breast cancer. By contrast, relatively few research projects were focused on other treatments and other cancers. While anthracycline and anthracycline-combined cardiotoxicity remain an important investigation area and the focus on anthracyclines may have been in part due to the substantial prior understanding of anthracycline-related cardiotoxicity or practical convenience, there is a persistent gap and opportunity to address the treatment effects of other therapies; for example, immune modulators, checkpoint inhibitors, radiation, immunotherapy, and dual/multi-agent therapies, which can have synergistic adverse effects. Knowledge of the underlying mechanisms of cardiotoxicities for these more recent therapies is lagging. Within the basic and translational research category, most research has centered on cardiac myocytes and relatively less effort has been focused on the other potential cells, such as vascular endothelial cells, cardiac fibroblasts, and myofibroblasts, macrophages, vascular and cardiac epithelial cells, among other potential cellular targets. Additionally, research has focused on cellular signaling or molecular signaling of remodeling and less on metabolic, energetic, and microvascular injury mechanisms.

Investigators submitting NIH research applications in this area should note that the NIH Center for Scientific Review (CSR) assigns grant applications to individual NIH Institutes and Centers (ICs) by matching research aims to IC mission. CSR also assigns the review study sections by matching the review requirements of the proposals with the review focus of the standing study sections. Because this research spans the missions of both NCI and NHLBI, the assignments are often not straightforward, especially if the aims overlap with the missions of both Institutes. Typically, if the proposed research aims focus on risk assessment/modeling, treatments and interventions, survivorship including clinical trials, they are likely to be assigned to NCI, whereas if the research focus is more on fundamental mechanistic understanding of cardiotoxicity, they are assigned to NHLBI. However, Institute assignment is not straightforward and both NCI and NHLBI support all 3 categories of grant proposals. As Institute and study section assignments may have a potential impact on the review and funding of the proposal, researchers proposing aims that span the missions of the 2 Institutes may benefit from early advice by the respective NIH program officers who oversee this research area to ensure that the applications are assigned to the appropriate Institute and study section.

Cancer treatment-related cardiotoxicity is a secondary effect of treatment or a derived condition from posttreatment. Relevant research requires an approach that combines the research expertise of not only cardiologists and oncologists, but potentially others, such as toxicologists, pharmacists, radiologists, and those with translational research experience, including, potentially, from the pharmaceutical industry. Recognizing the potential benefits of a multidisciplinary and collaborative research approach, the NCI and NHLBI are thus addressing this health challenge by close coordination, leveraging staff expertise and resources of both Institutes, to bring oncology and cardiology researchers together to more effectively advance cardio-oncology.

DISCLOSURE

The authors have nothing to disclose.

DISCLAIMER

The views expressed in this article are those of the authors and do not necessarily represent the views of the National Heart, Lung, and Blood Institute; the National Cancer Institute; the National Institutes of Health; or the U.S. Department of Health and Human Services.

REFERENCES

1. Miller KD, Nogueira L, Mariotto AB, et al. Cancer treatment and survivorship statistics, 2019. CA Cancer J Clin 2019;69(5):363–85.

2. American Cancer Society. Cancer Treatment & Survivorship Facts & Figures 2019-2021. Atlanta: American Cancer Society; 2019. https://www.cancer.org/content/dam/cancer-org/research/cancer-facts-and-statistics/cancer-treatment-and-survivorship-facts-and-figures/cancer-treatment-and-survivorship-facts-and-figures-2019-2021.pdf.

3. Miller KD, Fidler-Benaoudia M, Keegan TH, et al. Cancer statistics for adolescents and young adults, 2020. CA Cancer J Clin 2020;70(6):443–59. https://doi.org/10.3322/caac.21637.

4. Sasaki K, Strom SS, O'Brien S, et al. Relative survival in patients with chronic-phase chronic myeloid leukaemia in the tyrosine-kinase inhibitor era: analysis of patient data from six prospective clinical trials. Lancet Haematol 2015;2(5):e186–93.

5. Armstrong GT, Chen Y, Yasui Y, et al. Reduction in late mortality among 5-year survivors of childhood cancer. N Engl J Med 2016;374(9):833–42.

6. Mertens AC, Yasui Y, Neglia JP, et al. Late mortality experience in five-year survivors of childhood and adolescent cancer: the Childhood Cancer Survivor Study. J Clin Oncol 2001;19(13):3163–72.

7. Hudson MM, Ness KK, Gurney JG, et al. Clinical ascertainment of health outcomes among adults treated for childhood cancer. JAMA 2013;309(22):2371–81.

8. Mertens AC, Liu Q, Neglia JP, et al. Cause-specific late mortality among 5-year survivors of childhood cancer: the Childhood Cancer Survivor Study. J Natl Cancer Inst 2008;100(19):1368–79.

9. Herrmann J. Adverse cardiac effects of cancer therapies: cardiotoxicity and arrhythmia. Nat Rev Cardiol 2020;17(8):474–502.

10. Moslehi J, Lichtman AH, Sharpe AH, et al. Immune checkpoint inhibitor-associated myocarditis: manifestations and mechanisms. J Clin Invest 2021;131(5):e145186.

11. Alvi RM, Frigault MJ, Fradley MG, et al. Cardiovascular events among adults treated with chimeric antigen receptor T-cells (CAR-T). J Am Coll Cardiol 2019;74(25):3099–108.

12. Sorensen K, Levitt GA, Bull C, et al. Late anthracycline cardiotoxicity after childhood cancer: a prospective longitudinal study. Cancer 2003;97(8):1991–8.

13. Scully RE, Lipshultz SE. Anthracycline cardiotoxicity in long-term survivors of childhood cancer. Cardiovasc Toxicol 2007;7(2):122–8.

14. Ewer SM, Pham DD. Late-onset heart failure after treatment for breast cancer. Cancer 2020;126(1):19–21.

15. Armenian SH, Lacchetti C, Barac A, et al. Prevention and monitoring of cardiac dysfunction in survivors of adult cancers: american society of clinical oncology clinical practice guideline. J Clin Oncol 2017;35(8):893–911.

16. Zamorano JL, Lancellotti P, Rodriguez Muñoz D, et al. 2016 ESC position paper on cancer treatments and cardiovascular toxicity developed under the auspices of the ESC committee for practice guidelines: the task force for cancer treatments and cardiovascular toxicity of the European Society of Cardiology (ESC). Eur Heart J 2016;37(36): 2768–801.

17. Runowicz CD, Leach CR, Henry NL, et al. American cancer society/american society of clinical oncology breast cancer survivorship care guideline. J Clin Oncol 2016;34(6):611–35.

18. Miller JM, Meki MH, Ou Q, et al. Heart slice culture system reliably demonstrates clinical drug-related cardiotoxicity. Toxicol Appl Pharmacol 2020;406: 115213.

19. Abe JI, Yusuf SW, Deswal A, et al. Cardio-oncology: learning from the old, applying to the new. Front Cardiovasc Med 2020;7:601893.

20. Armenian SH, Lacchetti C, Lenihan D. Prevention and monitoring of cardiac dysfunction in survivors of adult cancers: american society of clinical oncology clinical practice guideline summary. J Oncol Pract 2017;13(4):270–5.

21. Oikonomou E, Anastasiou M, Siasos G, et al. Cancer therapeutics-related cardiovascular complications. Mechanisms, Diagnosis and treatment. Curr Pharm Des 2018;24(37):4424–35.

22. Lamore SD, Kohnken RA, Peters MF, et al. Cardiovascular toxicity induced by kinase inhibitors: mechanisms and preclinical approaches. Chem Res Toxicol 2020;33(1):125–36.

23. Herrmann J. Vascular toxic effects of cancer therapies. Nat Rev Cardiol 2020;17(8):503–22.

24. Anjos M, Fontes-Oliveira M, Costa VM, et al. An update of the molecular mechanisms underlying doxorubicin plus trastuzumab induced cardiotoxicity. Life Sci 2021;280:119760.

25. de Boer RA, Hulot JS, Tocchetti CG, et al. Common mechanistic pathways in cancer and heart failure. A scientific roadmap on behalf of the translational research committee of the heart failure association (HFA) of the european society of cardiology (ESC). Eur J Heart Fail 2020;22(12):2272–89.

26. Shelburne N, Adhikari B, Brell J, et al. Cancer treatment-related cardiotoxicity: current state of knowledge and future research priorities. J Natl Cancer Inst 2014;106(9).

27. Armenian SH, Hudson MM, Mulder RL, et al. Recommendations for cardiomyopathy surveillance for survivors of childhood cancer: a report from the International Late Effects of Childhood Cancer Guideline Harmonization Group. Lancet Oncol 2015;16(3):e123–36.

28. Curigliano G, Lenihan D, Fradley M, et al. Management of cardiac disease in cancer patients throughout oncological treatment: ESMO consensus recommendations. Ann Oncol 2020;31(2):171–90. https://doi.org/10.1016/j.annonc.2019.10.023.

29. Shelburne N, Simonds NI, Adhikari B, et al. Changing hearts and minds: improving outcomes in cancer treatment-related cardiotoxicity. Curr Oncol Rep 2019;21(1):9.

30. The search terms and method: ("cardiac toxicit*" OR "cardiovascular toxicity"~4 OR cardiotoxicity OR "cardiovascular adverse event*"~4 OR "cardiac complication*"~4) AND (chemotherap* OR radiothera* OR "cancer treatment*"~4 OR "cancer therap*"~4 OR "cancer radiation"~8). *OR* and *AND* are logical operators and terms within the quotations are word combinations. The '*' indicate a wild card allowing any words after the text. The '~' and number following it allow the preceding words within the quotations to be searched in any order along the text at a word length of upto the number indicated. The search was conducted on the 'Title', 'Abstract', and 'Specific Aims' fields of funded grants that are available in the NIH RePORTER database. Available at: https://reporter.nih.gov/) over the period 2011-2020 using an NIH in-house developed tool. Date accessed 7/29/2021.

31. NCTN: NCI's National Clinical Trials Network. Secondary nctn: nci's national clinical trials network. Available at: https://www.cancer.gov/research/infrastructure/clinical-trials/nctn Date. Accessed August 18, 2021.

32. AH-HA. Secondary AH-HA. Available at: https://clinicaltrials.gov/ct2/show/NCT03935282 Date. Accessed August 18, 2021.

33. RADCOMP. Secondary RADCOMP. Available at: https://clinicaltrials.gov/ct2/show/NCT02603341. Date accessed August 18, 2021.

34. WHI LILAC Study. Secondary WHI LILAC Study. Available at: https://sp.whi.org/studies/LILAC/Pages/Home.aspx Date. [Accessed 18 August 2021]. Accessed.

35. Asnani A, Moslehi JJ, Adhikari BB, et al. Preclinical models of cancer therapy-associated cardiovascular toxicity: a scientific statement from the american heart association. Circ Res 2021;129(1):e21–34.

36. Ohman RE, Yang EH, Abel ML. Inequity in Cardio-Oncology: Identifying Disparities in Cardiotoxicity and Links to Cardiac and Cancer Outcomes. J Am Heart Assoc 2021;10(24):e023852. https://doi.org/10.1161/JAHA.121.023852.

37. Fazal M, Malisa J, Rhee JW, et al. Racial and Ethnic Disparities in Cardio-Oncology: A Call to Action. JACC CardioOncol 2021;3(2):201–4. https://doi.org/10.1016/j.jaccao.2021.05.001.

38. Carnethon MR, Pu J, Howard G, et al. Cardiovascular Health in African Americans: A Scientific Statement From the American Heart Association. Circulation 2017;136(21):e393–423. https://doi.org/10.1161/CIR.0000000000000534.

39. Swenson CJ, Trepka MJ, Rewers MJ, et al. Cardio-vascular disease mortality in Hispanics and non-Hispanic whites. Am J Epidemiol 2002;156(10):919–28. https://doi.org/10.1093/aje/kwf140.

40. Society. AC. Cancer Facts & Figures for Hispanics/Latinos 2018-2020. 2018-2020.

41. Cousin L, Roper N, Nolan TS. Cardio-Oncology Health Disparities: Social Determinants of Health and Care for Black Breast Cancer Survivors. Clin J Oncol Nurs 2021;25(5):36–41. https://doi.org/10.1188/21.Cjon.S1.36-4.

42. Hasan S, Dinh K, Lombardo F, et al. Doxorubicin cardiotoxicity in African Americans. J Natl Med Assoc 2004;96(2):196–9.

43. Litvak A, Batukbhai B, Russell SD, et al. Racial disparities in the rate of cardiotoxicity of HER2-targeted therapies among women with early breast cancer. Cancer 2018;124(9):1904–11. https://doi.org/10.1002/cncr.31260.

44. Ending Structural Racism. Secondary Ending Structural Racism. Available at: https://www.nih.gov/ending-structural-racism/health-equity-research.

45. Fort DG, Herr TM, Shaw PL, et al. Mapping the evolving definitions of translational research. J Clin Transl Sci 2017;1(1):60–6.

46. Westfall JM, Mensah GA. T4 translational moonshot: making cardiovascular discoveries work for everyone. Circ Res 2018;122(2):210–2.

Printed and bound by CPI Group (UK) Ltd, Croydon, CR0 4YY

03/10/2024

01040365-0004